ANESTHESIOLOGY HANDBOOK

JOHNS HOPKINS ANESTHESIOLOGY HANDBOOK

Eugenie S. Heitmiller, MD
Associate Professor
Anesthesiology/Critical Care Medicine
Johns Hopkins University School of Medicine
Baltimore, Maryland

Deborah A. Schwengel, MD
Assistant Professor
Anesthesiology/Critical Care Medicine
Johns Hopkins University School of Medicine
Baltimore, Maryland

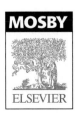

1600 John F. Kennedy Blvd.
Ste 1800
Philadelphia, PA 19103-2899

JOHNS HOPKINS ANESTHESIOLOGY HANDBOOK   ISBN: 978-1-4160-5916-5

Notice

Knowledge and best practice in this field are constantly changing. As new research and experience broaden our knowledge, changes in practice, treatment and drug therapy may become necessary or appropriate. Readers are advised to check the most current information provided (i) on procedures featured or (ii) by the manufacturer of each product to be administered, to verify the recommended dose or formula, the method and duration of administration, and contraindications. It is the responsibility of the practitioner, relying on their own experience and knowledge of the patient, to make diagnoses, to determine dosages and the best treatment for each individual patient, and to take all appropriate safety precautions. To the fullest extent of the law, neither the Publisher nor the Authors assume any liability for any injury and/or damage to persons or property arising out of or related to any use of the material contained in this book.

The Publisher

Library of Congress Cataloging-in-Publication Data

Johns Hopkins anesthesiology handbook / [edited by] Eugenie S. Heitmiller,
Deborah A. Schwengel.—1st ed.
    p. ; cm.
    ISBN 978-1-4160-5916-5
    1. Anesthesia—Handbooks, manuals, etc. I. Heitmiller, Eugenie S. II. Schwengel, Deborah A. III. Johns Hopkins University. School of Medicine. IV. Title: Anesthesiology handbook.
    [DNLM: 1. Anesthesia—Handbooks. WO 231 J65 2010]
RD82.2.J64 2010
617.9′6—dc22

                             2009015619

Acquisitions Editor: James Merritt
Developmental Editor: Andrew Hall
Publishing Services Manager: Linda Van Pelt
Project Manager: Priscilla Crater
Design Direction: Steven Stave

Printed in Canada

Last digit is the print number: 9 8 7 6 5 4 3 2 1

Working together to grow
libraries in developing countries

www.elsevier.com | www.bookaid.org | www.sabre.org

ELSEVIER   BOOK AID International   Sabre Foundation

Foreword

Boundless passion and enthusiasm, a fearless commitment to excellence, and a fundamental belief in challenging presumptions and striving to identify and answer fundamental questions in the mechanisms, prevention, and treatment of disease, in healthcare delivery and in the basic sciences, have been the hallmarks of Johns Hopkins Medicine in general and in the Department of Anesthesiology/Critical Care Medicine in particular. Over the past 30 years, our Department and our specialty have evolved from a profession centered around and limited to the practice of medicine in the operating room to one that extends to the perioperative environment and beyond. Indeed, along the way, in a relatively short period of time, we have spawned four new specialties: critical care medicine, pain management, patient safety, and safety outcome management, as well as the use of simulators in fundamentally rethinking medical education and quality of care.

Accompanying this explosion in the scope of anesthetic knowledge and practice has been a tidal wave of books, journals, and Web-based information about the clinical practice of anesthesiology and about the research that forms the basis of this practice. Sometimes difficult to answer are the basic questions: "what is important?", "how do I set up for a case?", "how do I finish a case?", "how do I maximize postoperative analgesia and recovery?", etc. Indeed, determining how to do these basic tasks is often overwhelming, particularly for physicians in training.

Over the years, much of the how-to clinical fundamentals and essential core information necessary for the safe practice of perioperative medicine and anesthesia were passed from faculty to student, resident to resident, and teacher to student via one-on-one didactic teaching in the operating room. With time, in our practice, this instruction also became increasingly formalized via an underground, grass-roots publishing and photocopying effort in which faculty and house staff created, edited, published, and internally distributed a manual or "cookbook" of how we provide anesthesia, critical care medicine, and pain management at the Johns Hopkins Medical Institutions.

One of the missions of Hopkins Medicine is to produce leaders in the field who will translate the foundation of a broad education in Medicine into improved health through patient care, research, and education. I believe that *The Johns Hopkins Anesthesiology Handbook* is part of this tradition and that it will be useful to many of our colleagues who practice anesthesia throughout North America and beyond. I am certain that this first edition is only the beginning of what will become a proud heritage.

This volume is the culmination of efforts of many individuals. I applaud my colleagues—the residents, fellows, and faculty of the Department of Anesthesiology and Critical Care Medicine—who made this book possible and who, I feel, are among the most creative and dedicated clinicians in this field.

Myron Yaster, MD
Richard J. Traystman Professor of Pediatric Anesthesia,
Critical Care Medicine, and Pain Management
Department of Anesthesiology/Critical Care Medicine
The Johns Hopkins University School of Medicine
Baltimore, Maryland

Preface

Consistently ranked as the #1 hospital in the United States and among the top 10 medical schools, the Johns Hopkins Medical Institutions and University have been prominently featured as institutions rich in history and dedicated to providing outstanding postgraduate medical training, cutting-edge research, and safe, quality patient care. The Department of Anesthesiology and Critical Care Medicine (ACCM) has long been committed to guiding the future development of our discipline and training the next generation of leaders in Anesthesiology.

Over the years, ACCM residents and attendings have worked together to develop summaries of "clinical pearls" for many of the anesthesia subspecialties; these lists of indications, dosages, treatments, and helpful guidelines are distributed on laminated cards for each rotation. In this Handbook, the content of those summaries has been consolidated into a concise pocket-sized reference. Although it was initially intended to be a tool for the Hopkins anesthesiology resident, we felt that the information provided herein might be useful to anesthesiology residents outside of Hopkins. Although much of what we need to know can be accessed online, an Internet-connected computer may not always be available or access may require too much time. The goal of this Handbook is to simplify the exercise of finding reference information, equations, and medication dosages. When we find tattered and well-worn copies of these books in call rooms, on anesthesia machines, and in scrub pants pockets, we will know that we have met our goal.

We would like to acknowledge several colleagues for their contributions to this Handbook. First and foremost, we are indebted to all of our contributors—the residents whom we strive to teach and the members of the faculty who served as chapter editors. We very much appreciate their efforts in providing this resource for future trainees. We are also indebted to our medical editors, Tzipora Sofare and Claire Levine, for their countless hours of reading, attention to detail, and top-notch editing; this handbook surely would not have been completed without their guidance, questioning, and prodding. We thank Dr. Ken Brady for simplifying our more complicated tables. We thank Dr. Myron Yaster, who had the original vision for a resident handbook such as this and secured the contract with Elsevier, for his perseverance and support. We likewise thank Dr. John Ulatowski, Chairman of the Department of Anesthesiology and Critical Care Medicine, who supported us in this endeavor. We appreciate his leadership and encouragement. Finally, we thank Andy Hall and our editorial staff at Elsevier for their advice and efforts in bringing the vision of this text to fruition.

Eugenie S. Heitmiller, MD
Associate Professor
Anesthesiology/Critical
   Care Medicine
Johns Hopkins University
   School of Medicine

Deborah A. Schwengel, MD
Assistant Professor
Anesthesiology/Critical
   Care Medicine
Johns Hopkins University
   School of Medicine

Table of Contents

Residency Basics

Sapna Kudchadkar, MD
Edited by Deborah Schwengel, MD

Welcome to anesthesiology! This chapter is intended to be an introduction for residents and medical students who are pursuing a career in this exciting and diverse field, and the information provided details various aspects of anesthesiology residency, from a general overview of the application process to important information about curriculum, procedural requirements, and certification examinations.

MEDICAL STUDENT ROTATIONS IN ANESTHESIOLOGY

Medical students are encouraged to elect an anesthesiology rotation to explore anesthesiology as a career option or to learn the scope of practice of anesthesiologists in modern medicine. Students are also given opportunities to learn some basic skills of airway management, vascular access, pain management, and general and regional anesthesia. They work alongside anesthesiology residents and faculty and attend a small-group learning series taught by the faculty specifically for medical students. Students are expected to work on call with the residents several times during their rotation, so that they can attend code and trauma calls with the on-call team. Advanced rotations are available for students interested in gaining more exposure to subspecialty areas of anesthesiology. ICU rotations are also encouraged for medical students who are considering careers in anesthesiology. Students who love working with their hands, are good at thinking on their feet, are good at multitasking, and are good at collaborating within a team are encouraged to consider a career in anesthesiology.

Once they gain sufficient experience to begin teaching someone else (usually toward the end of the CA1 year), residents are expected to teach medical students. In conjunction with their supervising faculty member, residents should teach students case-relevant medical knowledge, patient care, communication, and professionalism via various teaching methods that include:

- Discussing of plan for case.
- Discussing of how decisions are made.
- Tutoring students on procedural skills and allowing them to practice manual skills in appropriate situations.
- Students assisting residents and attendings in caring for patients.

APPLICATION TO ANESTHESIOLOGY RESIDENCY

On-line resources detail the anesthesiology residency application process. Most residency programs in the US utilize the Electronic Residency Application Service (ERAS) for receiving applications and the National Residency Match Program (NRMP). Information about individual programs can be located at their respective websites or at AMA-FRIEDA (www.ama-assn.org/go/freida). A general timeline for the residency application process is as follows:

> August—ERAS opens for application submissions.
> September—Residency programs begin to review applications.
> September to November—Programs begin to offer interviews.
> November—Dean's letter released to residency programs.
> October to January—Interviews are conducted.
> February—Rank Order List due in ERAS.
> March—Match Day.

The ERAS website (www.aamc.org/students/eras/) contains more detailed information.

PROGRAM REQUIREMENTS FOR GRADUATE MEDICAL EDUCATION IN ANESTHESIOLOGY

The American Board of Anesthesiology (ABA) defines the practice of anesthesiology as the practice of medicine dealing with but not limited to:

- Assessment of, consultation for, and preparation of patients for anesthesia.
- Relief and prevention of pain during and following surgical, obstetric, therapeutic, and diagnostic procedures.
- Monitoring and maintenance of normal physiology during the perioperative period.
- Management of critically ill patients.
- Diagnosis and treatment of acute, chronic, and cancer-related pain.
- Clinical management and teaching of cardiac and pulmonary resuscitation.
- Evaluation of respiratory function and application of respiratory therapy.
- Conduct of clinical, translational, and basic science research.
- Supervision, teaching, and evaluation of performance of personnel, both medical and paramedical, involved in perioperative care.

ANESTHESIA RESIDENCY BASICS

I. DURATION

- A minimum of 4 years of graduate medical education is necessary to train to become an anesthesiologist.
- Three of the 4 years must be dedicated to training in clinical anesthesia.

II. CURRICULUM

A. CLINICAL BASE YEAR (CBY)

Usually the PGY-1 year, this is a comprehensive 12-month education in the medical disciplines relevant to anesthesiology, including internal medicine and/or emergency medicine, surgery, pediatrics, critical care medicine, neurology, obstetrics and gynecology, family practice, or any combination of these specialties. A maximum of 1 month of anesthesiology training is permitted in the CBY.

B. CA-1 AND CA-2 YEARS

The first 2 years of anesthesiology training emphasize the fundamental aspects of the discipline.

1. Basic anesthesia training, encompassing all aspects of perioperative care under the direct supervision of faculty.
2. Training in the complex technology and equipment associated with the practice of anesthesiology.
3. Exposure to key subspecialty disciplines, including rotations in obstetric anesthesia, pediatric anesthesia, neuroanesthesia, cardiothoracic anesthesia, and pain management. Also required are rotations in critical care and the postanesthesia care unit.

C. CA-3 YEAR

A 12-month experience in complex and advanced anesthesia.

1. Exposure to a variety of difficult and complex anesthesia procedures and seriously ill patients.
2. Increased responsibility in providing perioperative anesthesia care.
3. Residents have the opportunity to choose specific advanced clinical experiences of special interest and to pursue basic science and/or clinical research.
4. Academic project at the discretion of the program director; must be completed by the end of the CA-3 year and is supervised by a faculty member.

REQUIREMENTS OF THE ACCREDITATION COUNCIL FOR GRADUATE MEDICAL EDUCATION (ACGME)

The ACGME exists to protect the process and quality of graduate medical education. An educational experience that is properly balanced with a service commitment must be provided. It is expected that each residency program provide the educational experiences necessary for a resident to develop into a competent and independent medical practitioner. Residency programs must adhere to specific duty-hour rules, and residents must demonstrate appropriate skills in each of the six following competencies:

1. **Patient care:** demonstrate compassionate, appropriate, and effective patient care for the treatment of health problems and promotion of health.
2. **Medical knowledge:** exhibit a comprehensive knowledge of the established and evolving biomedical, clinical, and cognate sciences and the application of this knowledge to patient care.
3. **Practice-based learning:** continue investigation and evaluation of their own patient care and appraisal, assimilation of scientific evidence, and improvements in patient care.
4. **Interpersonal and communication skills:** show skills that enable effective information exchange with patients, their families, and other health professionals.

RESIDENCY BASICS

5. **Professionalism:** commit to carrying out professional responsibilities while adhering to ethical principles and showing sensitivity to a diverse patient population.
6. **Systems-based practice:** manifest actions that demonstrate an awareness of and responsiveness to the larger context and system of healthcare and the ability to effectively utilize system resources to provide care that is of optimal value.

ACGME DUTY-HOUR RULES
1. Duty hours must be limited to 80 hours per week, averaged over a 4-week period, inclusive of all in-house call activities.
2. Residents must be provided with 1 day in 7 free from all educational and clinical responsibilities, averaged over a 4-week period, inclusive of call. Residents must have at least 4 days off in a 4-week block.
3. Adequate time for rest and personal activities must be provided and should consist of a 10-hour period provided between all daily duty periods and after in-house call.

CLINICAL EXPERIENCE
Programs are expected to provide residents with exposure to a large variety of surgical procedures and patients with a wide spectrum of disease processes to acquire a broad experience with different types of anesthetic management. The list below, published by the ACGME, represents the minimum clinical experience that should be obtained by a resident who is completing a training program in anesthesiology. Residents should keep logs of these experiences throughout their training.

- 40 anesthetics for vaginal delivery, with involvement in high-risk obstetrics
- 20 cesarean sections
- 100 anesthetics for children <12 years of age
    Including 15 <1 year of age, to include newborns <45 weeks postconceptual age
- 20 anesthetics for patients undergoing surgery with CPB
- 20 major vascular cases (including endovascular and excluding cardiac)
- 20 intrathoracic noncardiac cases
- 20 open craniotomy cases, including some for intracerebral procedures
- 50 epidural anesthetics for patients undergoing surgery
- 50 subarachnoid blocks for patients undergoing surgery
- 40 peripheral nerve blocks for patients undergoing surgery
- 25 new-patient evaluations for management of patients with acute, chronic, or cancer pain disorders
- Two contiguous weeks of experience in the PACU
- Documented involvement in the management of acute postoperative pain, including familiarity with patient-controlled intravenous techniques, neuraxial blockade, and other pain-control modalities

- Documented involvement in the systematic process of the preoperative management of the patient
- Sufficient instruction and clinical experience in caring for the geriatric patient
- Sufficient instruction and clinical experience in managing the needs of the ambulatory surgical patient
- Significant experience with complex procedures
    - Central vein catheter placement
    - Pulmonary artery catheter placement
    - Peripheral artery cannulation
    - Transesophageal echocardiography
    - Evoked potentials
    - Electroencephalography
- Significant experience with specialized techniques for airway management
    - Fiberoptic intubation
    - Double-lumen endotracheal tube placement
    - Laryngeal mask airway management

SUBSPECIALTY TRAINING

According to the American Society of Anesthesiologists (ASA), ~60% of all anesthesiology residency graduates pursue subspecialty training. These fellowship programs vary from 6 to 12 months in duration. ABA certification is currently available for cardiac anesthesia, critical care medicine, and pain management. A variety of subspecialty training programs is offered at various institutions, including but not limited to:
- Ambulatory anesthesia
- Cardiothoracic anesthesia
- Critical care medicine
- Neuroanesthesia
- Obstetric anesthesia
- Pain management
- Pediatric anesthesia
- Regional anesthesia
- Clinical research

ANESTHESIOLOGY BOARD CERTIFICATION

The ABA is the governing body that examines and certifies residents who complete training in an accredited anesthesiology residency program in the US. They also oversee maintenance of certification. Detailed application information, testing dates, and test content can be found at www.theaba.org.

PRIMARY CERTIFICATION

The ABA examination system consists of two distinct parts.

PART 1
The Written Examination
> Designed to evaluate a candidate's knowledge of basic and clinical sciences.
>
> Held once per year in the summer and must be passed to sit for Part 2, the oral examination.

Inservice Training Examination
> Offered annually for residents in training to gain experience with the examination content and style of questions.
>
> Scores are normalized for year of training so that residents can gauge their learning progress with others across the US.

PART 2
The Oral Examination
> Offered twice per year, this segment is designed to assess a candidate's ability to appropriately manage patients in clinical scenarios as defined by the ABA through demonstration of:

- Sound judgment in decision making and management of surgical and anesthetic complications
- Application of scientific principles to clinical problems
- Adaptability to managing unforeseen changes in clinical situations
- Demonstration of logical organization and effective presentation of information

SUBSPECIALTY CERTIFICATION
The ABA also awards certification in the subspecialties of Critical Care Medicine, Pain Medicine, and Hospice and Palliative Medicine.

REFERENCES
1. Accreditation Council for Graduate Medical Education, Program Requirements for Graduate Medical Education in Anesthesiology: Available at www.acgme.org. Accessed May 1, 2009.
2. American Board of Anesthesiology, Booklet of Information: Available at www.theaba.org. Accessed March 2007.
3. American Society of Anesthesiologists, May 1, 2009: Available at www.asahq.org/msd. Accessed May 1, 2009.

Safety

Haitham Al-Grain, MD, Stacy Hamid, MD, and John Marvel, MD
Edited by Bradford D. Winters, PhD, MD

I. ELECTRICAL SAFETY

A. IMPORTANCE

1. Increasing use of electronic surgical and anesthetic equipment in the OR has made electrical safety an important topic for anesthesiologists.
2. 40% of all hospital electrical accidents occur in the OR.
3. Basic electricity principles.

Ohm's Law: $E = I \times R$

where:

E = electromotive force, *volts* (drives electrons through an electrical circuit)

I = current, *amperes* (flow of electrons)

R = resistance to flow, *ohms*

B. ELECTRICAL SHOCK

1. May occur anytime an external electrical source comes in contact with an individual, leading to possible injury or death.
2. To receive a shock, a person must complete an electrical circuit, causing an electrical current to pass through him/her.
3. Electrical current through a human body can cause burns, disruption of normal cellular electrical activity, disturbances in normal brain function, and life-threatening cardiac dysrhythmias.

C. SEVERITY OF INJURY

1. Dependent on two factors.
a. Amount of current (measured in amperes).
b. Duration of time that current flows.

D. MACROSHOCK VERSUS MICROSHOCK

1. Macroshock.
a. High-flow current applied to the skin at two contact points, with the heart between those points and sufficient current to induce ventricular fibrillation.
b. At 60 Hz frequency (supplied by typical outlets), a current of 100 milliampere (mA) is necessary for macroshock to occur.
2. Microshock.
a. Low-flow current, as low as 20 microamperes (μA), when supplied directly through the heart via cardiac catheters or pacemaker wires, can induce ventricular fibrillation.

E. LINE ISOLATION MONITOR (LIM)
1. Electrical current basics
a. Outside the OR, an electrical potential exists between the "hot" wire (where current is flowing away from the power company) and the neutral wire, which takes current back to the power company, completing the circuit.
b. Because the neutral wire is "grounded" (connected to the earth, a good conductor), those who touch a "hot" wire will receive a shock if they are standing on the ground as they complete the circuit.
c. An extra low-resistance grounding wire exists on modern electrical systems to channel current away from a person (high resistance) who is in contact with the circuit.
2. OR electrical current and LIM
a. To provide an additional level of safety in the OR, all current is isolated from the ground by the use of an "isolation" transformer to separate the outside circuit (connected to the power company) from the ungrounded OR system circuit.
b. The LIM continuously measures current leakage in OR electrical systems.
c. When a piece of equipment with faulty wiring is plugged into such an ungrounded system, current will leak.
   i. If a leak is in macroshock range (>5 mA), the LIM will alarm.
d. LIM alarms only when the leak is in the macroshock range (mA).
e. LIM cannot detect low-flow current leaks (μA) that may lead to microshock.
f. LIM alarm does not cut the circuit, thereby allowing a faulty device to still function and present a threat.
g. If LIM alarms:
   i. The last piece of equipment plugged in should be unplugged (if safe to do so) and sent for inspection.
h. If LIM alarm remains active:
   i. Sequentially (in opposite order of activation) unplug nonvital equipment until LIM alarm stops.
   ii. If the faulty piece of equipment is not replaceable and removing it would bring harm to the patient (pt), minimize all other electrical equipment and send the offending instrument for repair after its use.

II. FIRE SAFETY AND PREVENTION
A. RISK OF FIRE
1. Risk of fire was greatly reduced with the advent of nonflammable volatile anesthetics, but fire still poses a significant hazard in the OR.
2. Electrocautery and other electrical devices near the oxygen-rich airway, flammable drapes, endotracheal tubes (ETTs), and alcohol-based skin antiseptic solutions make the threat of a disastrous OR fire very real.
3. Knowing how to prevent and treat fire injury, if necessary, is an important part of the anesthesiologist's knowledge base.

B. THE FIRE TRIANGLE

1. For a fire to occur, three components are necessary.
a. Heat (or ignition) source.
   i. Electrocautery.
   ii. Lasers.
   iii. Argon beam coagulators.
   iv. Lighted instruments.
b. Fuel.
   i. Drapes and gowns.
   ii. ETTs.
   iii. Prepping solutions (before drying).
   iv. Pt hair.
   v. Dressings.
c. Oxidizer.
   i. Oxygen is the most common oxidizer in the OR.
   ii. Nitrous oxide also supports combustion.
2. The three arms of the fire triangle should be prevented from coming together (Fig. 2.1).

C. PREVENTION—DISRUPTING THE FIRE TRIANGLE

1. Allow prep to completely dry before using electrocautery.
2. Do not allow heated light source to rest on drapes.
3. Reduce oxygen concentration (at least to <30%).
4. Use specialized, less flammable or nonflammable ETTs.
5. Place moistened pledgets around the ETT.

FIRE TRIANGLE

Four things must be present in order to produce fire:
- Enough **oxygen** to sustain combustion
- Enough **heat** to raise the material to its ignition temperature
- Some sort of **fuel** or **combustible material**
- **Chemical reaction**

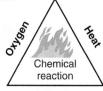

Take one of these four away, and the fire will be extinguished.

FIG. 2.1

Fire triangle.

D. TREATMENT OF AIRWAY FIRES
1. Turn off gases and disconnect the anesthetic circuit from the ETT.
2. Douse the region with saline.
3. Remove ETT—once fire is out (but not before!).
a. An ignited ETT can act like a "blowtorch" to the trachea and bronchi by directing oxygen-rich gases under pressure into the airways.
4. Reintubate pt.

E. TREATMENT OF DRAPE OR SKIN FIRES
1. Douse flame with saline or a nonflammable towel early if possible.
2. Remove all burning drapes and throw them to the floor.
3. Use the fire extinguisher that is appropriate for type of fire.

F. FIRE EXTINGUISHERS
1. Fire extinguishers are rated by the class of fire that they will extinguish.
a. Class A—used on paper, cloth, plastics.
b. Class B—used on oil and grease fires.
c. Class C—used on electrical equipment.
d. ABC—dry chemical acceptable for all three types of fires.
2. In the OR, a CO_2 fire extinguisher is used.
a. Will extinguish class B and C fires.
b. Expels a fog of cold CO_2 gas and snow.
c. Leaves no residue.
d. Range is only a few meters.
e. Cold fog is unlikely to injure pt.
3. Attempt to use a fire extinguisher only when the fire is small enough to manage.
4. Using a fire extinguisher (PASS).
a. **P**ull the pin.
b. **A**im at the base of the fire.
c. **S**queeze the handle.
d. **S**weep from side to side.
5. Evacuate area.
a. All OR workers should know evacuation routes.
b. Even when the fire is extinguished, smoke poses an additional hazard.

III. INDEXING SYSTEMS
A. MEDICAL GAS
1. Color coding system (USA). (Table 2.1)
2. Pin index system.
a. Shapes of connectors for cylinders (yokes) and lines (fittings) are specific to the gas to prevent misconnection.

B. MEDICATIONS
1. Volatile anesthetics (USA). (Table 2.2)

TABLE 2.1

MEDICAL GAS COLOR CODING SYSTEM (USA)

Oxygen	Green
Nitrous oxide	Blue
Air	Yellow
Carbon dioxide	Brown
Nitrogen	Dark blue

TABLE 2.2

VOLATILE ANESTHETIC COLOR CODING SYSTEM (USA)

Sevoflurane	Yellow
Isoflurane	Purple
Desflurane	Blue

TABLE 2.3

APPROXIMATE MAC FOR INCORRECT VA IN VAPORIZER

Vaporizer	Added Agent	Delivered MAC
Isoflurane	Desflurane or sevoflurane	Approximately the same or lower
Desflurane	Isoflurane or sevoflurane	Three times expected MAC
Sevoflurane	Desflurane or isoflurane	Approximately the same

MAC, Minimum alveolar concentration; *VA*, volatile anesthetic.

a. Newer units have specifically shaped ports and adapters for agent bottles to prevent filling with the wrong volatile anesthetic agent.
b. Some older vaporizers may have open sumps for filling with agent without an adapter.
   i. Vaporizer may be filled with wrong volatile anesthetic. (Table 2.3)
2. **IV medications.**
a. Nine classes of drugs commonly used in anesthesiology have a standard background color established for user-applied syringe labels. (Table 2.4)

IV. ENSURING CORRECT PATIENT AND PROCEDURE

A. IDENTIFICATION (ID) OF PTS

1. **Pts must be accurately identified using active forms of communication.**
a. ID bands must be physically present on pts.
2. **Use at least two pt identifiers in providing care to ensure that correct pt is receiving correct service or treatment on the correct side or site.**
a. Compare the two identifiers on ID band against the same two identifiers on requisition.
3. **Always use TWO pt identifiers when:**
a. Administering medications or blood products.

TABLE 2.4

STANDARD BACKGROUND COLORS FOR USER-APPLIED SYRINGE LABELS
(STANDARD D4774 OF THE AMERICAN SOCIETY FOR TESTING AND MATERIALS)

Drug Class	Color
Induction agents	Yellow
Tranquilizers	Orange
Muscle relaxants	Fluorescent red
Relaxant antagonists	Fluorescent red/white diagonal stripes
Narcotics	Blue
Narcotic antagonists	Blue/white diagonal stripes
Major tranquilizers	Salmon
Vasopressors	Violet
Hypotensive agents	Violet/white diagonal stripes
Local anesthetics	Gray
Anticholinergics	Green

b. Obtaining blood samples and other specimens for clinical testing.
c. Providing any treatments or procedures.
4. Inpatients—check ID band for name and history number.
5. Outpatients—ask pt (or accompanying person) to state pt's name and birth date.
6. In procedure areas, clinical personnel are responsible for:
a. Ensuring that all pts are appropriately identified and wearing the appropriate ID band.
b. Verifying identity of pt before initiating a procedure, sedation, or treatment for which an ID band is required.
7. An ID band that becomes damaged or must be removed because it interferes with pt care must be replaced and secured on the pt.
a. The nurse responsible for the pt must be notified.

B. INFORMED CONSENT
1. MUST be obtained prior to all invasive procedures and before blood or blood products are administered.
2. MUST outline, in detail, benefits and risks of procedure AND alternatives to treatment.
3. MUST honor pt's right to refuse treatment.
4. MUST be signed by pt or legal guardian and witnessed.
5. MUST include procedure, side, site, and/or level.

C. SAFE SURGERY CHECKLIST (Fig. 2.2)
1. This checklist strategy (a) includes a preanesthesia briefing, a time out, and a debriefing to reduce errors during surgery and other procedures through teamwork and communication, and (b) allows everyone involved a chance to air recommendations or concerns, creating a greater sense of teamwork.
2. Briefing (sign in)—before induction of anesthesia.

PRE-PROCEDURAL BRIEFING (SIGN IN)—PRIOR TO INDUCTION OF ANESTHESIA
- □ Patient has confirmed identity, procedure, and site.
- □ All documents match patient identifiers.
- □ Consent is accurate, complete and signed.
- □ Site correctly marked, or not applicable.
- □ History and physical in past 30 days; update note if H&P not done day of surgery.
- □ All allergies noted.
- □ Anesthesia safety check completed.
- □ Identify if difficult airway or aspiration risk; ensure equipment/assistance available.
- □ If risk of >500-mL blood loss (7 mL/kg in children), ensure adequate IV access and fluids or blood products.
- □ Discuss any safety, equipment, instrument, implant, or other concerns.
- □ Pulse oximeter on patient and functioning.
- □ Team introductions: first and last names, including roles; write names on board.
- □ Need for beta-blockade addressed.
- □ Need for glucose control addressed.
- □ Need for antibiotics and fluids for irrigation addressed.
- □ Any required blood products ordered and available.

TIME OUT—PRIOR TO START OF PROCEDURE (COMPLETE AND DOCUMENTED)
- □ Correct patient identity.
- □ Confirmation that the correct side and site are marked.
- □ Site mark visible after prep and draping.
- □ Consent form is accurate and read out loud.
- □ Agreement of all procedural team members on the procedure to be done.
- □ Correct patient position.
- □ Relevant images and results are properly labeled and appropriately displayed.
- □ Need for prophylactic antibiotics and re-dosing.
- □ Safety precautions based on patient history or medication use.
- □ Resolution of any conflicts in information.

DEBRIEFING (SIGN OUT)—END OF PROCEDURE PRIOR TO LEAVING OR
- □ Nurse verbally confirms with the team the name of the procedure recorded.
- □ Could anything have been done to make this case safer or more efficient?
- □ Ensure that instrument, sponge, and needle counts correct (or not applicable); if not follow hospital policy for incorrect counts.
- □ Complete any data collection forms.
- □ Ensure that the correct patient's name, history number, surgical specimen name, and laterality are on the specimen paperwork (must be verified by surgeon); ensure all blood transfusion documentation is in chart.
- □ Report any problems with surgical instruments.
- □ Plan for transition of care to postoperative unit:
  - Fluid management
  - Antibiotic dose and interval to be continued postoperatively
  - Pain management plan
  - Medications needed postoperatively, including beta blockers, glucose control, DVT prophylaxis
  - Tests/x-rays to be obtained

FIG. 2.2

Briefing and debriefing checklist to be performed before and after every procedure.

a. Pt confirms:
  i. Correct identity—name, medical record number, and date of birth on ID band and chart.
  ii. Correct procedure and site.
  iii. Consent form is complete and correct; describes procedure, side, and level when applicable.
b. Site marking is correct and marked as close to the incision as possible by person performing the procedure or part of his/her team.
c. Pulse oximeter is on pt and is functioning.

d. Allergies are checked.

e. If difficult airway or aspiration risk, appropriate equipment and assistance are available.

f. Blood availability is confirmed if appropriate; adequate IV access and fluids are planned.

g. Nurse confirms equipment, and implants are available.

3. Time out—just before skin incision or invasive procedure, with the healthcare provider(s) who will perform the procedure.

a. All team members introduce themselves by name and role.

b. Surgeon, anesthesia provider, and nurse verbally confirm pt, site, and procedure.

c. Anticipated critical events are discussed.

   i. Surgeon reviews critical or unexpected steps, operative duration, and anticipated blood loss.

   ii. Anesthesia team reviews any pt-specific concerns.

   iii. Nursing team confirms sterility and reviews any equipment issues.

d. Team confirms that antibiotic prophylaxis has been given within the last 60 min.

e. Essential imaging is displayed, and the name and number on radiologic studies are verified to be that of the pt.

f. Occurrence of the time out and the time that it was conducted are documented.

4. Debriefing (sign out) before pt leaves OR.

a. Nurse verbally confirms with the team:

   i. Name of the procedure recorded.

   ii. That instrument sponge and needle counts are correct (or not applicable).

   iii. That specimen is labeled correctly.

   iv. Any equipment problems to be addressed.

b. Surgeon, anesthesia provider, and nurse review the key concerns for recovery and management of pt.

D. ADVERSE-EVENT REPORTING

1. Adverse events are those that should not happen again.

2. Examples of adverse events.

a. Hospital-acquired infection.

b. Significant adverse drug event.

c. Transfusion-related hemolytic reaction.

d. Awareness during GA.

e. Equipment malfunctions that result in pt harm.

f. OR fires.

3. Questions to be addressed:

a. What happened?

b. Why did it happen?

c. Where did the system break down to allow this event to occur?

d. What will be done to reduce the probability of its happening again?

e. How will we know if these changes have worked?

f. How will we communicate the lessons learned from this investigation and any resulting changes in processes?

4. Debriefing may be used as a safety tool to identify opportunities for improvement.

5. Use after identification of a defect in the care process.

6. If an adverse event occurs:

a. Investigate event as soon as possible to understand why certain decisions were made.

b. Assemble a multidisciplinary group (e.g., nurse, physician, administrator, and pharmacist) for discussion.

c. Encourage participants to use blameless feedback and observations to support improvement (root-cause analysis or other similar tool).

d. Discussion can be brief (10–15 min) or prolonged (~2 wk), depending on complexity of issue.

e. Appoint someone to document debriefing.

f. Share key elements of learning within the department and institution to promote improvement.

2

SAFETY

V. INFECTION SAFETY: RISK AND CONTROL

A. RISK

1. Pts and healthcare workers are at risk for acquiring infections, both from pts and from other healthcare workers.

2. Viral infections, reflecting their prevalence in the community, are the most significant threat to healthcare workers.

B. STANDARD PRECAUTIONS

1. Used for the care of all pts.

a. Hand hygiene (hospital-approved hand sanitizer or handwashing).

   i. Before and after leaving pt's room.

   ii. Between pts.

   iii. After contact with pt care equipment and linens.

   iv. After removing gloves.

b. Gloves when touching any fluid.

c. Gown, mask, and eye protection during invasive procedures.

d. Needles should not be recapped.

   i. If recapping is necessary, use a one-handed scoop technique.

C. TRANSMISSION-BASED PRECAUTIONS

1. Used together with standard precautions.

2. Airborne infection precautions.

a. Used for microorganisms transmitted by airborne droplet nuclei (particles ≤5 μm in size) that can be dispersed over large distances by air currents.

b. Pt placement.
   i. Private room with negative air pressure, with 6 to 12 air changes per hour.
c. Standard respiratory protection.
   i. Worn for pulmonary tuberculosis and, if healthcare worker is not immune, for measles or varicella.
d. Powered air-purifying particulate respirators (PAPRS).
   i. Full-helmet/hood devices that use a variety of technologies, including electrostatic filters, to remove particulates such as aerosolized viruses and other microbiologic pathogens and biochemical/chemical agents that result from industrial accidents or bioterrorism.
   ii. They may be combined with a full protection suit, depending on the threat.
e. Pt transport.
   i. Place surgical mask on pt.

3. Droplet precautions.

a. Used for pts known or suspected to be infected with microorganisms transmitted by large-particle droplets (particles >5 μm) that can be generated during coughing, sneezing, talking, or by performing certain procedures.
b. Pt placement.
   i. Private room.
c. Respiratory protection.
   i. Wear a mask when working within 3 feet of pt.
d. Pt transport.
   i. Place surgical mask on pt.

4. Contact precautions.

a. Used for pts known or suspected to be infected or colonized with epidemiologically significant microorganisms, e.g., methicillin-resistant *Staphylococcus aureus* or vancomycin-resistant *Enterococcus* transmitted by direct contact with the pt or indirect contact with environmental surfaces or pt-care items.
b. Pt placement.
   i. Private room if possible.
c. Remove gloves and gown and apply hand hygiene (sanitizer or washing) before leaving pt's environment.
   i. Hand washing, not hand sanitizer, for contact with *Clostridium difficile*.
d. Pt transport.
   i. Precautions to minimize the risk of transmission should be executed.
e. Pt care equipment.
   i. Should be dedicated to a single pt (e.g., BP cuffs).

D. VIRAL INFECTIONS

1. Hepatitis A.

a. Self-limited illness.

b. Fecal-oral transmission.

c. Nosocomial transmission is rare.

d. Postexposure prophylaxis (PEP) by immune globulin IM.

e. Vaccine is not routinely recommended for healthcare workers.

2. Hepatitis B (HBV).

a. Risk for infection after percutaneous exposure is 37% to 62% if pt is positive for hepatitis B e antigen (HBeAg), and risk is 23% to 37% if pt is HBeAg negative.

b. Hepatitis B is a resilient virus and may still be infectious after 1 wk in dried blood on surfaces.

c. Vaccination is the primary strategy to prevent occupational transmission.

   i. Vaccine (3 doses IM) results in protective anti-hepatitis B surface antibodies (anti-HBs) in >90%.

   ii. Protective antibodies develop in 30% to 50% of nonresponders (i.e., anti-HBs <10 mIU/mL) with a second three-dose vaccine series.

d. PEP is with HBV hyperimmune globulin.

3. Hepatitis C.

a. Rate of seroconversion after accidental percutaneous exposure is 1.8%.

b. Hepatitis C may be transmitted through blood splashes to eye or via non-intact skin.

c. No vaccine or effective PEP exists for hepatitis C.

4. HIV infection and AIDS.

a. Rate of seroconversion after a percutaneous exposure is estimated to be 0.3%; after a mucous membrane exposure, it is 0.1%.

b. No cases of HIV transmission due to exposure of a small amount of blood on intact skin have been documented.

c. PEP after exposure with high risk of HIV transmission is recommended per CDC guidelines.

   i. CDC web site—http://www.cdc.gov/niosh/topics/bbp.

d. PEP should be initiated as soon as possible after exposure (<24 hr) for 4 wk.

VI. ENVIRONMENTAL EXPOSURE

A. RADIATION EXPOSURE

1. The magnitude of radiation absorbed is a function of three variables.

a. Total radiation exposure intensity and time.

b. Distance from the source of radiation.

c. The use of radiation shielding.

2. Radiation safety.

a. Lead aprons and thyroid collars leave exposed many vulnerable sites, which add to the total exposure.

b. Radiation exposure is inversely proportional to the square of the distance from the source; it becomes minimal at >36 in from the source.

2

SAFETY

    c. The US Regulatory Commission has established a limit of 5000 mREM/yr.

    d. Exposure of pregnant workers should be <500 mREM during pregnancy.

    e. Even very low levels of radiation exposure have stochastic biologic effects, which are cumulative and permanent.

      i. A stochastic effect occurs by chance and shows up years after exposure.

      ii. With increasing dose, the probability of the occurrence increases, but the severity does not.

      iii. Therefore the motto is, "as low as reasonably achievable."

B. WASTE ANESTHETIC GAS EXPOSURE

1. A large epidemiologic study found that the relative risk of spontaneous abortion for female physicians and nurses working in the OR was 1.4 and 1.3, respectively.

2. Some test data indicate that impairments of perceptual, cognitive, and motor skills may result from exposure to concentrations of nitrous oxide as small as 50 PPM.

3. Data from epidemiologic surveys suggest associations but have never proved causation.

4. Nitrous oxide inhibits methionine synthetase (by irreversibly oxidizing the cobalt atom of vitamin B_{12}, making it inactive), preventing the conversion of methyltetrahydrofolate to tetrahydrofolate.

5. High concentrations of nitrous oxide may result in anemia and polyneuropathy, but chronic exposure to trace levels does not appear to produce these effects.

6. The Occupational Safety and Health Administration (OSHA) is responsible for enacting job health standards, investigating work sites to detect violation of standards, and enforcing the standards by citing violators.

    a. OSHA currently does not have a standard for waste anesthetic gas exposure.

7. Standards for OR construction from the American Institute of Architects require 15 to 21 air exchanges per hour, with three exchanges bringing in outside air.

VII. FATIGUE AND SLEEP DEPRIVATION

A. EFFECTS

1. The effects of fatigue and sleep deprivation are a major concern for a variety of industries and professions, including airline pilots, truck drivers, and especially physicians.

2. At one time, extreme sleep deprivation and fatigue, especially during residency education, were seen as a "rite of passage" for medical professionals, testing their mettle and stamina.

3. Evidence has mounted in recent years that performance and safety for both pt and physician are negatively affected by extreme fatigue and sleep deprivation.

B. **ADVERSE EFFECTS OF FATIGUE AND SLEEP DEPRIVATION.**
1. Loss of attention and lack of recognition of early signs and symptoms of a developing problem.
2. Making a serious medical error (36% more likely when on a 24-hr vs. 16-hr shift).
3. Increased risk of occupational injury, such as a needle-stick injury.
4. Being involved in a motor vehicle accident on the way home (falling asleep at the wheel).

C. **GUIDELINES**
1. The American Council on Graduate Medical Education has recognized the potential impact that fatigue may have on both pt and physician safety and has established strict guidelines for resident physician work hours.
2. It is not yet clear whether these guideline changes have impacted pt or physician safety directly.
3. Interestingly, no work-hour restrictions have been instituted for attending-level physicians.

VIII. SUBSTANCE ABUSE
A. **A MAJOR PT CONCERN AND HAZARD FOR PHYSICIANS, PARTICULARLY ANESTHESIOLOGISTS**
1. Although anesthesiologists make up a small proportion of the entire physician population (3%-5%), by some accounts, our specialty may make up as much as one-third of all addicted physicians.
2. The percentage of addicted anesthesiologists ranges from 1% to 2% in some surveys to as high as ≥16% in others.
a. These data are heavily biased owing to their reliance on self-reporting.
3. Comprehensive drug screening programs for physicians and nurses in the workplace are uncommon; hence, the actual addiction rate is unknown.
a. Virtually all experts agree that the problem is grossly underestimated.
b. Substance abuse is a grave threat to an anesthesiologist's safety.
   i. The relative risk of dying from a drug overdose is 2.79 (95% CI, 1.87–4.15) when compared with that of other physicians.
c. Easy access to potent and extremely addictive medication has often been cited as a likely contributing factor.
   i. Medication diversion may harm pts as well; if an anesthesiologist is personally using a controlled substance (e.g., narcotic or sedative) signed out for a particular pt, that pt is potentially deprived of adequate pain relief or anxiolysis.

d. Studies indicate that anesthesiologists preferentially abuse narcotics, whereas psychiatrists tend to abuse benzodiazepines.
e. The potential threat to pt safety inherent in having an intoxicated provider rendering care is tremendous.
f. Judgment and vigilance are greatly impaired under such conditions, and grave harm may occur.
g. Unfortunately, quality data that report the impact of healthcare-provider substance abuse on pt safety are lacking.

B. COMMONLY ABUSED MEDICATIONS
1. Alcohol.
2. Marijuana.
3. Propofol.
4. Isoflurane.
5. Benzodiazepines.
6. Fentanyl and other narcotics.

REFERENCES
1. Barash PG, Cullen BF, Stoelting RK: Clinical anesthesia, 5th ed. Philadelphia, Lippincott Williams & Wilkins, 2006.
2. Safety event investigation tool. Available at http://pathology2.jhu.edu/CQI/TEXTFILES/SAFETY_Investigation_Tool.pdf. Accessed June 15, 2007.
3. Johns Hopkins Hospital/University. Available at http://www.hopkinsmedicine.org/hnf/hnf_5017.htm. Accessed June 16, 2007.
4. The Johns Hopkins Cutting Edge. Available at http://www.hopkinscf.org/docs_shared/CuttingEdge_June06.pdf. Accessed June 18, 2007.
5. The Joint Commission of Hospital Accreditation Organizations. Available at http://www.jcipatientsafety.org/22782/. Accessed June 15, 2007.

Documentation, Economics, and Legal Issues

Adam Carinci, MD, Danesh Mazloomdoost, MD, Darcy Towsley, MD, and Adam Schiavi, MD, PhD
Edited by Jerry Stonemetz, MD

I. DOCUMENTATION

A. DOCUMENTATION COMPLIANCE AND PROFESSIONAL FEE BILLING

1. Billing compliance has become a source of increasing concern for anesthesiologists due to complexities of billing and perceived lack of guidance on how to bill for specific clinical services that do not readily conform to government billing rules. These complexities include:

a. Correctly defining anesthesia time and discontinuous anesthesia time.

b. Documenting medical necessity for monitored anesthesia care cases.

c. Distinguishing monitored anesthesia care from general anesthesia care.

d. Properly billing for specialized services such as acute pain and critical care.

e. Distinguishing between consultations and visits.

2. Four elements are required for anesthesia service billing.

a. Pt identifier.

b. Provider name(s).

c. Anesthesia times.

d. Procedure and diagnostic information.

3. Pt identifier.

a. Each pt must have a unique identifier that discretely represents the pt, in compliance with HIPAA mandates.

b. Typically, these identifiers are medical record numbers or account numbers that are unique from the social security number or date of birth.

4. Provider name.

a. In addition to the primary anesthesiologist's identity, all other providers and the duration of their presence must be included in the billing statement.

b. Providers could include CRNAs, residents, surgeons, and other physicians involved in the case.

   i. In academic settings, the payment concurrency rule of the Center for Medicare Services (CMS) states that an attending physician who supervises two residents can receive only 50% of the compensation for each case.

   ii. This is specific for anesthesiology and has seriously affected the financial health of anesthesia teaching departments.

5. Anesthesia times.

a. *Anesthesia start time* begins after preoperative assessment and placement of lines or blocks in the preoperative area.

   i. Transport to the OR, if properly documented, may constitute the anesthesia start time; otherwise, start time commences at the moment the pt enters the OR with the anesthesiologist present.

b. *Anesthesia end time* corresponds to the moment the anesthesiologist is no longer in personal attendance of the pt, when care has been turned over to PACU or ICU staff.

   i. Documentation of a sign-out is required to indicate transition of care.

6. Procedure and diagnostic information.

a. The procedure title and postoperative diagnoses must be noted on the anesthesia billing record.

b. As CPT codes are required to bill for a case, either the anesthesiologist must designate the procedure and corresponding CPT code, or details of the case must be documented for the coding personnel to assign appropriate CPT codes.

c. Minor mismatches can yield dramatic losses in revenue or fraudulent charges if proper CPT codes are not assigned.

B. HIPAA

1. Mandated as Public Law 104–191 in 1996.

2. Enacted as a result of broad changes espoused by the Clinton Administration.

3. Essentially a three-pronged approach to improve healthcare to:

a. Ensure that preexisting conditions are no longer a valid reason for denying health insurance to any pt.

b. Simplify claim submission, based on recognition that at least 25% of the healthcare dollar is spent on non-value-added administrative costs.

c. Increase funding to combat fraud and abuse in Medicare billing.

   i. The recommendation for this third arm of the legislation came from results of Operation Restore Trust (ORT), an initiative that sought, found, and aggressively prosecuted fraudulent Medicare billing, which resulted in heavy fines and penalties.

   ii. Consequently, with passage of HIPAA, more than $1 million was allocated to combat this perceived significant problem. Money was earmarked to facilitate the Office of the Inspector General (OIG) in investigating claims of fraudulent billing and went predominantly to reward whistle-blowers who reported episodes of fraud and abuse.

4. HIPAA elicits specific concerns for anesthesia providers, and anesthesia billing is typically one of the highlighted areas of the yearly OIG Workplan, a document released by the OIG that indicates the specific areas that will be investigated in the coming year.

a. Anesthesia is highlighted primarily because billing is so complex, and areas that receive perennial review by the OIG involve time discrepancies and supervision lapses of the anesthesia care team.

5. One particular concern is the stance of the CMS that mistakes in billings constitute an attempt at fraud.
   a. If a mistake is made that results in fewer charges, no consequence or penalty is levied.
   b. However, a mistake that results in increased charges is considered to be a fraudulent claim, and the claimant may be subjected to a $10,000 fine per occurrence plus the requirement to reimburse the charges with any interest that may have accrued.
   c. Based on heavy criticism and feedback, CMS modified the approach to assigning penalties. If an entity can demonstrate that it makes a concerted effort to combat fraud and abuse (e.g., a compliance program), then mistakes are not penalized as heavily. Charges and interest still apply, but the onerous assignment of penalties is removed.

C. BILLING COMPLIANCE PROGRAMS
1. A compliance program need not be perfect to be implemented.
   a. According to the ASA, "Ultimately, the issue is whether the practice is *implementing* the compliance program, by educating its physicians and staff regarding billing standards, identifying problems, and taking corrective action, not whether the compliance program is comprehensive in scope."
   b. To assist anesthesiology groups in navigating complexities of billing compliance and to identify specific risk areas, the OIG has published the OIG Compliance Program for Individual and Small Group Practices.
      i. It highlights seven components that the OIG deems essential to a sound compliance plan (Box 3.1).

D. THE JOINT COMMISSION
1. US-based non-profit organization (previously known as Joint Commission on Accreditation of Healthcare Organizations) founded in 1951.
2. Mission—to continuously improve the safety and quality of care provided to the public through the provision of healthcare accreditation and related services that support performance improvement in healthcare organizations.

BOX 3.1

COMPONENTS OF OIG COMPLIANCE PROGRAM FOR INDIVIDUAL AND SMALL GROUP PRACTICES

Implementation of written policies and standards of conduct
   Designation of a compliance officer or contact
   Development of a training and education program
   Creation of accessible lines of communication to keep practice employees updated about compliance activities
   Performance of internal audits to monitor compliance
   Enforcement of standards through well-publicized disciplinary directives
   Prompt corrective action to detected offenses

DOCUMENTATION, ECONOMICS, AND LEGAL ISSUES

3

3. Surveyors are sent to evaluate healthcare organizations' practices and facilities for accreditation.
a. Since January 1, 2006, surveys are unannounced.
b. Organizations deemed to be in compliance with all applicable standards are granted accreditation.
c. To be accredited, organizations must meet the Medicare and Medicaid certification requirements, which are necessary for gaining reimbursement from Medicare and managed-care organizations.
4. National Patient Safety Goals—initiated in 2003 (Box 3.2).
a. Promote specific improvements in pt safety.
b. Highlight problematic areas in healthcare.
c. Describe evidence and expert-based solutions to these problems.
d. Focus on system-wide solutions wherever possible.
e. Updated annually.

BOX 3.2

NATIONAL PATIENT SAFETY GOALS AND ASSOCIATED REQUIREMENTS

Goal 1—Improve accuracy of pt identification.
- Use at least two pt identifiers.

Goal 2—Improve effectiveness of communication among caregivers.
- Use "read back" technique when receiving verbal orders or critical test results.
- Standardize a "do not use" list of abbreviations, symbols, and acronyms.
- Act to improve on timeliness of reporting critical care results.
- Implement a standardized approach to "handoff" communication.

Goal 3—Improve safety of using medications.
- Standardize and limit the number of drug concentrations used.
- Identify a list of look-alike/sound-alike drugs.
- Label all medications, medication containers, and solutions.

Goal 7—Reduce the risk of healthcare-associated infections.
- Comply with current CDC guidelines for hand hygiene.
- Manage as sentinel events all identified cases of unanticipated death/loss of function associated with healthcare-associated infection.

Goal 8—Accurately and completely reconcile medications across the continuum of care.
- Use a process for comparing a pt's current medications with those ordered while under care of the organization.
- Provide a complete list of medications to the next provider when referring, transferring, or discharging pts.

Goal 9—Reduce the risk of pt harm that results from falls.
- Implement a fall-reduction program.

Goal 13—Encourage active involvement by pts in their own care as a pt safety strategy.
- Define means for pts and their families to report concerns about safety.

Goal 16—Improve recognition and response to changes in a pt's condition.

Gaps in numbering indicate either nonapplicability to hospital setting or retirement of goal.

5. Joint Commission checklist for OR areas.
a. Verify that all staff members have ID badges.
b. Check for food or drink in workrooms.
c. Remove boxes from floors.
d. Ensure that all equipment is at least 18 in from sprinkler heads.
e. Remove any door wedges.
f. Verify that oxygen tanks are properly secured.
g. Replace any full sharps disposal containers.
h. Check document bins to ensure that pt information is not visible.
i. Ensure that workrooms are kept clean.
j. Check staff for proper attire.
   i. Head covers.
   ii. No visible undergarments.
   iii. No jewelry.
   iv. Eye protection when warranted.
k. Check for unattended controlled medications.
l. Ensure that soda lime has not expired.
m. Verify proper labels on all drugs.
   i. Propofol label should include date and time.
n. Discard any expired medications.

II. ECONOMICS
A. PROFESSIONAL FEES
1. A surgical procedure generates three bills:
a. Facility fee.
   i. Hospital/surgical center overhead, equipment, human support services (nursing, staffing, etc.).
b. Surgeon's professional fee (profee).
c. Anesthesiologist's profee.
2. Anesthesiologist's profee is based on the total units a case is worth according to the following formula developed by the ASA Committee on Economics:

$$Units_{tot} = BU + TU + QCU$$

where:

$$BU = Base\ Units\ (type\ of\ procedure\ done)$$

$$TU = Time\ Units\ (length\ of\ procedure)$$

$$QCU = Qualifying\ Circumstance\ Units\ (special\ circumstances,\ procedures, techniques\ of\ case)$$

3. To calculate the final anesthesia profee, a conversion factor (CF), which is based on the insurance provider's prenegotiated value for a total unit, is applied to the total units:

$$U_{tot} \times CF = Anesthesia\ profee$$

4. Base Units.

a. Include:

    i. Preoperative assessment.

    ii. Preparation time.

    iii. Intraoperative management.

    iv. Postoperative course.

b. Base Units are based on CPT codes for each case, which were developed by the AMA as a means by which to categorize physician services.

c. Every surgical procedure has a surgical CPT code and a corresponding anesthesiology CPT code.

d. While knee arthroscopy may have several surgical CPT codes, only one anesthesiology CPT code corresponds to all of those procedures.

e. CMS and ASA negotiate the relative value units (RVUs) for each anesthesiology CPT code.

5. Time Units.

a. TUs reflect the length of the procedure.

b. Anesthesiology time begins when the provider is preparing the pt for anesthesia services, including transport if it is adequately documented.

    i. Transport time should include some level of monitoring documentation.

c. Anesthesiology time does not include preoperative assessment, preoperative line or block placement (these count toward QCU), or room preparation.

d. Typically, 1 TU equals 15 min or a fraction thereof, but some insurance carriers may allow 1 TU as 10 min.

6. Qualifying Circumstance Units.

a. QCUs fall under two categories: special pt considerations (emergency, deliberate hypotension, hypothermia) and specific procedures as indicated for the case (arterial catheter, central venous catheter, pulmonary artery catheter, regional block, transesophageal echocardiography).

b. The ASA Relative Value Guide defines the value of QCUs by a quantum of units or a flat fee charge.

7. Conversion Factor.

a. Reimbursement of the CF is insurance–payer-dependent and is negotiable between the payer and the anesthesiology physician group.

b. The national mean CF among non-government payers is ~$45.85 to $57.85/unit according to the annual ASA survey of anesthesia fees.[1]

8. Other considerations.

a. *Obstetrics billing*, until recently, has lacked a standard formula.

b. In 2002, the ASA Committee on Economics made a generalized recommendation that professional charges reflect the intensity and time involved in any neuraxial labor analgesia, as in any of the following models[2]:

    i. BU + Pt contact time (insertion, management, adverse events, removal) + TU (running the neuraxial analgesia).

  ii. BU + TU < Maximum cap.
  iii. Single fee.
  iv. Incremental time-based fee (e.g., 0–2 hr, 2–6 hr, >6 hr).
c. *Pain physicians* and *intensivists* charge procedural fees plus a consultant fee, per the Evaluation and Management Coding guidelines developed by the AMA and published in the CPT guidebook. The basic format consists of:
  i. CPT code for the visit/procedure.
  ii. Place or type of service provided (e.g., office visit).
  iii. Content of the service (e.g., comprehensive H&P).
  iv. Nature of the presenting problem.
  v. Time required to provide the service.
d. *Emergency airway consults* incur a procedure fee defined in the CPT guidebook.
  i. Typically, an emergency intubation will be coded as a procedure worth 6 units, provided that a minimum amount of data is collected on the pt and the procedure.
e. Reimbursement model promotes greatest revenue generation with multiple short cases versus a long single case.
  i. Unfortunately, reimbursement is not oriented significantly toward difficulty of anesthesia, wherein charges are increased with complexity of pt comorbidities.
  Example:
  Profee charges for pt undergoing upper abdominal incisional hernia repair. Pt has severe comorbidities that require placement of an arterial line during the procedure. The surgical CPT code is 49560, and the anesthesia CPT code is 00756, which corresponds to a BU value of 7 units. The procedure takes 3 hr, which corresponds to 12 TUs. An arterial line is a QC that may be charged as 4 units, and a pt who has ASA IV status may qualify as a QC of 2 additional units (though frequently not paid by insurance).
  Total charges would be calculated as follows:

$$\text{BU (7)} + \text{TU (12)} + \text{QCU (4 + 2 = 6)} = \text{Total units (25)}$$

  Using a CF of $50/unit results in a total charge of $1250.
  It must be remembered that charges do not equate to payment. Payment is based on contractual agreement with insurance companies, which define their own CF and payment rules.
9. **Practice models.**
a. Anesthesiology practice groups fall within a spectrum in which:
  i. At one extreme, a fee is collected for every case for which the anesthesiologist bills individually (fee-per-case).
  ii. At the opposite extreme, every anesthesiologist is compensated based on the income of the group (salaried).
b. In the former:
  i. Junior members may receive undesirable cases in terms of workload or compensation.

  ii. However, this model may also offer an incentive for efficiency and productivity.
 c. In the latter:
   i. Salaries may be distributed equitably or based on seniority.
   ii. However, no financial incentive exists to accept heavier cases or to turnover more quickly.
 d. Helpful tips when evaluating whether to join a practice.
   i. Determine where the practice falls on the fee-per-case-versus-salaried spectrum.
   ii. Ask for the blended-unit value, or the average CF, of all insurance carriers used by the practice.

B. GENERAL COST OVERVIEW OF ANESTHESIA EQUIPMENT, SUPPLIES, AND MEDICATIONS

1. Healthcare currently accounts for ~14% of the gross domestic product.
2. Anesthesia providers have represented 3% to 5% of total healthcare costs in the US.[3]
3. Anesthesiologists are under increasing pressure to limit expenses.
 a. A large percentage of anesthesia groups are receiving subsidies.
 b. Consequently, they need to align incentives with hospitals.
 c. Reducing expenses is a great mechanism by which to deliver value back to the hospital.
4. Complicated decisions are required on an individual basis regarding which pts are suitable for ambulatory surgery, which preoperative studies are needed, which anesthetics to use, and which monitors are needed.
5. Although anesthesia drug expenses represent a small portion of total perioperative costs, the great number of doses actually administered contributes substantially to the aggregate total cost to the institution in actual dollars.
 a. It is estimated that the 10 highest expenditure drugs account for >80% of anesthetic drug costs at some institutions.
 b. Cost of anesthetic drugs must include costs of additional equipment (e.g., special vaporizers or extra infusion pumps) and associated maintenance.
6. Other indirect costs that are commonly overlooked.
 a. Increased setup time.
 b. Increased room turnover time.
 c. Extended PACU recovery time.
 d. Additional expensive drugs required to treat side effects.
7. It is estimated that reducing fresh gas flows from 5 L/min to 2 L/min wherever possible would save ~$100 million annually in the US.
8. See Table 3.1 for costs of specific supplies.

TABLE 3.1	
COSTS OF SPECIFIC SUPPLIES	
EQUIPMENT (TYPICAL OR)	
Anesthesia machine	$35,000–$45,000
Sonosite/puncture ultrasound	$30,000
Bronchoscope	$8000
Central line kit	$27.00–$45.00
Arterial line catheter	$6.00
Laryngeal mask airway	$10.00
Endotracheal tube	$5.00–$20.00
Epidural tray	$17.00
Spinal tray	$9.00
MEDICATIONS (TYPICAL CASE SETUP)	
Premedications	
Midazolam (2 mg/2 mL)	$0.94
Scopolamine (0.4 mg/1 mL)	$3.45
Narcotics	
Fentanyl (250 mcg/5 mL)	$0.69
Remifentanil (2 mg/2 mL)	$47.15
Hydromorphone (4 mg/1 mL)	$3.15
Morphine (10 mg/1 mL)	$1.40
Induction Agents	
Thiopental (500 mg/20 mL)	$13.14
Propofol (20-mL bottle)	$7.42
Propofol (50-mL bottle)	$18.54
Ketamine (500 mg/5 mL)	$14.39
Etomidate (20 mg/10 mL)	$12.06
Neuromuscular Blockers	
Succinylcholine (200 mg/10 mL)	$1.90
Vecuronium (10 mg/10 mL)	$5.71
Rocuronium (50 mg/5 mL)	$26.64
Pancuronium (10 mg/10 mL)	$2.92
Other Medications	
Lidocaine (100 mg/5 mL)	$0.59
Atropine (1 mg/1 mL)	$0.53
Epinephrine (1-mg/1-mL ampule)	$0.62
Dolasetron (12.5 mg/0.625 mL)	$26.23

III. LEGAL ISSUES

A. **FOUR PRINCIPLES OF MEDICAL ETHICS (BY GILLON) PROVIDE A SIMPLE, ACCESSIBLE, AND CULTURALLY NEUTRAL APPROACH TO THINKING ABOUT ETHICAL ISSUES IN HEALTHCARE**

1. *Autonomy*—obligation to let others make their own decisions through deliberative thought.
2. *Beneficence*—obligation to do good or to provide net benefit over harm to pts.
3. *Non-malfeasance*—obligation to do no harm.

4. *Justice*—obligation to respect people's rights, distribute resources fairly, and respect morally acceptable laws.

B. OBTAINING CONSENT FOR ANESTHESIA CARE
1. All pts must provide adequate written informed consent for anesthesia care prior to any treatment/intervention.
2. Information provided to pt must include anesthetic plan, alternatives, and risks.
3. Separate written consent should be included for Jehovah's Witnesses or other restrictive religious beliefs, and for the pt with DNR orders.

C. LEGAL ASPECTS OF CONSENT AND RIGHT TO REFUSE TREATMENT
1. US Code §1395cc (a)—Patient self-determination act of 1990: All pts admitted to a hospital must be made aware of their right to prepare advance directives and refuse life-prolonging treatment.
2. The principle of autonomy states that the competent pt has the right to determine what shall be done to his/her body.
a. Mandated by common law principles of autonomy and self-determination, which are the foundations of the consensual nature of medicine.
b. Mandated by constitutional rights—the 14th Amendment's protection of liberty interests and the 1st Amendment's protection of religious rights.
3. The US Supreme Court observed, "The logical corollary of the doctrine of informed consent is that the pt generally possesses the right not to consent, that is, to refuse treatment."
4. Failure to implement a valid advanced directive can lead to legal action (e.g., battery).
5. Consents have no time limit for a specific procedure as long as the risks are the same.
a. The only exception is consent for sterilization, which has a 30-day expiration.
b. From an anesthetic point of view, serial consents are allowed for planned repeated procedures such as electroconvulsive shock therapy and radiation oncology for which a pt comes several times per week as part of a planned treatment.
c. We typically do not allow for serial consents for bone marrow procedures and lumbar punctures because usually a longer period of time passes between procedures, and the clinical condition of the pt changes; therefore the risks may change.
6. Emergency procedures (level I traumas) do not require consent.
a. Emergencies not immediately life threatening may not require consent if two physicians decide that the procedure is warranted and consent is not obtainable.
7. No difference exists between the surgical and anesthesia consent processes.

a. Full discussion of risks and benefits must occur.

b. Surgical consent does not imply anesthesia consent.

8. Telephone consent requires a witness; parent or legal guardian must give consent.

9. Impaired adults are treated in the same manner as children are treated—a legal health guardian must provide consent.

D. ADVANCE DIRECTIVES

1. Technology and advanced therapeutics in medicine increase the physician's ability to prolong pts' lives by sustaining bodily function without a cure, concomitantly increasing the probability of prolonging suffering and a lingering death.

2. The advance directive is a written statement or pro forma document executed by a competent adult that provides others with information about their wishes concerning the nature and extent of medical care to be provided should they lose their decision-making capacity.

3. Classified as instructional (living wills and do not resuscitate (DNR) orders) and proxy (assignment of a person as durable power of attorney).

4. Medical professionals should follow pts' advance directives and not allow their moral beliefs or personal preferences to influence them.

a. They should also be aware of any local laws that govern their responsibilities vis à vis advance directives.

E. REFUSAL OF BLOOD PRODUCTS

1. Pts of the Jehovah's Witness faith.

a. Will not accept RBC transfusion.

b. Belief: "Jehovah requires that we abstain from blood. This means that we must not take into our bodies in any way at all other people's blood or even our own blood that has been stored."

c. Basis: "As for the believers from among the nations, we have sent out, rendering our decision that they should keep themselves from what is sacrificed to idols as well as from blood and what is strangled and from fornication" (*Acts 21:25*).[4]

d. Believers vary in what they will accept. Discuss with pt the use of:
    i. Cell saver.
    ii. FFP.
    iii. Platelets.
    iv. Cryoglobulin.
    v. Albumin.

e. Discuss with surgeon limits to the procedure and triggers to abort procedure.
    i. Hb—acceptable lower limit.
    ii. Estimated blood loss—acceptable upper limit.
    iii. Hemodynamic instability.
    iv. Determine at what point surgery can or cannot be aborted.

f. Techniques for optimizing Hb and reducing blood loss during surgery.

      i. Preoperative erythropoietin to optimize Hb.

      ii. Acute hemodilution.

      iii. Cell saver.

      iv. Antifibrinolytics.

      v. DDAVP.

g. Minors.

    i. In some jurisdictions, parents/guardians may not legally withhold blood or blood products from a minor.

    ii. If the parent/guardian refuses blood or blood products for the minor, the responsible physician should, prior to the procedure, discuss the risks, benefits, and alternatives with the minor's surrogate and should be judicious about the need for blood or blood products.

    iii. Teenagers represent a gray area.

       • It is recommended that consent be discussed privately with a teenager away from the influence of parents.

       • May need to consult with a psychiatrist to assist in defining clarification.

F. DNR

1. DNR specifically applies to the performance of CPR to resuscitate.

2. CPR includes any form of artificial respiration, open/closed chest compressions, and defibrillation to provide oxygen to the heart and brain until return of spontaneous circulation and breathing.

3. "Do Not Resuscitate" or "No Code Order" specifies that medical personnel are not to provide CPR to a person experiencing a cardiac arrest.

4. Does not include medical treatments in the pre-arrest phase, BP support with medications, or the administration of IV fluids.

5. Does NOT mean "do not treat" or to discontinue any form of life-sustaining medical treatment or procedure.

6. In any arrest situation, death is uncertain; therefore pt consent to receive CPR is usually presumed unless otherwise specified by a DNR order.

7. Attending physician writes DNR order after consultation with competent pt or the pt's legal proxy, and it becomes a permanent part of the medical record until revoked.

G. DNR IN THE OR

1. Routine anesthesia care involves practices and procedures that are viewed as resuscitative. Any directive that limits these procedures must be reviewed and modified as necessary to maintain, suspend, or modify the DNR order.

2. The anesthesiologist frequently does not know the circumstances in which a DNR order was written. Therefore communication is essential with the pt, family, primary care team, and surgical team prior to induction of anesthesia, and discussion should be documented.

3. If pt rescinds DNR status for a procedure, the postoperative time period and the circumstances in which the DNR is to be reinstated must be specified preoperatively.
4. Automatic suspension of DNR orders in the perioperative period violates pts' rights.
5. A pt should not be refused appropriate operative management simply because the perioperative physicians are uncomfortable with DNR status.
6. Any modifications to the advance directives must be documented in the medical record.
7. If the DNR is modified, the point at which the original, preexisting directive is to be reinstated must be clarified and documented.
8. Should irreconcilable conflicts arise, the anesthesiologist may withdraw from care (providing an alternative) and/or voice concerns to the appropriate institutional body (ethics council or compliance office).

REFERENCES

1. Bierstein K: Fees paid for anesthesia services. ASA Newsletter 2005; 69(8):30–33. Available at http://www.asahq.org/Newsletters/2005/08-05/PM0805.pdf. Accessed January 16, 2008.
2. Hannenberg AA: Toward fair and reasonable fees in obstetrical anesthesia. ASA Newsletter 2001; 65 (12). Available at http://www.asahq.org/Newsletters/2001/12_01/hannenberg.htm. Accessed January 16, 2008.
3. Abenstein JP, Warner MA: Anesthesia providers, patient outcomes and costs. Anesth Analg 82:1273–1283, 1996.
4. New World Translation of the Holy Scriptures Online Bible. www.watchtower.org/e/bible/ac/chapter_021.htm. Accessed May 3, 2009.

SUGGESTED READING

American Society of Anesthesiologists: Perioperative DNR guidelines. Available at www.ASAhq.org/publicationsAndServices/standards/09.html. Accessed June 7, 2007.
Barash PG, Cullen BF, Stoelting RK: Clinical anesthesia. Philadelphia: Lippincott, Williams & Wilkins, 2006.
Basanta WE: Advance directives and life-sustaining treatment: A legal primer. Hematol Oncol Clin North Am 16:1381–1396, 2002.
Baum JA: Low flow anaesthesia: The sensible and judicious use of inhalation anaesthetics. Acta Anaesthesiol Scand 111:264, 1997.
Beauchamp TL, Childress JF: Principles of Biomedical Ethics, 3rd ed. New York: Oxford University Press, 1989.
Draft OIG Compliance Program for Individual and Small Group Physician Practices. Federal Register, June 7, 2000; 65(13):36818–36835. Available at http://oig.hhs.gov/authorities/docs/cpgphysiciandraft.pdf. Accessed January 16, 2008.

Ewanchuk M, Brindley PG: Ethics review: Perioperative do-not-resuscitate orders—Doing "nothing" when "something" can be done. Critical Care 2006;10:219. Available at http://ccforum.com/content/pdf/cc4929.pdf. Accessed January 16, 2008.

Guarisco KK: Managing do-not-resuscitate orders in the perianesthesia period. J Perianesth Nur 19:300–307, 2004.

Gillon R: Medical ethics: Four principles plus attention to scope. BMJ 309(6948):184–188, 1994.

Johnstone RE, Martinec CL: Costs of anesthesia. Anesth Analg 76:840, 1993.

Johnstone R, Jozefczyk KG: Costs of anesthetic drugs: Experiences with a cost education trial. Anesth Analg 78:766, 1994.

Semo JJ: Anesthesia billing compliance: A practical approach. ASA Newsletter 1999; 63(12). Available at http://www.asahq.org/Newsletters/1999/12_99/bill1299.html. Accessed January 16, 2008.

Watchtower: Official Web Site of Jehova's Witnesses. Available at www.watchtower.org. Accessed February 13, 2009.

Woolley S: Children of Jehovah's Witnesses and adolescent Jehovah's Witnesses: what are their rights? Arch Dis Child 90:715–719, 2005.

Preoperative Evaluation

Enyinnaya R. Nwaneri, MD, and Ramola Bhambani, MD
Edited by Eugenie Heitmiller, MD, and Jerry Stonemetz, MD

I. GENERAL OVERVIEW

A. **PREOPERATIVE H&P MUST BE PERFORMED WITHIN 30 DAYS OF THE SCHEDULED PROCEDURE (REGULATION OF THE JOINT COMMISSION)**

B. **OBJECTIVES OF PREOPERATIVE EVALUATION**
1. To understand the impact and risk of coexisting medical diseases on anesthesia and surgical procedures.
a. To assign ASA status (Box 4.1).
2. To establish a management plan for perioperative anesthetic care.
3. To obtain informed consent.
4. To establish a good doctor-pt relationship.
5. To allay pt anxiety.

C. **ANESTHESIOLOGY CONSULTATIONS**
1. Whenever possible, pts should see their internists, cardiologists, or other specialists prior to an anesthetic preoperative evaluation, and all records from the specialists should be available on the day of the preoperative assessment.
2. Recommendations for preoperative assessment, depending on medical condition and surgical procedure, are displayed in Figure 4.1.
a. Pts who are not coming to the anesthesiology preoperative evaluation clinic and who are not an "A" category in the algorithm in Figure 4.1 should be evaluated by their primary care physician.
b. Charts for "B" and "C" class pts should be completed at least 72 hr prior to surgery.
  i. Otherwise, inadequate time is allowed for review, increasing risk of cancellation due to inadequate testing.
c. Low-risk medical conditions—healthy with no medical problems (ASA I) or well-controlled chronic conditions (ASA II).

BOX 4.1

ASA STATUS

Class I Healthy pt (no physiologic, physical, or psychologic abnormalities)
Class II Pt with mild systemic disease without limitation of daily activities
Class III Pt with severe systemic disease that limits activity but is not incapacitating
Class IV Pt with incapacitating systemic disease that is a constant threat to life
Class V Moribund pt not expected to survive 24 hr with or without the procedure
Class VI Brain-dead pt whose organs are being removed for donor purposes

If the procedure is performed as an emergency, an "E" is added to the ASA status.

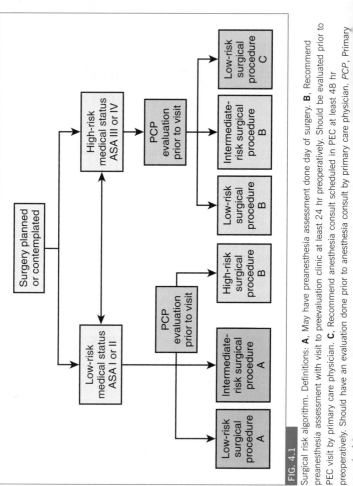

FIG. 4.1

Surgical risk algorithm. Definitions: **A,** May have preanesthesia assessment done day of surgery. **B,** Recommend preanesthesia assessment with visit to preevaluation clinic at least 24 hr preoperatively. Should be evaluated prior to PEC visit by primary care physician. **C,** Recommend anesthesia consult scheduled in PEC at least 48 hr preoperatively. Should have an evaluation done prior to anesthesia consult by primary care physician. *PCP,* Primary

d. High-risk medical conditions—multiple medical comorbidities not well controlled (ASA III) or extremely compromised function secondary to comorbidities (ASA IV).

e. Low-risk surgical procedure—poses minimal physiologic stress (e.g., minor outpatient surgery).

f. Intermediate-risk surgical procedure—medium-risk procedure with moderate physiologic stress and minimal blood loss, fluid shifts, or postoperative changes.

g. High-risk surgical procedure—high-risk procedure with significant fluid shifts, possible blood loss, and perioperative stress.

D. DOCUMENTED ASSESSMENT

1. A preinduction assessment must be documented on the anesthetic or sedation record immediately prior to administration of any anesthetic or sedative medications for a procedure.

II. HISTORY

A. REVIEW CHART IF AVAILABLE; THEN INTERVIEW PT.

1. The anxious pt is reassured if the physician knows the pt's history.

B. LIST ALL MEDICATIONS AND DOSAGE SCHEDULES.

1. Pay particular attention to use of monoamine oxidase inhibitors (MAOIs).

a. Meperidine can produce a hypertensive crisis in pts receiving MAOIs.

C. LIST ALL ALLERGIES TO MEDICATION, FOODS, AND LATEX; DOCUMENT DETAILS OF REACTION.

1. Allergy to egg, lecithin, or soybean oil should be noted and may affect use of propofol.

D. ANESTHETIC HISTORY

1. Adverse reactions (pt or related family) to anesthetic agents.

a. Malignant hyperthermia.

b. Volatile agent-induced hepatitis.

c. Prolonged paralysis (abnormal plasma cholinesterase).

d. Acute intermittent porphyria.

   i. Thiopental can precipitate a fatal episode of acute intermittent porphyria.

e. Syncopal episode, tachycardia, or palpitations may be side effects associated with injection of LA with epinephrine.

2. If available, check previous anesthesia records for problems (or successes) with:

a. Premedication, anesthetic agents.

b. Vascular access or placement of invasive catheters for monitoring.

c. Ventilatory issues.

  i.   Ease of mask ventilation.
  ii. Laryngoscopy view.
  iii. Size and type of laryngoscope blade.
  iv. Size of ETT used.
  v.   Evidence of difficult airway; method for securing airway.
  vi. History of dental injury.
  vii. Temporomandibular joint disease.
d. CV instability.
  i.   Intraoperative ischemia.
  ii. CHF.
e. Postoperative issues.
  i.   Stridor or croup (in children).
  ii. ICU admissions.
  iii. Prolonged emergence.
  iv. Need for reintubation.
  v.   Awareness during GA.
  vi. PONV.

E. SURGICAL HISTORY
1. Symptoms and implications of disease for which surgery is planned as well as previous surgical procedures.

III. PHYSICAL EXAM
A. GENERAL
Assessment prior to anesthesia/sedation focuses on vital signs, airway, and cardiopulmonary examination but may include all systems, depending on clinical status of the pt and planned procedure. Abnormalities discovered on preoperative physical may require further workup.

B. VITAL SIGNS AND GENERAL CONSIDERATIONS
1. Height, weight, and vital signs.
2. General appearance (e.g., frail, obese, appearance for stated age).
3. Level of mental function (e.g., awake, alert, oriented, confused, uncooperative).
4. Location of painful sites.

C. AIRWAY EXAMINATION (SEE CHAPTER 6, *AIRWAY*)
1. Mallampati score.
2. Mouth opening (finger breadths).
3. Temporomandibular distance (finger breadths).
4. Neck range of motion (normal, limited, or fixed; flexion and extension).
5. Dentition (loose teeth, caps, decayed teeth, dentures, missing teeth).
6. Presence of a beard.

D. HEART
1. HR.

2. Extra heart sound (S3, S4).
3. Irregular heartbeat or ectopic beats.
4. Heart murmur.

E. LUNGS
1. Quality of breath sounds.
2. Presence of rhonchi, rales, or wheezes.

F. NEUROLOGIC (FOR PTS WITH UNDERLYING NEUROLOGIC DISEASE)
1. Extremity weakness.
2. Areas of sensory loss.
3. Mental functioning (as above).

G. VASCULAR
1. Jugular venous distention.
2. Carotid artery bruits.
3. Assessment of IV access sites.

H. ASSESSMENT FOR REGIONAL TECHNIQUE
1. For pts undergoing central neuraxial blocks (spinals and epidurals) or peripheral nerve blocks:
a. Examine area of planned block to ensure that it is free from infection and anatomic abnormalities.
b. Examine pt for evidence of bleeding disorder (petechiae, purpura)
2. Pts with preexisting neurologic deficits should have a documented neurologic exam before use of any regional technique.

IV. LABORATORY STUDIES
A. GENERAL
1. Lab studies should be selected on basis of pt's medical condition and surgical procedure.
2. For all pts scheduled for low- or intermediate-risk surgery, only the following labs are necessary:
a. Hb/Hct on any menstruating female.
b. Urine pregnancy test the morning of surgery on any menstruating female.
c. ECG on any pt over the age of 50, unless provided with a previous normal tracing within 1 year. If pt has history of cardiac disease or the previous ECG tracing is remarkable for abnormal findings, a comparison tracing should be obtained within 1 mo of surgery.

B. CBC (HEME-8)
1. History of anemia or other blood disorder (e.g., sickle cell disease), coagulopathy, malignancy, chronic disease states.
2. Hb for following pts having outpatient procedures:

a. Infants <60 wk postgestation.
b. Menstruating females.

C. COAGULATION STUDIES

1. PT.
a. For known bleeding disorders in pt or family member.
b. History of easy bruising or excessive bleeding.
c. Coumadin use (INR).
d. Liver disease.

2. PTT.
a. Order if pt has history of heparin use.

3. Bleeding time.
a. If history indicates possible increased bleeding risk despite normal PT and PTT (e.g., pts on aspirin).
b. Bleeding time is not a reliable test.
c. May want to consider platelet function assay.

D. METABOLIC PANELS

1. Basic metabolic panel.
a. Renal disease.
   i. Check serum potassium level on the morning of surgery for renal failure pts.
b. Diuretic use.
   i. Pts receiving potassium supplementation.
c. Digoxin or chronic steroid therapy.
d. Glucose the morning of surgery for diabetics or pt with significant history of hypoglycemia.

2. Comprehensive metabolic panel.
a. Chronic renal disease.
b. CV disease.
c. Hepatic disease.
d. Intracranial disease.

E. ECG

1. History of CV disease.
a. Coronary artery disease.
b. Valvular disease.
c. History of dysrhythmias.
d. Hypertension.
e. Poor exercise tolerance.
f. If pt has any cardiac history or the previous tracing is remarkable for abnormal findings, a comparison tracing is required within 1 month of surgery.

2. Pt >50 yr, unless a normal tracing obtained 1 yr previous is provided.

3. Diabetics >20 yr of age.

4. Morbid obesity, looking for signs of right heart strain (Pickwickian syndrome).

F. PREGNANCY TEST
1. Menstruating females who have not undergone sterilization procedures.

G. CXR
1. Pts with symptoms or signs of current cardiopulmonary disease.
2. Pts with pulmonary dysfunction and no previous CXR for 1 yr.

H. PULMONARY FUNCTION TEST (PFT)
1. For evaluation of severity of lung disease in pts with significant pulmonary symptoms.
2. Evaluation of response to bronchodilators.
3. For pts with undiagnosed dyspnea or shortness of breath.

V. EVALUATION BY SYSTEM

A. CV
1. Noncardiac surgical pts with coronary artery disease are at risk for perioperative morbidity and mortality from ischemic cardiac events (Table 4.1).
2. Perioperative cardiac events such as MI, unstable angina, CHF, and dysrhythmias are the leading causes of perioperative deaths (Table 4.2).

TABLE 4.1

STRATIFICATION OF CARDIAC RISK FOR NONCARDIAC
SURGICAL PROCEDURES

Cardiac Risk*	Noncardiac Surgical Procedure
High cardiac risk (often >5%)	Emergency major operations, particularly in the elderly
	Aortic and other major vascular procedures
	Peripheral vascular procedures
	Anticipated prolonged surgical procedures associated with large fluid shifts and/or blood loss
Intermediate cardiac risk (generally <5%)	Carotid endarterectomy
	Head and neck procedures
	Intraperitoneal and intrathoracic procedures
	Orthopedic surgery
	Prostate surgery
Low cardiac risk† (generally <1%)	Endoscopic procedures
	Superficial procedures
	Cataract surgery
	Breast surgery

*Combined incidence of cardiac death and nonfatal MI.
†These procedures generally do not require further preoperative cardiac testing. (From Eagle KA, Berger PB, Calkins H, et al: J Am Coll Cardiol 2002;39[3]:542–553, with permission.)

PREOPERATIVE EVALUATION

4

TABLE 4.2

PREDICTORS OF CARDIAC RISK BASED ON UNDERLYING CARDIOVASCULAR DISEASE

Degree of Cardiac Risk	Clinical Predictors
Major	Unstable coronary syndromes
	MI in past 30 days
	Unstable or severe angina
	Stable angina in sedentary pt
	Decompensated CHF
	Significant dysrhythmias
	High-grade AV block
	Symptomatic ventricular dysrhythmias with underlying heart disease
	Supraventricular dysrhythmias with uncontrolled ventricular rate
	Severe valvular disease
Intermediate	Mild angina pectoris
	Previous MI by history or pathologic Q waves
	Compensated or previous CHF
	Diabetes mellitus
Minor	Advanced age
	Abnormal ECG (LV hypertrophy, left bundle-branch block, ST-T abnormalities)
	Rhythm other than sinus (e.g., atrial fibrillation)
	Low functional capacity (e.g., inability to climb one flight of stairs with a bag of groceries)
	History of stroke
	Uncontrolled systemic hypertension

CHF, Congestive heart failure; *AV,* atrioventricular; *MI,* myocardial infarction; *ECG,* electrocardiogram; *LV,* left ventricular. (From Eagle KA, Berger PB, Calkins H, et al: J Am Coll Cardiol 2002;39[3]:542–553, with permission.)

3. Functional capacity can be expressed in MET (metabolic equivalent of the task) values (Table 4.3).
a. A single MET represents oxygen consumption at rest.
b. Poor functional capacity is defined as an exercise capacity of <4 METs.
4. **Cardiology consultation may be necessary in conjunction with further studies.**
a. Exercise stress testing to assess functional capacity, ECG changes, and hemodynamic response (Box 4.2).
b. Radionuclide imaging to assess myocardial perfusion, infarction, and function.
    i. Thallium test.
        • Areas of thallium redistribution upon delayed imaging are considered to represent myocardium at risk.
        • A fixed defect (unchanged distribution with time) is believed to represent scar tissue (an old MI).

TABLE 4.3	
ESTIMATED ENERGY REQUIREMENTS FOR VARIOUS ACTIVITIES	
Metabolic Equivalents (METs)	Activity
1	Can you take care of yourself?
	Can you eat, dress, and use the toilet?
	Can you walk indoors around the house?
	Can you walk a block or two on level ground at 2–3 mph (3.2–4.8 km/hr)?
4	Can you do light work around the house like dusting or washing dishes?
	Can you climb a flight of stairs or walk up a hill?
	Can you walk on level ground at 4 mph (6.4 km/hr)?
	Can you run a short distance?
	Can you do heavy work around the house such as scrubbing floors or moving heavy furniture?
	Can you participate in moderate recreational activities such as golfing, bowling, dancing, doubles tennis, or throwing a baseball or football?
>10	Can you participate in strenuous sports such as swimming, singles tennis, football, basketball, or skiing?

(From Eagle KA, Berger PB, Calkins H, et al: J Am Coll Cardiol 2002;39[3]:542–553, with permission.)

4

PREOPERATIVE EVALUATION

BOX 4.2
TREADMILL TEST RESPONSES PREDICTIVE OF SEVERE MULTI-VESSEL AND/OR LEFT MAIN CORONARY ARTERY DISEASE
ELECTROCARDIOGRAPHIC RESPONSES
ST-segment response
Downsloping
Elevation
ST-segment depression exceeding 2.5 mm
Serious ventricular dysrhythmias occurring at low heart rates (120–130 bpm)
Early onset (first 3 min) of ischemic ST-segment depression or elevation
Prolonged duration in the post-test recovery period (≥8 min) of ischemic ST-segment depression
NONELECTROCARDIOGRAPHIC CRITERIA
Low achieved heart rate (≤120 bpm)
Hypotension* (≥10 mm Hg fall in systolic BP)
Rise in diastolic BP (≥110–120 mm Hg)
Low achieved rate-pressure product (≤15,000)
Inability to exercise beyond 3 min

*In the absence of antihypertensive medications or hypovolemia of any cause.
(From Goldschlager N: Ann Intern Med 1982;97:383, with permission.)

- Coronary stenoses of >90% will likely produce perfusion abnormalities at rest, whereas stenoses of ≥50% may be detected only with increased stress or exercise.
  ii. Technetium-99m sestamibi.
  - Occurrence of regional wall motion abnormalities and the inability to increase LV ejection fraction during exercise suggest myocardial ischemia.
  iii. Pharmacologic stress test with radionuclide imaging may be useful in pts who are unable to complete an exercise stress test.
  - Dipyridamole or adenosine is used for coronary dilation.
  - The presence of areas of redistribution correlates well with increased perioperative cardiac risk.
c. Echocardiography.
  i. Evaluates global and regional ventricular function, pericardial effusions, and congenital abnormalities.
  ii. Transesophageal echocardiography may be necessary to assess valvular function, mural or atrial thrombi, and aortic aneurysms.
  iii. Stress echocardiography may be useful if a prior stress ECG is nondiagnostic, if baseline ECG is abnormal, or if atypical symptoms are present.

B. RESPIRATORY
1. Asthma.
a. Pt who reports an exacerbation or a new episode of wheezing within 4 wk prior to surgery may need to have elective procedure postponed.
b. Pt with poorly controlled asthma may need to be referred to primary care physician or pulmonologist to optimize condition prior to surgery.
c. Pertinent history.
  i. How often do you have to use your inhaler?
  ii. Have you experienced any recent wheezing?
  iii. How frequent are your ED visits or hospital admissions due to asthma?
  iv. Did you ever receive steroids?
  v. Have you ever been intubated because of your asthma?
2. COPD.
a. The most common pulmonary disorder encountered in anesthetic practice.
b. Pertinent history.
  i. Are you using supplemental oxygen? How much?
  ii. What is your smoking history?
  iii. Are you short of breath?
  iv. Have you experienced any changes in dyspnea?
  v. Do you have a productive cough on most days of 3 consecutive months?
  vi. Have you been producing more sputum recently?
c. Preoperative management of COPD.
  i. Cessation of smoking for at least 2 mo.
  ii. Bronchodilator therapy (i.e., inhaled β-2 adrenergic agonists, glucocorticoids, ipratropium bromide).

iii. Possibly antibiotics in pts with chronic bronchitis exacerbations.

iv. Referral to a pulmonologist or the pt's primary care physician to optimize respiratory status.

3. Smoking.

a. Pt may wheeze when intubated.

b. Smokers have a higher risk of atelectasis due to secretions.

c. Smokers may experience increased cough postoperatively.

d. Pertinent history.

    i. How many packs/years?

    ii. Do you smoke currently?

    iii. Did you smoke today?

    iv. Do you have a chronic/active cough? Is it productive?

e. Preoperative management for smokers.

    i. Decrease or stop use of cigarettes at least 2 mo prior to surgery to:

- Decrease secretions.
- Improve ciliary and small airway function.
- Reduce pulmonary complications.
- Reduce carboxyhemoglobin levels, which increases oxygen availability to the tissues.

4. Upper respiratory infections (URI).

a. URI can increase risk of mucous plugging, atelectasis, and desaturation.

b. No contraindication to GA in pts with a history of URI (clear runny nose) who are afebrile and have a benign lung exam.

c. May need to postpone case if URI is accompanied by:

    i. Purulent (yellow or green) rhinorrhea.

    ii. Productive cough.

    iii. Fever.

    iv. Rhonchi, wheezing, or history of significant asthma.

5. Obstructive sleep apnea (OSA).

a. Increases risk for airway collapse and susceptibility to the respiratory depressant and airway effects of sedatives, opioids, and inhaled anesthetics.

b. Severity of OSA should be carefully assessed preoperatively to anticipate intraoperative management and postoperative disposition to a monitored bed or ICU.

c. Pertinent history.

    i. Do you snore?

    ii. Do you experience daytime somnolence?

    iii. Have you been told that you stop breathing while you are sleeping?

    iv. Do you have difficulty breathing during sleep?

    v. Do you find yourself waking up frequently during sleep?

    vi. Have you ever had a sleep study? If so, what were the results?

    vii. If OSA has been formally diagnosed:

- Is OSA mild or severe?
- Is CPAP or BiPAP used?

d. Physical exam in pts with OSA may show:
   i. Increased BMI (>95th percentile for age).
   ii. Increased neck circumference.
   iii. Inability to visualize the soft palate.
   iv. Large tongue.
   v. Tonsillar hypertrophy.
e. Physical features of pediatric OSA are often different from adult OSA (see Chapter 13, *Pediatrics*).
f. Preoperative management.
   i. Consider preoperative initiation of CPAP.
   ii. Consider negative inspiratory positive-pressure ventilation for pts with severe OSA who do not respond adequately to CPAP.
   iii. Plan for monitored bed after surgery, depending on procedure and need for postoperative opioids.

6. Tests/studies for pts with pulmonary disease.
a. CXR may be indicated:
   i. If concern about infection (i.e., URI, pneumonia).
   ii. If wheezing or crackles on lung exam or a history of pulmonary dysfunction (i.e., COPD) with no previous CXR for 1 yr.
b. Baseline ABG rarely needed but may be helpful:
   i. In pts with severe OSA to determine extent of CO_2 retention and compensation.
   ii. To determine the adequacy of ventilation and arterial oxygenation for pts with COPD.
   iii. For asthmatic pts with active bronchospasm who present for emergency surgery.
c. PFT if pulmonary symptoms are significant.
   i. Pts with severe COPD and PFT results <50% of predicted are at greatest risk for postoperative pulmonary complications.
d. Sleep study results for pts with OSA.

C. CNS
1. Seizures.
a. Benzodiazepines are known to increase the seizure threshold.
b. Use sevoflurane with caution in pts with seizures.
   i. Seizures have been associated with sevoflurane use in children and adults.
c. Pertinent history.
   i. When was your last seizure?
   ii. How well controlled are your seizures on your current regimen?
d. Check drug levels if pt is on phenytoin, carbamazepine, or phenobarbital, particularly if seizures are not well controlled or if concerned about medication toxicity.

2. Myasthenia gravis.
a. Muscle relaxants may render pts with myasthenia too weak to be extubated and requiring postoperative mechanical ventilation.

b. Pertinent history.
   i.   Have you had any recent attacks?
   ii. What muscle groups are typically affected?
   iii. How is your breathing?
   iv. How well controlled are your symptoms on your current regimen?
c. Physical exam for signs of weakness.
   i. Ocular.
      • Ptosis.
      • Diplopia.
   ii. Bulbar.
      • Dysarthria.
      • Difficulty with chewing and swallowing.
      • Proximal muscle weakness in the neck and shoulders.
      • Respiratory muscle weakness.
d. Plasmapheresis and administration of IV immunoglobulin may be indicated preoperatively in myasthenic pts with respiratory and oropharyngeal weakness.

3. Parkinson disease (PD).
a. Avoid phenothiazines, butyrophenones (droperidol), and metoclopramide because of antidopaminergic activity that can exacerbate symptoms in pts with PD.
b. Pertinent history.
   i. What are your symptoms?
   ii. How well controlled are your symptoms on your current medication regimen?

4. Multiple sclerosis.
a. The stress of surgery and anesthesia may worsen the symptoms of a pt with multiple sclerosis or reset their baseline functioning to a level less than it was preoperatively.
b. Elective surgery should be avoided during an exacerbation.

5. Cerebrovascular disease.
a. Pts with cerebrovascular disease are at risk for a cerebrovascular event.
b. Optimal BP control in the preoperative and perioperative period is essential.
c. Pertinent history.
   i.   Have you ever had a stroke or a transient ischemic attack (TIA)?
   ii. What type of stroke did you have?
   iii. Do you have any residual neurologic deficits?
   iv. Are you on anticoagulation medication?
   v.   When was your last dose?
   vi. How well controlled is your BP?
d. Pts with cerebrovascular disease should be examined for the presence of carotid bruits.
e. Obtain ultrasound of carotid arteries to assess for occlusive disease if history of TIA or stroke.

   f. Coagulation studies (i.e., PT, PTT, INR) to confirm reversal of anticoagulation and antiplatelet therapy in pts with a history of stroke or TIA who are on chronic therapy.

6. Intracranial mass and/or increased ICP.

a. Pertinent history.

     i. Have you had recent problems with headaches and/or seizures?

     ii. Any changes in your cognitive function?

     iii. Any new neurologic deficits?

     vi. Signs/symptoms of elevated ICP, for example, nausea/vomiting.

     v. Personality changes, altered level of consciousness.

     vi. Changes in breathing patterns.

     vii. History of shunt placement.

b. CT and MRI scans/reports in pts with intracranial masses to assess for possible intracranial hypertension (i.e., evidence of brain edema, a midline shift of >0.5 cm, increased ventricular size).

7. Other.

a. Injury to spinal cord, cerebral palsy, mental retardation.

b. Chronic pain, neuropathy/paresthesias.

c. Myopathy, muscular dystrophy, multiple sclerosis.

d. Syncope.

e. Hearing or vision loss.

D. RENAL

1. ~5% of the population has renal disease, and renal dysfunction increases morbidity and mortality.

2. Definition of acute renal failure.

a. Increase in serum creatinine by 0.5 mg/dL, increase in serum creatinine by 50%, or serum creatinine >2 mg/dL.

b. The degree of residual renal function is best estimated by creatinine clearance.

c. Postoperative renal dysfunction is associated with GI bleeding, respiratory infection, and sepsis.

d. Etiologies of acute renal dysfunction.

     i. Prerenal.

       • Decreased circulating volume (hypovolemia) or a perceived decrease in circulating volume (decreased cardiac output or hypotension).

       • Early correction usually results in reversal of dysfunction, but continued renal hypoperfusion may result in renal damage.

     ii. Intrarenal.

       • Most common cause is acute tubular necrosis due to ischemia.

       • Other causes are toxins, acute glomerulonephritis, and interstitial nephritis.

     iii. Postrenal.

       • Obstructive lesions—renal calculi, neurogenic bladder, prostatic disease, or tumor.

e. Clinical features of renal insufficiency or failure.
  i. Hypervolemia.
  ii. Hypertension.
  iii. Peripheral edema.
  iv. Potassium retention.
  v. Impaired excretion of drugs.

3. Chronic renal disease.
a. Etiologies of chronic renal disease.
  i. Hypertension.
  ii. Diabetes mellitus.
  iii. Chronic glomerulonephritis.
  iv. Tubulointerstitial disease.
  v. Renovascular disease.
  vi. Polycystic kidney disease.
b. Clinical features of chronic renal disease.
  i. Cardiac: hypervolemia, hypertension, CHF, edema, accelerated atherosclerosis, coronary artery disease, pericarditis, and pericardial effusions.
  ii. Metabolic: hyperkalemia, hypermagnesemia, hyponatremia, hypocalcemia, hyperphosphatemia, metabolic acidosis, glucose intolerance, hypertriglyceridemia.
  iii. Hematologic: chronic anemia, platelet dysfunction.
  iv. GI: increased gastric volume and acid production, delayed gastric emptying, N/V, peptic ulceration.
  v. Neurologic: mental changes, encephalopathy, coma, peripheral and autonomic neuropathies.
  vi. Increased susceptibility to infection.

5. Pertinent history.
a. Symptoms.
  i. Polyuria.
  ii. Polydipsia.
  iii. Dysuria.
  iv. Oliguria.
  v. Edema.
  vi. Dyspnea.
b. Schedule and site of hemodialysis should be noted and coordinated with elective procedures so that pt can be dialyzed the day before surgery.

6. Physical exam.
a. Arteriovenous fistula should be evaluated for patency (check for presence of a thrill or bruit).
b. IV access and BP determinations should be performed on limb opposite to fistula.

7. Laboratory studies.
a. Urine and serum indices—to distinguish pre/intra/postrenal etiologies.
b. Urinalysis unless pt is anuric.

      i. Abnormal findings due to renal disease are proteinuria, pyuria, hematuria, casts, and abnormal specific gravity.

      ii. Urine electrolytes, osmolality, and urine creatinine indicate volume status and concentrating ability and are used to help differentiate between prerenal and intrarenal disease.

c. BUN is an insensitive measure of GFR, because it is influenced by volume status, cardiac output, diet, and body habitus.

      i. Ratio of BUN to creatinine is normally 10–20:1.

      ii. Disproportionate elevation of the BUN may reflect hypovolemia, low cardiac output, GI bleeding, or steroid use.

d. Serum creatinine normally is 0.6 to 1.2 mg/dL but is affected by pt's skeletal muscle mass and activity level.

e. Creatinine clearance is used to estimate GFR and provides the best estimate of renal reserve (normal is 80–120 mL/min).

      i. It can be estimated with the following equation: $[140 - \text{age (yr)}] \times \text{wt (kg)}] \div [72 \times \text{serum creatinine (mg/dL)}]$.

      ii. Multiply total by 0.85 for women.

f. Serum Na^+, K^+, Cl^-, and HCO_3^- concentrations are usually normal until renal failure is advanced.

g. The fractional excretion of sodium (FENa) calculation can be used to distinguish prerenal from renal disorders.

h. FENa = $[(\text{urinary } Na^+ \times \text{plasma creatinine}) \div (\text{plasma } Na^+ \times \text{urinary creatinine})] \times 100$.

      i. <1 = prerenal disease.

      ii. >2 = renal disease.

      iii. This equation is not accurate for pts treated with diuretics.

i. The risks and benefits of proceeding with elective surgery should be carefully considered if serum $[Na^+]$ is >150 mEq/L or $[K^+]$ is >5.9 mEq/L.

j. Hematologic studies may show anemia and coagulation abnormalities.

k. ECG may indicate myocardial ischemia/infarction, pericarditis, and electrolyte abnormalities.

l. CXR may show fluid overload, pericardial effusion, infection, uremic pneumonitis, or cardiomegaly.

8. Optimization of renal pt.

a. Pts on hemodialysis should be dialyzed before surgery.

b. If the pt is on continuous renal replacement therapy (CRRT), the decision to continue intraoperatively must be based on the reason for the CRRT, the duration of the procedure, and the type of procedure.

c. Most pts will be able to tolerate discontinuation of CRRT before surgery and reinstitution afterward.

d. Major surgical procedures or prolonged surgical procedures may require intraoperative CRRT.

E. ENDOCRINE

1. Diabetes.

a. The most commonly encountered endocrine disorder in the perioperative setting.
b. Blood glucose usually increases during and after surgery because of the release of stress hormones.
c. Control of blood glucose in the perioperative setting is essential for wound healing and minimizing infection risk.
d. Pertinent history.
   i. Have you been diagnosed with other problems associated with your diabetes (i.e., eyes, kidneys, feeling in your hands and feet)?
   ii. How well controlled are your blood sugars on your current regimen?
   iii. Do you have GERD or heartburn?
e. Pts with type I diabetes with chronic hyperglycemia can develop limited-mobility joint syndrome.
f. Diabetics are more likely to exhibit labile hemodynamics (hypotension requiring vasopressor therapy, bradycardia that is resistant to atropine) while anesthetized.
g. ECG in diabetics >age 20 yr.
   i. Diabetics have an increased incidence of ST-segment and T-wave segment abnormalities and silent myocardial ischemia and infarction on preoperative ECG.
h. Obtain blood glucose immediately before and after surgery.
i. Hb A1C levels may also be obtained preoperatively.
j. BUN and creatinine may be indicated to assess the degree of renal insufficiency.

2. Adrenal cortical disorders or chronic steroid therapy.
a. Pts who have been treated with steroids for >1 mo in the past 6 to 12 mo for the treatment of various nonendocrine medical disorders may require an intraoperative dose of IV "stress dose" steroids.
   i. For short, minor procedures, continuation of the usual oral steroid dose is usually sufficient.
b. Pts with true adrenal insufficiency must receive supplemental corticosteroid and/or mineralocorticoid replacement preoperatively.
   i. 50 to 100 mg hydrocortisone preoperatively and 100 mg q 8 hr for 1 to 3 postoperative days, depending on the surgical stress, is most commonly used.
c. Serum chemistries may be indicated in pts with adrenal disorders.
   i. Pts with Cushing syndrome tend to have hypokalemic metabolic alkalosis, resulting from mineralocorticoid activity of glucocorticoids.

3. Thyroid dysfunction.
a. Elective surgical procedures should be postponed until pt is clinically and chemically euthyroid with medical treatment.
b. Obtain pertinent history (Box 4.3).
c. Large goiters with potential upper airway compression increase risk of difficult airway.

4

PREOPERATIVE EVALUATION

> **BOX 4.3**
>
> **PERTINENT HISTORY QUESTIONS FOR THYROID DYSFUNCTION**
>
> Do you suffer from any symptoms of thyroid disease such as:
>
> | For Hyperthyroidism | For Hypothyroidism |
> |---|---|
> | Tachycardia | Bradycardia |
> | Weight loss | Weight gain |
> | Heat intolerance | Cold intolerance |
> | Muscle weakness | Muscle fatigue |
> | Diarrhea | Lethargy |
> | Hyperactive reflexes | Constipation |
> | Anxiety | Hypoactive reflexes |
> | Tremors or feeling nervous | Depression |

   i. CXR or CT of the chest may be indicated to determine whether pt with a large goiter has airway compromise (i.e., tracheal deviation/collapse).
d. Review TSH, T_3, total and free T_4 for pts with symptomatic thyroid dysfunction to determine need for medical management.
   i. These studies should be normal prior to surgery.
e. Evaluate ECG in pts with hyperthyroidism to assess for sinus tachycardia or atrial fibrillation, as compared with bradycardia or a junctional rhythm in pts with hypothyroidism.

F. HEPATIC
1. Alcoholic cardiomyopathy should always be considered in pts with a history of alcohol abuse.
2. Risk assessment (Tables 4.4).
3. Pertinent history.
a. History of jaundice, pruritus, malaise, anorexia, bleeding.
b. History of hepatitis or cirrhosis.
c. Exposure to drugs, alcohol, and hepatic toxins.
4. Physical examination.
a. Look for stigmata of liver disease.
   i.   Hepatosplenomegaly.
   ii. Jaundice/scleral icterus.
   ii. Ascites.
   iii. Peripheral edema.
   iv. Spider angiomata.
   v.   Testicular atrophy.
   vi. Caput medusae.
   vii. Hemorrhoids.
   viii. Asterixis.
   ix. Gynecomastia.
   x.   Temporal wasting.

TABLE 4.4

MODIFIED CHILD-PUGH SCORING SYSTEM FOR HEPATIC FAILURE

Parameter		Modified Child-Pugh Score Points	
	1	2	3
Albumin (g/dL)	>3.5	1.8–3.5	<2.8
Prothrombin time			
Seconds prolonged	<4	4–6	>6
International normalized ratio	<1.7	1.7–2.3	>2.3
Bilirubin (mg/dL)*	<2	2–3	>3
Ascites	Absent	Slight-moderate	Tense
Encephalopathy	None	Grade I-II	Grade III-IV

TOTAL POINTS	CLASS	1-YEAR SURVIVAL	2-YEAR SURVIVAL
5–6	A	100%	85%
7–9	B	81%	57%
10–15	C	45%	35%

*For cholestatic diseases (e.g., primarily biliary cirrhosis), the bilirubin level is disproportionate to the impairment in hepatic function, and an allowance should be made. For these conditions, assign 1 point for a bilirubin level <4 mg/dL, 2 points for a bilirubin level of 4–10 mg/dL, and 3 points for a bilirubin level >10 mg/dL. (Adapted from Pugh RNH, Murray-Lyon IM, Dawson JL, et al: Br J Surg 1973;60:646–649.)

b. Also look at other system involvement due to hepatic dysfunction, as mentioned above.
5. Laboratory tests/studies.
a. Hepatic function.
    i. Serum bilirubin.
    ii. Albumin.
    iii. PT.
    iv. Total protein.
b. Transaminases.
c. Alkaline phosphatase.
d. Hematologic studies.
e. Hepatitis serologies.
f. Assessment of cardiac/pulmonary/renal status.
    i. ECG, CXR, renal function tests may be needed based on age, disease severity, and duration of hepatic disease.

G. GI
1. Upper GI bleed.
a. Etiology.
    i. Esophagitis.
    ii. Gastritis.
    iii. Gastric or duodenal ulcer.
    iv. Varices.
    v. Mallory-Weiss tear.

b. Assume pt is at risk for aspiration.

c. Check Hb prior to induction, especially if pt has active bleeding.

2. Aspiration risk.

a. Pts who are at high risk of pulmonary aspiration.

   i. Gastric volume >25 mL (0.4 mL/kg) and gastric pH < 2.5.

b. Pts who should receive GI prophylaxis include those with:

   i. Symptoms related to passive reflux of gastric fluid such as acid taste or sensation of refluxing liquid into the mouth.

   ii. Abnormal pharyngeal or esophageal anatomy (e.g., large hiatal hernia, Zenker diverticulum, scleroderma).

   iii. External pressure on the stomach (ascites, pregnancy, obesity).

   iv. Full stomach (have eaten immediately prior to emergency surgery).

   v. Pts who may have reduced gastric emptying (diabetes, stress, pain).

   vi. Pts with bowel obstruction.

   vii. Pts with upper GI bleed.

b. Medications used for aspiration prophylaxis.

   i. H_2 blockers.

     • Decrease gastric acid secretion.

     • Inhibit further acid production.

     • Do not affect gastric contents already in the stomach.

     • Do not facilitate gastric emptying.

   ii. Metoclopramide.

     • Stimulates gastric emptying.

     • Shortens gastric emptying time.

     • Increases lower esophageal sphincter tone.

     • May have antiemetic effects.

     • Does not affect gastric pH.

     • Cannot clear large volumes of food in a few hours.

     • Often used in combination with an H_2 blocker for high-risk pts.

   iii. Antacids.

     • Increase gastric fluid pH to >2.5.

     • Increase gastric fluid volume.

     • Are immediately effective and alter the acidity of existing gastric contents.

     • Useful in emergency situations.

   iv. Proton pump inhibitors.

     • Thought to be as effective as H_2 blockers.

3. Carcinoid tumors.

a. Secrete serotonin and bradykinin.

b. Pts with significant symptoms should be on octreotide to avoid carcinoid syndrome and crisis.

c. Increased incidence of peptic ulcer disease with carcinoid tumor.

H. HEMATOLOGY AND ONCOLOGY

1. Abnormal coagulation.

a. May be acquired, inherited, or result from medical therapy.

b. Pts on chronic anticoagulation may be instructed to stop taking their medications prior to surgery.

c. Pts who must continue their anticoagulation therapy (i.e., pts with artificial heart valves) are typically admitted to the hospital preoperatively and placed on a heparin infusion, which is discontinued 4 to 6 hr prior to surgery.

d. The risk of epidural hematoma may preclude the use of central neuraxial blocks in pts receiving anticoagulation therapy or who have platelet deficiency/abnormalities.

e. The anesthesiologist should assess the need for blood products in the preoperative and intraoperative setting.

f. Pertinent history.
   i. Do you have a history of bleeding or easy bruising?
   ii. When was your last dose of anticoagulation therapy?
   iii. Have you received any transfusions in the past?
   iv. Do you accept blood transfusions?

g. Physical examination.
   i. Pts should be examined for sites of oozing and/or bruising.

h. Laboratory studies.

i. CBC, PTT, PT/INR, platelet count.

2. Anemia.

a. History of anemia.
   i. Examine mucous membranes for pallor.
   ii. Obtain Hb.

b. Hematology consults are recommended in pts with sickle cell disease (i.e., SS, SC).
   i. Obtain Hb and % HbS if sickle cell anemia (goal: Hb $\geq$ 10 g/dL or % HbS < 30).

3. History of radiation and/or chemotherapy.

a. If pt has received cardiotoxic medications, obtain echocardiogram results for ventricular function.

b. CBC, PTT, PT/INR, platelet count.

VI. PREOPERATIVE INSTRUCTIONS

A. FASTING (NPO) GUIDELINES (Box 4.4)

B. HOME MEDICATIONS (Table 4.5)

1. In general, all medications should be continued on the day of surgery, taken with a sip of water prior to coming to the hospital. This includes:

a. CV medications (β blockers, antiarrhythmics, digoxin, Ca^{++}-channel blockers, ACE inhibitors, statins).
   i. Perioperative β blockade should be initiated in pts at risk for perioperative myocardial ischemia.
   ii. Pts can continue to take aspirin up to morning of surgery unless surgeon asks that it be held.

4

PREOPERATIVE EVALUATION

BOX 4.4

FASTING (NPO) GUIDELINES

- Clear liquids: 2 hr.
- May have up to 8 oz of clear liquid such as water, carbonated beverages, apple juice or other clear juices (no pulp), black coffee or tea without milk or creamer, plain gelatin.
- Breast milk: 4 hr.
- Infant formula for ages <1 yr: 6 hr.
- Solid foods or non-clear liquids, milk, or candy: 8 hr.

TABLE 4.5

HOME MEDICATIONS

Class of Medications	Medication	Recommendations
Oral hypoglycemic agents	Glucophage (Metformin)	Hold morning dose on day of surgery.
	Pioglitazone (Actos)	Hold morning dose on day of surgery.
	Glyburide (DiaBeta, Micronase)	
	Tolazamide (Tolinase)	
	Rosiglitazone (Avandia)	
	Glimepiride (Amaryl)	
	All others	
Diuretics	Furosemide tablets (Lasix) HCTZ	Hold morning of surgery, *unless* prescribed for CHF; these pts should take their morning dose of diuretics.
Insulin	NPH, regular	Hold insulin morning of surgery. Bring insulin with pt to hospital.
Herbal supplements		Stop all herbal supplements at least 24 hr prior to surgery.

As a general rule, for pts scheduled for surgery with anesthesia, we recommend that all medications be continued on the day of surgery and taken with a sip of water prior to coming to the hospital. Exceptions to this recommendation are summarized in the table. *HCTZ*, Hydrochlorothiazide; *NPH*, neutral protamine Hagedorn.

---

b. GERD medications.
c. Asthma medications, including inhalers, montelukast (Singulair), and steroids.
   i. If steroids have been prescribed for asthma in the past 6 mo and/or if the pt had active wheezing within the past 2 mo, 1 mg/kg prednisone daily starting 3 days prior to procedure, with a dose on day of surgery, should be prescribed.
d. Medications for neurologic conditions such as seizure or PD should be continued throughout the perioperative period, including the morning of surgery.
   i. Cases have been reported in which pts with PD have difficulty ventilating in the postoperative period due to weakness and rigidity

in the setting of decreased blood levels of their anti-parkinsonian medications (which are known to have a notoriously short half-life).

e. Medications for psychiatric conditions (e.g., antidepressants, antipsychotics) are generally continued perioperatively.

f. Anti-thyroid medications should be continued through the morning of surgery because of their short half-life.

C. MEDICATIONS TO BE HELD THE DAY OF SURGERY (OR EARLIER)

1. Anticoagulants may need to be discontinued up to 2 wk prior to surgery.

2. Oral hypoglycemics (sulfonylureas and metformin) are typically held on the day of surgery or at least 8 hr preoperatively because of their long duration of action and the risk of lactic acidosis.

a. Pts who are unable to discontinue metformin preoperatively should be monitored for the development of lactic acidosis in the perioperative period.

b. Oral hypoglycemics can be restarted postoperatively when the pt is taking drugs by mouth.

c. Metformin can be restarted postoperatively if hepatic and renal functions remain adequate.

3. Insulin should be held the morning of surgery.

a. Pts should be instructed to bring their insulin with them to the hospital.

4. Diuretics should be held the morning of surgery unless prescribed for CHF.

a. If prescribed for CHF, pt should take morning dose of diuretics.

5. Herbal supplements should be stopped at least 24 hr prior to surgery.

VII. PREMEDICATION

A. SEDATION

1. Benzodiazepines.

a. Primary class of medications used for preoperative sedation.
   i. Midazolam.
   ii. Lorazepam (Ativan tablet).

b. Commonly used for sedation and anxiety relief prior to elective surgery.

c. Will also suppress recall of events that occur following their administration.

d. Disadvantages.
   i. Excessive and prolonged sedation in some pts (usually associated with high doses).
   ii. Possible interference with the release of cortisol in response to stress.

2. Practical considerations with sedation administration.

a. Oral and/or IV sedation should not be administered until nurse confirms that pt has signed surgical consents in the chart, the surgical site has been signed, and the anesthesiologist has completed the preoperative evaluation.

b. Pt must be on a stretcher before any sedation can be administered.

c. Supplemental oxygen must be available to be administered to all pts who receive sedation.

d. Once a dose of sedation has been administered in the preoperative area, pt must be closely observed.

3. Preoperative sedation in specific pt populations.

a. May be helpful in asthmatic pts whose asthma has an emotional component.

b. Avoided in pts with elevated ICP because resultant respiratory depression can lead to hypercapnia and further increase in ICP.

c. Preoperative sedation and opioids are avoided in pts with significant OSA.

   i. Pts tend to be highly sensitive to CNS depressant effects that result in hypoventilation and/or upper airway obstruction.

d. Preoperative sedation with opioids and benzodiazepines is usually avoided in pts with myasthenia gravis because of increased sensitivity to respiratory depressants.

e. Diphenhydramine is useful for premedication and sedation in pts with tremor.

B. ANALGESIA

1. Opioids are the primary class of medications used for preoperative analgesia.

a. Morphine.

b. Fentanyl.

c. Hydromorphone.

2. Preoperative use of opioids.

a. Analgesia in pts with preoperative pain.

b. Analgesia prior to insertion of invasive monitoring catheters or the institution of a regional anesthetic.

c. Administration may decrease the need for parenteral analgesics in the early postoperative period.

3. Disadvantages of preoperative opioids.

a. Respiratory depression.

b. Nausea or vomiting.

c. Delayed gastric emptying.

d. Pruritus.

e. Biliary tract spasm.

f. Orthostatic hypotension.

C. ANTIEMETICS

1. Pts with high risk of PONV.

a. Females.

b. Pts with a history of motion sickness or prior PONV.

c. Use of general rather than regional anesthesia.

d. Administration of opioids.

2. Surgical procedures with high risk of PONV.

a. Gynecologic operations.

b. Ophthalmologic operations.

c. Plastic surgery.

d. Orthopedic shoulder surgery.

e. Breast surgery.

3. Antiemetics used to prevent PONV (see Chapter 16, *Postoperative Issues*).

a. Serotonin antagonists (ondansetron, dolasetron).

b. Butyrophenones (droperidol).

c. GI prokinetics (metoclopramide).

d. Phenothiazines (perphenazine).

4. Disadvantages of preoperative administration of antiemetics.

a. Increased cost (particularly with serotonin antagonists).

b. Increased risk of dysphoria and sedation (particularly with butyrophenones).

c. Orthostatic hypotension.

4. Some pts will have PONV even with antiemetic prophylaxis.

VIII. SPECIFIC PERIOPERATIVE ISSUES FOR PEDIATRIC PTS

A. CRITERIA FOR CHILDREN HAVING A PROCEDURE AS AN OUTPATIENT

1. Full-term infants (defined as ≥37 wk postconception at birth) without significant medical problems who are at least 48 wk postconception at the time of scheduled procedure.

2. Premature infants (defined as <37 wk postconception at birth) who are ≥60 wk postconceptual age at the time of scheduled procedure.

3. Premature infants who are between 52 and 60 wk postconceptual age and have no medical problems.

4. Infants who have required supplemental or apnea monitoring must be symptom-free, have required no supplemental oxygen or monitoring for at least 6 mo, and be ≥60 wk postconception at the time of scheduled procedure.

5. Older children with significant medical problems should be evaluated as candidates for outpatient surgery on a case-by-case basis.

B. PREOPERATIVE TESTING IN PEDIATRIC PTS

1. Healthy children are not required to undergo routine testing if their procedure is expected to cause minimal blood loss.

2. Obtain preoperative Hb levels for infants who are <60 wk postconception or who have a history of anemia and are having outpatient procedures with GA.

3. Type and screen per surgeon request.

PREOPERATIVE EVALUATION

a. Pediatric cardiac surgery pts who weigh <20 kg generally need 1 unit of RBCs and 1 unit of thawed FFP (or one unit whole blood) for the pump prime in addition to the needs for the case.

4. **All menstruating pediatric pts should undergo preoperative pregnancy testing.**

C. PREOPERATIVE CONSULTS IN PEDIATRIC PTS

1. **Anesthesia consults may be indicated in children who have significant medical conditions that can influence the safe delivery of anesthesia. These conditions include:**
a. Abnormal airway anatomy or syndrome with known difficulty airway.
b. History of significant life-threatening intraoperative or perioperative complication.
c. Cystic fibrosis.
d. Symptomatic heart disease or heart failure.
e. Organ transplant pts.
f. Renal failure.
g. Hemoglobinopathies.
h. Scoliosis.
i. Skeletal dysplasia.
j. Neuromuscular disorders.
k. Metabolic disorders.
l. Pts who are oxygen dependent or receiving home ventilator therapy.
m. Former premature infants with ongoing oxygen requirement or severe chronic lung disease.

2. **Pts with known congenital heart disease must have a recent cardiac evaluation by a cardiologist.**

REFERENCES

American Society of Anesthesiologists Task Force on Perioperative Management of Patients with Obstructive Sleep Apnea. Practice Guidelines for the Perioperative Management of Patients with Obstructive Sleep Apnea. Anesthesiology 2006;104:1081–1093.

American Society of Anesthesiologists Task Force on Preanesthesia Evaluation. Practice Advisory for Preanesthesia Evaluation. Anesthesiology 2002;96:485–496.

American Society of Anesthesiologists Task Force on Preoperative Fasting. Practice Guidelines for the Preoperative Fasting and Use of Pharmacologic Agents to Reduce the Risk of Pulmonary Aspiration: Application to Healthy Patients Undergoing Elective Procedures. Anesthesiology 1999;90:896–905.

Barash PG, Cullen BF, Stoelting RK: Clinical Anesthesia, 5th ed. Philadelphia: Lippincott Williams & Wilkins, 2006.

Dunn PF: Clinical Anesthesia Procedures of the Massachusetts General Hospital, 7th ed. Philadelphia: Lippincott Williams & Wilkins, 2007.

Eagle KA, Berger PB, Calkins H, et al: ACC/AHA guideline update for perioperative cardiovascular evaluation for noncardiac surgery—executive summary: A report of the ACC/AHA Task Force on Practice Guidelines (Committee to Update the 1996 Guidelines on Perioperative Cardiovascular Evaluation for Noncardiac Surgery). J Am Coll Cardiol 2002;39(3):542–553.

Goldschlager N: Use of the treadmill test in the diagnosis of coronary artery disease in patients with chest pain. Ann Intern Med 1982;97:383.

Miller RD: Miller's Anesthesia, 6th ed. Philadelphia: Churchill Livingstone, 2005.

Morgan GE, Mikhail MD, Murray MJ: Clinical Anesthesiology, 4th ed. New York: McGraw-Hill Companies, 2006.

Pugh RNH, Murray-Lyon IM, Dawson JL, et al: Transection of oesophagus for bleeding of oesophageal varices. Br J Surg 1973;60:646–649.

Stoelting RK, Miller RD: Basics of Anesthesia, 4th ed. Philadelphia: Churchill Livingstone, 2000.

Vann M: Preoperative assessment and perioperative management of systemic disease. In Glidden RS: Anesthesiology. Baltimore: Lippincott Williams & Wilkins, 2003.

4

PREOPERATIVE EVALUATION

Equipment and Monitoring

Maria Birzescu, MD, E. David Bravos, MD, and David Nieglos, MD
Edited by Robert S. Greenberg, MD

Nearly everything that anesthesiologists do involves equipment, and it is the practitioners' responsibility to ensure that equipment that they are planning to use is functional. Equally important is knowing how to use the equipment before it is needed.

I. STANDARD MONITORS

The ASA has created standards for basic anesthetic monitoring (www. asahq.org) that focuses on oxygenation, ventilation, circulation, and temperature (when changes in body temperature are intended, anticipated, or suspected). To comply with these standards, basic monitoring usually comprises the following.

A. OXYGEN ANALYZER

1. Measures oxygen concentration in the anesthesia breathing circuit.
2. Set to alarm at a low oxygen concentration limit to prevent hypoxic mixture from being delivered to pt.

B. PULSE OXIMETER

1. Most commonly used monitor for assessing peripheral oxygenation (SpO_2).
2. Measures differential absorption of two wavelengths of light (red and infrared) by oxygenated and deoxygenated Hb.
a. Carboxyhemoglobin can lead to a falsely high SpO_2.
b. Methemoglobin will cause SpO_2 to trend toward 85%, regardless of the arterial oxygen saturation (SaO_2).
3. Requires pulsatile blood flow.

C. ELECTROCARDIOGRAM

1. ECG tracing is a recording of the summed electrical vectors produced during depolarization and repolarization of the heart.
2. Representation of the cardiac cycle as seen by ECG includes P wave (atrial depolarization), QRS complex (ventricular depolarization), and T wave (ventricular repolarization) (Fig. 5.1).
3. Five-electrode configuration system allows monitoring of six different ECG leads (I, II, III, aVR, aVF, V5).
4. The ground electrode (green lead on the five-lead configuration) is required for ECG tracing and can be placed anywhere on the body.
5. Electrical axis of lead II parallels the atria, resulting in the greatest P wave voltages of any surface lead, thus enhancing diagnosis of dysrhythmias and detection of inferior wall ischemia.
6. Lead V is most sensitive for detection of anterior and lateral ischemia.
a. By monitoring leads II and V5 simultaneously, the most information can be obtained.

5

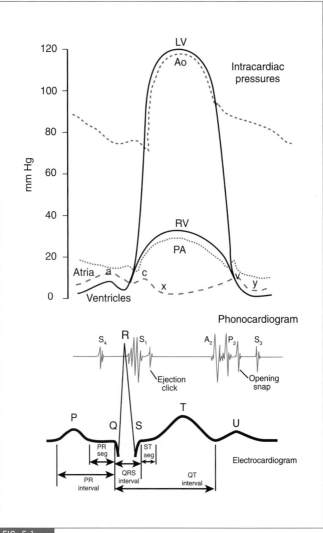

FIG. 5.1

Representation of the cardiac cycle as seen by vascular catheter pressure tracings from LV, aortic, RV, pulmonary arterial, and atrial tracings (*upper panel*) with phonocardiogram (*middle panel*) and electrocardiogram signals (*lower panel*). *LV*, left ventricle, *AO*, aorta; *RV*, right ventricle; *PA*, pulmonary artery. *(From: Johns Hopkins Hospital: The Harriett Lane Handbook, 18th ed. Philadelphia: Mosby, 2008. p 174.)*

D. CAPNOGRAPHY
1. Measures end-tidal carbon dioxide (E_TCO_2) quantitatively and produces a waveform.
2. Detection of CO_2 confirms placement of an ETT in the trachea.
a. Lack of E_TCO_2 may indicate an esophageal intubation or extremely poor cardiac output.
3. Gradient between E_TCO_2 and $PaCO_2$ (usually 2–5 mm Hg) reflects alveolar dead space.
4. Causes of elevated E_TCO_2.
a. Hypoventilation.
b. Increased CO_2 production.
   i. Malignant hyperthermia.
   ii. Shivering.
   iii. Catecholamine release.
c. Exhausted CO_2 absorbent or streaming around/through absorbent.
d. Incompetent inspiratory or expiratory valve (anesthesia circuit).
e. Inadvertent administration of CO_2.
5. Causes of decreased E_TCO_2.
a. Conditions that result in decreased pulmonary perfusion will increase alveolar dead space, which dilutes expired CO_2 and decreases E_TCO_2. Conditions include:
   i. Pulmonary embolism (air, clot, fat).
   ii. Low cardiac output.
   iii. Hypotension.
   iv. Severe bronchospasm.
   v. Right-to-left intracardiac shunt.
6. Two types of capnographs rely on the absorption of infrared light by CO_2.
a. *Flow-through* capnograph measures CO_2 passing through an adaptor placed in the breathing circuit.
b. *Aspiration* capnograph continuously suctions gas from the breathing circuit into a sample cell.
   i. In small infants, the volume of suction exceeds the tidal volume; therefore some dead space is sampled, leading to a falsely low E_TCO_2.
7. Respiratory patterns of E_TCO_2 aid in diagnosis and recognition of ventilation abnormalities (Fig. 5.2).

E. BP MEASUREMENT
1. Noninvasive.
a. Palpation.
   i. Palpate arterial peripheral pulse.
   ii. Inflate BP cuff proximal to palpated pulse until pulse is no longer palpable.
   iii. Release cuff pressure 2–3 mm Hg per heartbeat.
   iv. Pressure at which pulse becomes palpable again is systolic pressure.

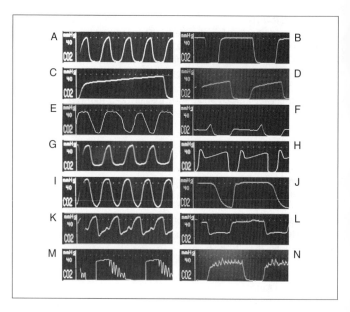

    v. Diastolic pressure cannot be determined from this method, and systolic pressure is usually underestimated by roughly 10 mm Hg.

  b. Doppler probe.

    i. Uses same technique as palpation method but instead of palpating pulse, a Doppler probe is used to detect arterial flow over the peripheral artery.

    ii. Only systolic pressure can be determined by this method.

  c. Auscultation.

    i. Uses same techniques as palpation method, but systolic and diastolic pressure can be determined by Korotkoff sounds.

      • Korotkoff sounds are generated by turbulent flow that occurs with partial occlusion of the artery.

    ii. BP cuff is placed on upper arm and is inflated until a pulse is no longer palpable (typically the radial pulse).

    iii. A stethoscope is placed over the brachial artery, and BP cuff is slowly deflated 2 to 3 mm Hg per heartbeat.

    iv. As cuff pressure falls below systolic pressure, arterial wall is partially opened, allowing turbulent flow to pass, which is audible through the stethoscope.

    v. Onset of Korotkoff sounds coincides with the systolic BP, and the offset of sounds coincides with diastolic BP.

  d. Oscillometric.

FIG. 5.2

Examples of capnograph waves. **A**, Normal spontaneous breathing. **B**, Normal mechanical ventilation. **C**, Prolonged exhalation during spontaneous breathing. As CO_2 diffuses from the mixed venous blood into the alveoli, its concentration progressively rises. **D**, Increased slope of phase III in a mechanically ventilated patient with emphysema. **E**, Added dead space during spontaneous ventilation. **F**, Dual plateau (i.e., tails-up pattern) caused by a leak in the sample line. The alveolar plateau is artifactually low because of dilution of exhaled gas with air leaking inward. During each mechanical breath, the leak is reduced because of higher pressure within the airway and tubing, explaining the rise in the CO_2 concentration at the end of the alveolar plateau. This pattern is not seen during spontaneous ventilation because the required increase in airway pressure is absent. **G**, Exhausted CO_2 absorbent produces an inhaled CO_2 concentration greater than zero. **H**, Double peak for a patient with a single-lung transplant. The first peak represents CO_2 from the transplanted (normal) lung. CO_2 exhalation from the remaining (obstructed) lung is delayed, producing the second peak. **I**, Inspiratory valve stuck open during spontaneous breathing. Some backflow into the inspired limb of the circuit causes a rise in the level of inspired CO_2. **J**, Inspiratory valve stuck open during mechanical ventilation. The "slurred" downslope during inspiration represents a small amount of inspired CO_2 in the inspired limb of the circuit. **K** and **L**, Expiratory valve stuck open during spontaneous breathing or mechanical ventilation. Inhalation of exhaled gas causes an increase in inspired CO_2. **M**, Cardiogenic oscillations, when seen, usually occur with sidestream capnographs for spontaneously breathing patients at the end of each exhalation. Cardiac action causes to-and-fro movement of the interface between exhaled and fresh gas. The CO_2 concentration in gas entering the sampling line therefore alternates between high and low values. **N**, Electrical noise resulting from a malfunctioning component. The seemingly random nature of the signal perturbations (~3/sec) implies a nonbiologic cause. *(From Moon RE, Camporesi EM: Respiratory monitoring. In: Miller RD, (ed): Miller's Anesthesia, 6th ed. Philadelphia: Churchill Livingstone, 2005.)*

5

EQUIPMENT AND MONITORING

i. Based on arterial pulsations that cause oscillations in cuff pressure (Fig. 5.3).
ii. The oscillations are relatively smaller in amplitude above the systolic BP and increase when nearing systolic BP with cuff deflation.
iii. They reach their maximum amplitude at mean arterial pressure, then decrease again with continued cuff deflation toward diastolic BP.

2. Invasive.

a. Arterial catheter.
   i. Indications.
      • Continuous beat-to-beat BP monitoring (see Fig. 5.1).
      • Anticipated wide swings in BP.

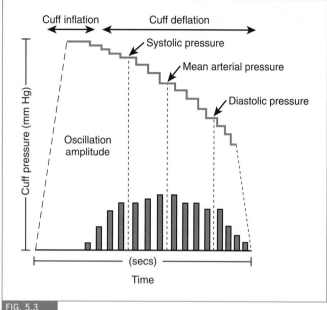

FIG. 5.3

Noninvasive BP determination sequence using oscillometry.

- Systolic variability of >10 mm Hg between expiration and inspiration is associated with hypovolemia due to rapid blood loss or large fluid shifts.
- Frequent ABG measurements.
- Inability to obtain a noninvasive BP measurement.
- Use of arterial waveform for diagnostic purposes (i.e., for timing of intraaortic balloon pump) (see Fig. 9.2).

b. Central venous catheterization.
  i. Indications.
    - CVP monitoring.
    - Placement of sheath for pulmonary artery catheterization.
    - Transvenous pacing.
    - Temporary hemodialysis.
    - Vasoactive or caustic drug (e.g., high-dose potassium, TPN) administration.
    - Long-term drug administration.
    - Aspiration of air emboli.
    - Inability to obtain adequate peripheral IV access.
    - Repeated blood sampling when arterial catheter not available.

BOX 5.1

INDICATIONS FOR PULMONARY ARTERY CATHETERIZATION

CARDIAC DISEASE

- LV dysfunction
- Recent MI
- Unstable angina
- Valvular heart disease
- Assessment of heart failure (e.g., cardiomyopathy, pericardial tamponade, cor pulmonale)

PULMONARY DISEASE

- Acute respiratory failure (e.g., adult respiratory distress syndrome)
- Assessment of pulmonary edema (cardiogenic vs. noncardiogenic)
- Pulmonary hypertension (primary vs. secondary)

COMPLEX FLUID MANAGEMENT

- Assessment of shock etiology (e.g., hypovolemic vs. cardiogenic)
- Sepsis
- Acute renal failure
- Acute burns
- Hemorrhagic pancreatitis

SPECIFIC SURGICAL PROCEDURES

- Coronary artery bypass grafting
- Valve replacement
- Heart transplantation
- Pericardiectomy
- Aortic crossclamping (e.g., aortic aneurysm repair)
- Sitting craniotomies
- Portal systemic shunts

HIGH-RISK OBSTETRICS

- Severe toxemia
- Placental abruption

---

ii. CVP waveform as it relates to the ECG is shown in Fig. 5.1.
c. Pulmonary artery catheterization (PAC).
   i. Indications (Box 5.1).
      • Currently controversial, following ICU studies that demonstrated no benefit and possible harm from PAC.
      • PAC monitoring appears appropriate in pts undergoing procedures with a high risk of complications from hemodynamic changes.
         - Proficiency of the clinicians and institution with PAC monitoring should be considered.
   ii. Insertion of PAC is guided by changes in waveform as the PAC passes through the right atrium, tricuspid valve, right ventricle, pulmonary valve, and into the pulmonary artery (see Fig. 5.1).

5

EQUIPMENT AND MONITORING

F. BRAIN OXIMETRY USING NEAR-INFRARED SPECTROSCOPY

1. Monitors regional saturation of Hb in the brain (rSO_2).
2. Sensors (right and left) placed on forehead emit light of specific wavelengths and measure the light reflected back to the sensor.
3. Measures venous and capillary blood oxygenation in addition to arterial blood saturation.
4. Reading represents the average saturation of all regional microvascular Hb.
5. Normal reading is 70% to 80%.
6. Severe hypoxia, cardiac arrest, cerebral embolization, cerebral hypoperfusion, and deep hypothermia are associated with significant decreases in rSO_2.
7. Particularly important during cardiac surgery using CPB.
a. Allows surgeons, anesthesiologists, and perfusionists to diagnose and correct any events that could lead to strokes.

G. ASSESSMENT OF NMB: PERIPHERAL NERVE STIMULATORS

1. Different responses to nerve stimulation can be seen, depending on the type of NMB and the pattern of stimulation used.
2. Train-of-four (TOF) and tetany are most often used.
3. Percent of receptor blockade can be roughly estimated by the number of twitches present.
a. 3 twitches → ~75% block.
b. 2 twitches → ~80% block.
c. 1 twitch → ~90% block.
4. Two of the most common muscles stimulated are the adductor pollicis and the orbicularis oculi.
a. Twitches in the adductor pollicis can be seen by stimulation of the ulnar nerve.
b. Twitches in the orbicularis oculi can be seen by stimulation of the facial nerves.
c. In general, muscles have different sensitivities to NMBs.
d. More centrally located muscles, including the laryngeal muscles and diaphragm, are quicker to respond to NMBs than are more peripheral muscles.
e. In addition, the orbicularis oculi is relatively more resistant compared with the adductor pollicis.
f. The best areas on which to place the pads of the nerve stimulator are those that isolate the nerve and will not directly stimulate the muscle.
   i. For the orbicularis oculi, pads should be placed superolateral and inferolateral to the lateral canthus.
   ii. For the ulnar nerve, pads should be placed just proximal and distal to the ulnar nerve as it travels through the groove between the medial epicondyle and the medial aspect of the olecranon process of the arm.

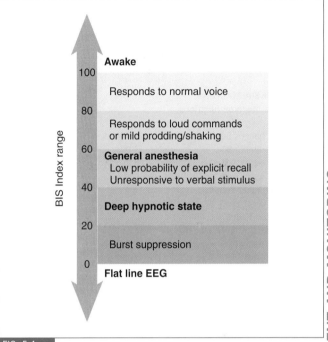

FIG. 5.4

BIS index range. The general association between clinical state and BIS values is shown. The goals established for each patient should govern titration of anesthetics to BIS ranges. These goals and associated BIS ranges may vary over time and in the context of patient status and treatment plan.

H. BISPECTRAL INDEX (BIS) (Fig. 5.4)
1. BIS is a variable, derived from EEG recordings, that correlates the readings to produce a numerical value to determine a pt's hypnotic state while under anesthesia.
a. This value can then be used as a surrogate for the likelihood of determining awareness during GA.

I. TEMPERATURE MONITORING
1. Monitoring temperature is essential when changes in body temperature are anticipated.
a. Changes can be due to the ambient temperature and can be induced by general and/or regional anesthesia.

2. Hypothermia can lead to shivering, which can cause increased myocardial work, decreased metabolism of drugs, and/or coagulopathy.
a. It has also been associated with increased risk of surgical site infection.
3. Central core temperature is best monitored by placement of probes in the bladder, nasopharynx, distal esophagus, or ear canal.

J. ANESTHESIA MACHINE
1. Anesthesia machine functions.
a. Blends gas to produce anesthesia.
b. Vaporizer changes liquid agent to a vapor and delivers it into O_2 in continuous amounts.
c. Provides life support for pt rendered apneic.
d. Removes CO_2 or excess anesthetic vapor.
2. Six machine components.
a. High-pressure system.
b. Low-pressure system.
c. Breathing circuit (including CO_2 absorber).
d. Manual ventilation.
e. Mechanical ventilation.
f. Scavenging system.
3. Safety features of anesthesia machines.
a. Designed to prevent delivery of wrong gas.
b. Non-interchangeable connections.
c. Pin index system (tanks and yokes).
d. Color coding of lines and tanks.
e. Flowmeter dial size.
f. Fail-safe valve shuts off or decreases N_2O flow if low oxygen pressure, and the machine will alarm at a pressure ≤30 psi.
g. Oxygen and N_2O flow control valves are linked mechanically or pneumatically by a proportioning system to help prevent delivery of an hypoxic mixture.
h. Hypoxic mixture is possible when third gas such as helium is used; therefore analyzer is mandatory.
4. Machine quick facts.
a. Read floats from the top, except for ball, which is read in the middle.
b. Pipeline pressure = 50 to 55 psi.
c. O_2 tank—1900 psi reduced to 45 psi.
d. N_2O tank—745 psi reduced to 45 psi.
e. Flow control valves for each gas control rate of flow.
5. Anesthesia machine checkout.
a. The anesthesia machine must be comprehensively checked each day before the first pt, and a shortened checkout must be completed before each subsequent pt (Table 5.1).
b. The checkout procedures differ somewhat between brands and models of machines (e.g., Draeger Fabius/Tiro and Ohmeda Aestiva) (Figs. 5.5

TABLE 5.1

SUMMARY OF CHECKOUT RECOMMENDATIONS BY FREQUENCY

Item to be Completed	Completed Daily Prior to First Patient	Completed Prior to Each Procedure
Item #1. Verify that auxiliary oxygen cylinder and self-inflating manual ventilation device are available and functioning.	X	
Item #2. Verify that patient suction is adequate to clear the airway.	X	X
Item #3. Turn on anesthesia delivery system and confirm that AC power is available.	X	
Item #4. Verify availability of required monitors, including alarms.	X	X
Item #5. Verify that pressure is adequate on the spare oxygen cylinder mounted on the anesthesia machine.	X	
Item #6. Verify that the piped gas pressures are ≥50 psig.	X	
Item #7. Verify that vaporizers are adequately filled and, if applicable, that the filler ports are tightly closed.	X	
Item #8. Verify that no leaks exist in the gas supply lines between the flowmeters and the common gas outlet.	X	
Item #9. Test scavenging system function.	X	
Item #10. Calibrate, or verify calibration of, the O_2 monitor, and check the low oxygen alarm.	X	
Item #11. Verify that carbon dioxide absorbent is not exhausted.	X	X
Item #12. Breathing system pressure and leak testing.	X	
Item #13. Verify that gas flows properly through the breathing circuit during both inspiration and exhalation.	X	X
Item #14. Document completion of checkout procedures.	X	X
Item #15. Confirm ventilator settings and evaluate readiness to deliver anesthesia care. (ANESTHESIA TIME OUT)	X	

Adapted from Recommendations for Pre-Anesthesia Checkout Procedures by the Sub-Committee of the ASA Committee on Equipment and Facilities, 2008.

5

EQUIPMENT AND MONITORING

DRAEGER FABIUS/TIRO PREOPERATIVE CHECKLIST
Checking the Flow Control/Metering System
☐ Activate ManSpont mode.
☐ Fully open O_2 metering valve. O_2 flow of at least 10 L/min present.
☐ Fully open N_2O metering valve. N_2O flow of at least 10 L/min present.
☐ Turn off O_2 supply. Remove O_2 connector and close O_2 cylinder valve. Ensure that O_2 Low Supply Pressure Alarm LED is blinking and that N_2O does not flow.
☐ Restore O_2 supply: N_2O flow is present.
☐ Set O_2 metering valve to 1.5 L/min. N_2O flow = 3–5 L/min.
☐ Close O_2 metering valve: No N_2O flow.
☐ Open AIR flow control valve. Air flow of at least 10 L/min present.
☐ Close all metering valves.
Oxygen Sensor Calibration
☐ Remove O_2 sensor housing from inspiratory valve dome.
☐ Calibrate O_2 sensor and flow sensor.
☐ Replace O_2 sensor.
☐ Set O_2 metering valve to ~3 L/min.
☐ Verify O_2 concentration of ~100%.
☐ Close O_2 metering valve.
Anesthetic Vaporizer
☐ Fastening: Latched down firmly and set vertically.
☐ Handwheel: In zero position and engaged.
☐ Filling level between min. and max.
☐ Interlock: Locking function OK (when present).
☐ Key-indexed filling system: Sealing key/pin inserted and closed tight (when present). Filler opening locked shut.
☐ Quik Fil or Funnel filling system: Locking screw tight (when present).
☐ Operational light lit on desflurane vaporizer.
Checking Condition of CO_2 Absorbent
☐ Color change is seen in no more than half the canister CO_2 of absorbent.
Leak-testing Fresh Gas Circuit
☐ Test with vaporizer handwheel set to zero.
☐ Go to Standby; press Leak Test soft key. Follow instructions on screen.
   If the system leaks (i.e., pressure drops):
   • Check that all plug-in, push-fit, and screw connectors fit tightly.
   • Replace any missing or damaged seals. If necessary, call local Authorized Service Organization or Draeger Service.
Inspiratory and Expiratory Valves (Compact Breathing Systems)
☐ Press the ManSpont key and confirm.
☐ Set APL-valve to MAIN position and adjust to 30 cmH_2O.
☐ Press O_2 flush.
☐ Breathing bag for manual ventilation fills.
☐ Inspiratory and expiratory valve discs move freely when breathing bag is squeezed and released.
Pressure-limiting Valve (Compact Breathing Systems)
☐ Set APL valve to MAN and 30 cmH_2O. Set fresh gas flow to 20 L/min.
☐ Press the ManSpont key and confirm.
☐ When pressure waveform on the Breathing Pressure Trace window stabilizes (e.g., flat line), flip APL-valve to SPONT to release pressure.
☐ Peak pressure display on monitor reads 24–36 cmH_2O.

FIG. 5.5
Checkout procedures for Draeger Fabius/Tiro anesthesia machine.

Checking Ventilator Operation
- [ ] Connect a breathing bag to Y-piece to act as test lung.
- [ ] Press Pressure Control Key and confirm.
- [ ] Check that ventilation measurements are displayed.
- [ ] Check that ventilator piston is cycling.
- [ ] Monitor operation of inspiratory and expiratory valve discs.
- [ ] Check that breathing bag (test lung) on Y-piece is ventilating.
- [ ] Press Standby key and confirm.

FIG. 5.5—cont'd

and 5.6); however, the same general steps are taken with each machine.

c. General inspection of anesthesia machine and work area.
d. Verify that backup ventilation equipment (self-inflating bag) is present.
e. Turn machine power switch on.
f. Check high-pressure system—pipelines and tanks.
  i. Pipeline pressure must read 50 to 55 psi.
  ii. Open oxygen tank and verify that it is at least half full (>1000 psi).
  iii. Full O_2 tank = 1800 to 2200 psi.
  iv. Full N_2O tank = 745 psi.
  v. Full air tank = 1800 psi.
g. Check low-pressure system.
  i. Turn off all flowmeters.
  ii. Check vaporizers and fill if necessary.
  iii. Negative-pressure suction bulb test.
h. Test flowmeters.
  i. Test flow in all flowmeters.
  ii. Attempt to create hypoxic O_2/N_2O mixture.
i. Check and adjust scavenging system.
  i. Ensure that scavenger is connected.
  ii. Turn off flow and ensure that scavenger bag is empty.
  iii. Activate oxygen tank flush valve and ensure that scavenger bag distends.
  iv. Ensure that CO_2 absorber is less than $\frac{1}{2}$ purple.
j. Calibrate oxygen monitor.
  i. Calibrate at room air; once connected, calibrate with oxygen flow and ensure that FIO_2 reads >90%.
k. Check status of breathing system.
  i. Set selector to bag or manual.
  ii. Check integrity of circuit.
  iii. Attach filter or humidifier to be used during the case.
l. Perform leak test of breathing system.
  i. Set flows to zero, close APL (adjustable pressure-limiting) valve, occlude Y-piece.

AESTIVA PREOPERATIVE CHECKLIST

Every day before the first patient
- [ ] Inspect the system. Look for damage, necessary drugs and equipment, correct breathing circuit setup, and hazardous conditions.
- [ ] Turn on the system.
- [ ] Set the ventilator controls to decrease alarms.
- [ ] Do the pipeline and cylinder tests. Look for sufficient pressure and no high pressure leaks (cylinders).
- [ ] Do the flow control tests:
  - Minimum flows: O_2 25–75 mL/min, all other gases no flow.
  - Link system: Increase N_2O flow to drive up O_2 flow, Decrease O_2 flow to drive down N_2O flow. The O_2 flow is $\geq$ nominal 25%
  - O_2 supply failure alarm. Alarm operates when O_2 pressure is decreased below set limit. Air flow continues. All other gases stop.
- [ ] Do the vaporizer back pressure tests:
  - Set O_2 flow to 6 L/min.
  - Turn on one vaporizer at a time.
  - Make sure that the O_2 flow stays above 5 L/min.
- [ ] Do a low-pressure leak test.
- [ ] Do the alarm tests:
  - Make sure all monitors operate correctly.
  - Make sure the sensor operates correctly. It shows approximately 21% O_2 in room air and 100% SO_2 after two min in pure O_2.
  - Make sure these ventilator alarms operate correctly: high and low O_2; low minute volume; high airway pressure; apnea and low airway pressure; sustained airway pressure.

Every time a different clinician uses the system
- [ ] Do a low-pressure leak test.

Before every patient
- [ ] Look for damage, necessary drugs and equipment, correct breathing circuit setup, and hazardous conditions.
- [ ] Check vaporizer installation:
  - Make sure the top of each vaporizer is horizontal (not on crooked).
  - Make sure each vaporizer is locked and cannot be removed.
  - Make sure the alarms and indicators operate correctly (Tec 6 vaporizer).
  - Make sure you cannot turn on more than one vaporizer at the same time.
- [ ] Do the breathing system tests:
  - Make sure the one way valves and auxiliary equipment (humidifier, etc.) operate correctly.
  - With a circle breathing-circuit module, push the drain button for $\geq$10 sec to remove condensate.
  - Ventilator circuit leak test.
  - Bag/Manual circuit leak test.
  - Bag/Manual circuit APL valve test.
  - Circuit leak test.
- [ ] Set the appropriate controls and alarms limits for the case.

FIG. 5.6

Checkout procedures for Ohmeda Aestiva anesthesia machine.

    ii. Pressurize circuit to 30 cm H_2O.

    iii. Ensure that circuit holds pressure with flows again at zero.

    iv. Open APL and confirm that pressure decreases.

    v. On the Draeger machines, this is accomplished by attaching the circuit Y-piece to the center pole and following the directions on the ventilator screen.

m. Test ventilation systems and unidirectional valves.

    i. Place second breathing bag on Y-piece.

    ii. Set appropriate ventilator settings for next pt.

    iii. Switch to automatic ventilation mode.

    iv. Ensure that ventilator is delivering a volume and rate that are reasonable for the pt.

n. Check, calibrate, or set alarm limits of monitors.

o. Check final status of anesthesia machine and workstation.

    i. Some use mnemonics to avoid forgetting anything:

    ii. SOAP (suction, oxygen, airway, pharmaceuticals).

    iii. MIDAS (machine/monitors, inhaled agents/IV, drugs, airway, suction).

The Airway

Kanupriya Kumar, MD, Ira Lehrer, DO, and Ankit Patel, DO
Edited by Lauren Berkow, MD

I. NORMAL AIRWAY ANATOMY AND INNERVATION (Fig. 6.1)

A. PEDIATRIC AIRWAY
1. Vocal cords at level of C_3-C_4.
2. Prominent occiput.
3. Large tongue.
4. Large, omega-shaped epiglottis (straight blades tend to be better).
5. Narrowest point is *below* the vocal cords (at the cricoid cartilage).

B. ADULT AIRWAY
1. Vocal cords at level of C_4-C_5.
2. Narrowest point is *at* the vocal cords.

C. CARTILAGES
1. Paired—arytenoids, corniculates, cuneiform.
2. Unpaired—thyroid, cricoid (the only true ring), epiglottic.

D. INNERVATION
1. Trigeminal nerve (cranial nerve [CN] V).
a. The first (ophthalmic) and second (maxillary) branches provide sensory input from the nose.
2. Glossopharyngeal nerve (CN IX).
a. Sensory from the posterior third of the tongue, tonsils, and nasopharynx.
3. Vagus nerve (CN X).
a. Superior laryngeal nerve.
   i. Internal laryngeal nerve—sensory from tongue to vocal cords.
   ii. External laryngeal nerve—sensory from supraglottic mucosa and motor to the cricothyroid muscle (adductor/tensor).
b. Recurrent laryngeal nerve.
   i. Motor to all of the laryngeal muscles, except cricothyroid muscle.
   ii. Sensory from below vocal cords.

II. EVALUATION FOR DIFFICULT AIRWAY (Fig. 6.2)

A. HISTORY OF DIFFICULT INTUBATION IS BEST PREDICTOR
1. Notes in the chart or previous anesthesia records detailing difficult ventilation or intubation.
2. Pt description of difficult or awake intubation.
3. History of obstructive sleep apnea.
4. Presence of disease states associated with difficult airway (Box 6.1).

B. EXAM
1. Risk factors for difficult bag-mask ventilation.

6

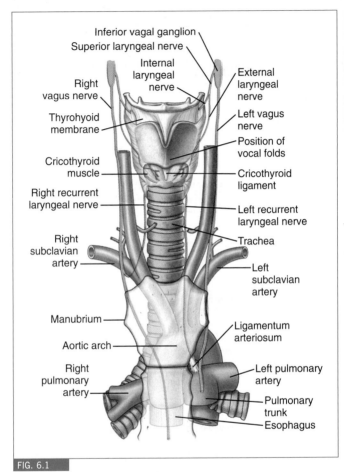

FIG. 6.1

Normal airway anatomy and innervation.

a. Presence of beard (may hide receding chin; difficult mask fit due to beard).
b. Obesity: Body mass index >26 kg/m^2.
c. Edentulous.
d. Limited neck movement (unable to touch chin to chest or extend neck).

2. Risk factors for difficult intubation.

a. Mouth opening.
   i. <2 cm or fingerbreadths between lips, teeth, or gums (if edentulous) in an adult.

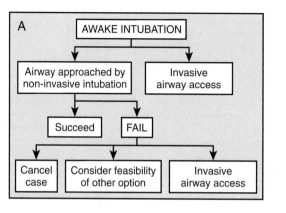

FIG. 6.2

Algorithm for evaluation of difficult airway. *(Adapted from American Society of Anesthesiologists Task Force on Management of the Difficult Airway. Practice guidelines for management of the difficult airway: An updated report by the American Society of Anesthesiologists Task Force on Management of the Difficult Airway. Anesthesiology 2003;98[5]:1269–1277.)*

6

THE AIRWAY

      ii. Prominent overbite (maxillary incisors anterior to mandibular incisors).
- b. Mallampati classification (Fig. 6.3).
  - i. Originally described by Mallampati, modified later by Samsoon and Young.
  - ii. Performed with pt sitting up with head in neutral position and tongue protruding.
  - ii. Class III and Class IV associated with difficult intubation.
- c. Thyromental distance (TMD) (Fig. 6.4).
  - i. Distance from thyroid notch to mental prominence with neck fully extended.
  - ii. TMD ≥3 fingerbreadths (6 cm) is normal for most adults.
  - iii. TMD ≤2 cm—may have difficulty visualizing larynx with laryngoscopy.
- d. Neck.
  - i. Full range of motion allows for the alignment of the three axes—oral, pharyngeal, laryngeal.
  - ii. 35° of extension from horizontal is normal.
  - iii. Short, thick neck or neck extension <35° may be predictor of difficult visualization of larynx.

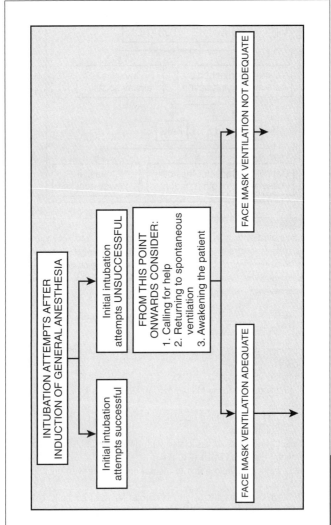

FIG. 6.2—cont'd

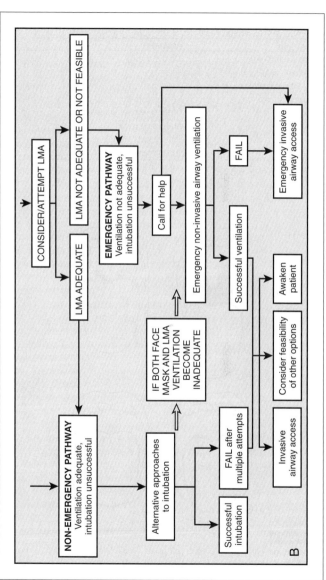

BOX 6.1	
DISEASE STATES ASSOCIATED WITH DIFFICULT AIRWAY MANAGEMENT	
CONGENITAL	ACQUIRED
Pierre-Robin syndrome	Morbid obesity
Treacher-Collins syndrome	Acromegaly
Goldenhaar syndrome	Infections involving the airway (Ludwig angina)
Mucopolysaccharidoses	Rheumatoid arthritis
Achondroplasia	Obstructive sleep apnea
Micrognathia	Ankylosing spondylitis
Down syndrome	Tumors involving the airway
	Trauma (airway, cervical spine)

(Data from Barash PG, Cullen BF, Stoelting RK [eds]: Clinical Anesthesia. Philadelphia: Williams & Wilkins, 2001; and from Benumof JL: Airway Management: Principles and Practice. St. Louis: Mosby, 1996.)

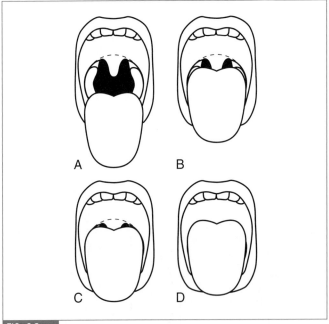

FIG. 6.3

Mallampati classification. A, Class I: soft palate, uvula, fauces, pillars visible. No difficulty. B, Class II: soft palate, uvula, fauces visible. No difficulty. C, Class III: soft palate, base of uvula visible. Moderate difficulty. D, Class IV: only hard palate visible. Severe difficulty. *(From Hagberg CA, Ghatge S: Does the airway examination predict difficult intubation? In: Fleisher LA [ed]: Evidence-Based Practice of Anesthesiology. Philadelphia, Saunders, 2004.)*

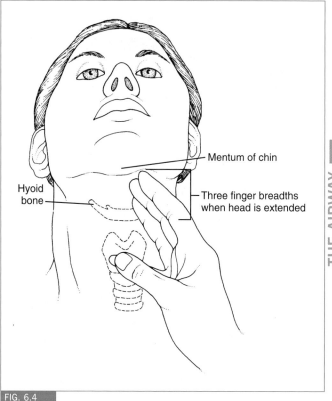

Hyoid bone

Mentum of chin

Three finger breadths when head is extended

FIG. 6.4

Thyromental distance. *(From Lutes M, Hopson LR: Tracheal intubation. In: Roberts JR, Hedges JR, Chanmugam AS, et al [eds]: Clinical Procedures in Emergency Medicine, 4th ed. Philadelphia: Saunders, 2004.)*

III. MANAGEMENT OF A DIFFICULT MASK AIRWAY

A. SIZE
1. Use correct size oral airway.

B. VENTILATION
1. Use two-handed mask ventilation, with an assistant if necessary, to ventilate pt.

C. IF ALONE, OPTIONS INCLUDE:
1. Performing two-handed mask ventilation with the pop-off valve closed and releasing the mask seal to allow for passive exhalation.

2. Performing two-handed mask ventilation with the ventilator turned on.
3. Placing LMA.

IV. AIRWAY DEVICES

A. ENDOTRACHEAL TUBE (ETT)
1. Anode—reinforced with wire designed for laser application.
2. RAE (Ring-Adair-Elwyn)—available in nasal and oral forms, with preformed bend to prevent kinking or obstruction.
a. Used for oral, head, and neck surgery (e.g., tonsillectomy, adenoidectomy, palate surgery).
3. Endotrol—contains an embedded string or wire to manipulate distal tip anteriorly.

B. SUPRAGLOTTIC AIRWAY
1. Airway device is placed blindly into oropharynx and ventilatory lumen seats above glottic opening.
a. Can be used as rescue device when ventilation is difficult or impossible.
b. Can be used as a conduit for fiberoptic intubation.
c. Can be used as primary airway (pt breathes spontaneously).
d. Should not be used in pts at risk for aspiration.

V. METHODS OF INTUBATION

A. AFTER INDUCTION OF ANESTHESIA
1. Laryngoscopy.
a. Allows visualization of vocal cords using laryngoscope device usually consisting of handle (power source) and blade.
b. Laryngoscope blade types.
    i. Macintosh blade—curved blade inserted into the vallecula anterior to epiglottis to indirectly lift epiglottis.
    ii. Miller blade—straight blade placed under epiglottis to lift epiglottis directly.
    iii. Rigid intubating scopes (Dedoscope, Hollinger scope).
c. Cormack and Lehane grades of laryngoscopy (Fig 6.5).
    i. Grade I: entire laryngeal aperture visualized.
    ii. Grade II: posterior portion of the laryngeal aperture visualized.
    iii. Grade III: visualization of the epiglottis only.
    iv. Grade IV: epiglottis not visualized.
        • Grades III and IV considered difficult laryngoscopy, often require blind placement of tube.
d. Maneuvers to improve view at laryngoscopy.
    i. Use of alternate blade (larger size, different type).
    ii. Change in head position (more or less elevation, shoulder roll).
    iii. External laryngeal manipulation (external pressure on neck downward or rightward, often improves view).
2. Rapid-sequence intubation.

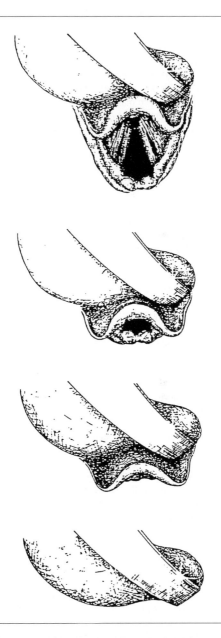

FIG. 6.5

Cormack-Lehane grades of laryngoscopy. *(From Cormack RS, Lehane J: Difficult tracheal intubation in obstetrics. Anaesthesia 1984;39:1105.)*

a. For pts at risk of aspiration (trauma, recent meal, severe gastroesophageal reflux).
b. Preoxygenation and cricoid pressure (Sellick maneuver).
c. Rapid induction followed by short-acting muscle relaxant (usually succinylcholine), with no mask ventilation once asleep.
d. Intubation with styletted ETT.
e. Release of cricoid pressure after tube placement confirmed.

B. **AWAKE INTUBATION—AIRWAY BLOCKS (Fig. 6.6)**
1. **Glossopharyngeal nerve (innervates posterior tongue and oropharynx).**
a. After negative aspiration, 2 to 3 mL 1% to 2% lidocaine is injected into base of posterior tonsillar pillars bilaterally using a 25 G needle (spinal needle works well).
2. **Superior laryngeal nerve (sensory internal branch innervates the upper larynx to the level of the vocal cords; motor external branch innervates cricothyroid muscle).**
a. With pt supine and neck extended, thyrohyoid membrane is located.
b. Hyoid bone is displaced laterally toward side to be blocked.
c. 25 G needle is inserted inferior to greater cornu and advanced 2 to 3 mm.
d. Slight loss of resistance is noted as needle passes through thyrohyoid membrane.
e. After negative aspiration, 2 to 3 mL 1% to 2% lidocaine is injected bilaterally.
f. Note: As this block is in area of carotids, provider must be certain to aspirate prior to and during injection.
3. **Recurrent laryngeal nerve (sensory below the vocal cords; motor for vocal cords, inferior larynx and all intrinsic laryngeal muscles, except for cricothyroid).**
a. This nerve is blocked with transtracheal injection using a 20 or 22 G angiocatheter inserted through cricothyroid membrane.
b. After aspiration for air to confirm tracheal placement, needle is removed, leaving only the catheter.
c. 3 to 5 mL of 2% to 4% lidocaine is injected at end inspiration.
d. Angiocatheters are used preferably to needles for this block because pt may cough during injection, and a soft catheter is less likely to damage trachea.

C. **FIBEROPTIC INTUBATION**
1. **General.**
a. May be performed before or after induction of anesthesia.
b. Best performed in awake pts with known difficult airway or risk factors for difficult mask ventilation and in pts with unstable necks.
c. Use of antisialagogue (0.2 mg glycopyrrolate or 0.1 to 0.2 mg atropine IV) is recommended 15 min prior to topicalization of airway.
d. Oxygen supplementation during topicalization.

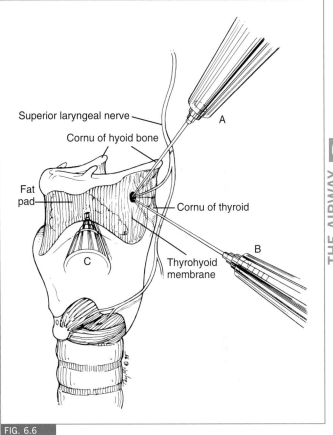

FIG. 6.6

Awake intubation—airway blocks. *(From Hagberg CA: Benumof's Airway Management, 2nd Ed. Mosby. Philadelphia, 2007.)*

   i. Nasal cannula in nose or mouth, face mask oxygen, or circle system attached to nasal airway with ETT adaptor should be considered.

e. Sedated and/or topicalized pts are at risk for aspiration.

2. Preparation for oral route.

a. Can be introduced directly into the mouth or through an airway device.

   i. Ovassapian or Williams airway.

   ii. Supraglottic airway (e.g., LMA).

b. Oropharyngeal topical anesthesia.

i. Materials: Nebulizer and 1 amp (5 mL) 4% lidocaine (total dose: 200 mg).
ii. Technique: With pt sitting, allow pt to breathe nebulized mixture delivered by nebulizing face mask or oral pipe until all lidocaine is used; 10 to 15 min should be allowed for full effect.
c. Oral topicalization.
i. 1 to 2 in of 5% lidocaine ointment should be applied on both sides of tongue blade (lidocaine lollipop), and pt allowed to suck on it.
ii. Oropharynx is sprayed with aerosolized lidocaine, progressively farther back in posterior oropharynx.
iii. Provider must be mindful of amount of lidocaine delivered to prevent toxicity.

3. Preparation for nasal route.
a. Nasal topicalization.
i. Which nares pt can breathe through more easily is determined, as this may be the one in which the ETT is more easily inserted; however, topicalization of both nares increases success.
ii. Cotton-tipped applicators soaked in one tube of 2% lidocaine jelly +10 mg phenylephrine (1 mL) as a slurry are gently inserted into the nares, starting along the medial (septal) portion to anesthetize septal area first.
iii. Applicators are left in place for 2 to 3 min for topical effect.
iv. Some anesthetists use cocaine rather than this slurry.
b. Dilation of nares.
i. Remove swabs and dilate with progressively larger nasal airways, starting with 6.5 mm and increasing size up to 8.5 mm, coated with lidocaine jelly/phenylephrine slurry.
ii. Advancing against resistance should be avoided to prevent trauma; if resistance is encountered, change to other side.
iii. Optional—2% lidocaine can be injected through nasal airway to topicalize back of oropharynx. When cough reflex is absent, oropharynx should be well topicalized.
c. ETT preparation.
i. Softening ETT in warm saline may aid in passage through nares.
ii. May require the use of longer ETTs (microlaryngeal tubes) if smaller internal diameter sizes are used.

D. FOB TECHNIQUE (Table 6.1)
1. Oral.
a. Load ETT onto FOB.
b. Place FOB directly into mouth or through Williams or Ovassapian airway.
c. Advance FOB through glottis and vocal cords until carina is visualized.
d. Slide ETT off of FOB into trachea; confirm placement as FOB is removed.

TABLE 6.1

FOB AND ETT SIZES

FOB Size	Diameter (mm)	Will Accommodate ETT Size
Pediatric	2.2	3.0 mm ID or larger, 28 F DLT
Adult medium	3.1–4.1	5.0 mm ID or larger, 37 F DLT
Adult large	5.2	6.0 mm ID or larger, will not fit inside DLT or Aintree catheter

ID, Internal diameter; *F*, French; *DLT*, double-lumen tube.

TABLE 6.2

LMA AND ETT SIZES

LMA Size	Pt Weight (kg)	Will Accommodate ETT Size (ID) (mm)
Size 1	<5	3.5
Size 1.5	5–10	4.0
Size 2	10–20	4.5
Size 2.5	20–30	5.0
Size 3	30–50	6.0
Size 4	50–70	6.0
Size 5	70–100	7.0

LMA, Laryngeal mask airway; *ETT*, endotracheal tube; *ID*, internal diameter.

6

THE AIRWAY

2. **Nasal.**
a. Place warmed ETT into dilated nares (ETT balloon is completely deflated).
b. ETT size depends on size of pt's nares.
   i. In nares dilated to 7.5 nasal airway, 6.5 ETT should pass.
   ii. In nares dilated to 8.0 nasal airway, 7.0 ETT should pass.
c. Place FOB inside ETT and advance until glottis, vocal cords, and carina are visualized.
d. Advance ETT through nares over FOB until placed into trachea.
3. **Converting an LMA to an ETT using FOB guidance (Table 6.2).**
a. Place Aintree catheter (Cook Critical Care, Inc.) over 3.5 to 4.1 mm FOB (5.0 mm FOB will not fit inside catheter).
b. Lubricate outside of Aintree catheter to facilitate passage through LMA.
c. Place Aintree/FOB unit through LMA until vocal cords and carina are visualized.
d. Pass Aintree/FOB unit into trachea; remove FOB, leaving catheter in place.
e. Deflate and remove LMA.
f. Slide ETT over Aintree catheter into trachea and remove catheter.
g. Can also place ETT directly through LMA into trachea, either blindly or with FOB guidance, but LMA must be left in place.
h. ETT size that will fit inside LMA depends on LMA size and vendor (see Table 6.2)

> BOX 6.2
>
> ### ALTERNATIVE METHODS OF INTUBATION
>
> - Light-wand intubation
> - Laryngeal mask airway (LMA) assisted intubation; intubating LMA (marketed as Fastrach)
> - Bougie-assisted intubation (Eschmann stylet, gum elastic bougie)
> - Blind nasal intubation
> - Retrograde wire-assisted intubation
> - Video laryngoscopes (Storz video laryngoscope, AirTraq, Glidescope, Mcgrath scope)
> - Combitube
> - Surgical laryngoscopes (Dedoscope, Hollinger scope)

E. ALTERNATE INTUBATION TECHNIQUES (Box 6.2)

1. Devices that allow alternative techniques to direct laryngoscopy or fiberoptic intubation are commercially available and may be useful for difficult airway management.

F. SURGICAL AIRWAY (Fig. 6.7)

1. **Transtracheal jet ventilation through the cricothyroid membrane.**
   a. 14 or 16 G IV catheter is placed through cricothyroid membrane.
   b. Jet ventilation through catheter is performed until chest rise is obtained.
   c. Oxygenation and capnography must be carefully monitored.
   d. Risk of barotrauma, pneumothorax, pneumomediastinum.
2. **Cricothyrotomy.**
   a. Emergent airway placed through cricothyroid membrane.
   b. Open technique for adults.
      i. Scalpel to make incision.
      ii. Clamp to spread the tissues.
      iii. 5.0 uncuffed ETT to secure airway.
   c. Kits are commercially available for percutaneous technique.
   d. This is a temporary airway, which must be converted to formal tracheostomy.
3. **Tracheostomy.**
   a. Performed by ENT surgeons.

G. COMPLICATIONS OF INTUBATION

1. Injury to lips, gums, soft tissues in mouth.
2. Bleeding.
3. Damage or dislodgement of teeth.
4. Aspiration of gastric contents.
5. Hypoxia (due to loss of airway or inability to ventilate).
6. Damage to vocal cords.
7. Airway edema (true or false vocal cords).

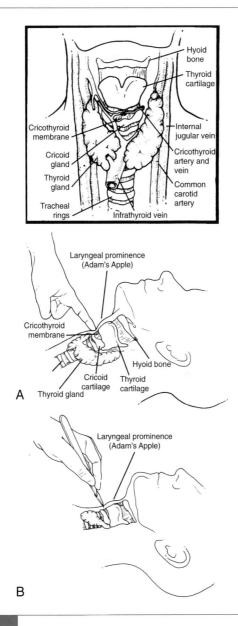

FIG. 6.7

Surgical airway technique. A, Palpate and identify cricothyroid membrane. B, Make a vertical incision through the skin.

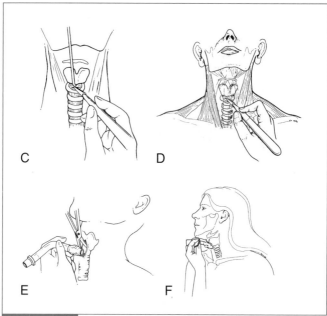

FIG. 6.7—cont'd

C, Expose the trachea and make an incision into the trachea. Push the tracheal hook into the trachea and provide upward traction. D, Enlarge the tracheal incision to accommodate an endotracheal or tracheostomy tube. E, Advance an endotracheal tube (e.g. 5.0 mm uncuffed tube for an adult) or cricothyrotomy tube into tracheal opening. F, Aiming downward, advance tube into trachea and confirm placement by the presence of end tidal carbon dioxide, breath sounds, and chest rise. *(From Mace SE, Hedges JR: Cricothyrotomy and translaryngeal jet ventilation. In: Roberts JR, Hedges JR, Chanmugam AS, et al [eds]: Clinical Procedures in Emergency Medicine, 4th ed. Philadelphia: Saunders, 2004.)*

VI. EXTUBATION

A. PT MUST MEET ALL EXTUBATION CRITERIA

1. Awake and alert to ensure airway protection.
2. Respiratory rate <30 to 35.
3. Stable BP and pulse, no significant inotropic support.
4. Adequate gas exchange (baseline oxygen saturation or >93%; not significantly acidotic or hypercapnic by arterial blood gas, if applicable).

5. Adequate NMB reversal (strong grip, sustained head lift).
6. Negative inspiratory force >20 mm Hg.
7. Vital capacity >15 mg/kg.

B. EXTUBATION COMPLICATIONS
1. Hypoventilation when the stimulus of the ETT is removed, leading to hypercarbia, hypoxia.
2. Postextubation airway edema, which may lead to stridor or laryngospasm.
3. Aspiration.
4. Negative pressure pulmonary edema.
a. If pt attempts to breathe against a closed glottis or other upper airway obstruction.
5. Vocal cord injury.

REFERENCES CONSULTED
Barash PG, Cullen BF, Stoelting RK (eds): Clinical Anesthesia. Philadelphia: Williams & Wilkins, 2001.

Benumof JL: Airway Management: Principles and Practice, St. Louis: Mosby, 1996.

Berkow L: Strategies for airway management. Best Pract Res Clin Anaesthesiol 2004;18(4):531–548.

Samsoon GLT, Young JRB: Difficult tracheal intubation: A retrospective study. Anaesthesia 1997;42:487–490.

6

THE AIRWAY

General Anesthetic Care

Akara Forsythe, MD, Jeremy Goetz, DO, Leo Hsiao, DO,
and Stephen Yang, MD
Edited by Theresa Hartsell, MD, PhD, and Elizabeth Martinez, MD

I. INTRAVENOUS ANESTHETICS (Table 7.1)

The goal of using IV anesthetics for induction is to provide a smooth transition to an unconscious state while maintaining hemodynamic stability. Some agents commonly used for induction of GA may often be utilized for maintenance of anesthesia or, at lesser doses, for sedation.

II. VOLATILE ANESTHETICS (VAs) (Tables 7.2 and 7.3)

7

Inhalational induction with VAs provides an alternative means of induction for pediatric pts and for pts in whom maintenance of spontaneous ventilation is employed to reduce risk of airway compromise or obstruction.

A. DEFINITIONS

1. Minimum alveolar concentration (MAC)—concentration required to produce immobility in 50% of individuals exposed to a noxious or painful stimulus.
2. MAC ED_{95}—concentration required to produce immobility in 95% of individuals exposed to a supramaximal painful stimulus, typically $1.3 \times$ MAC.
3. MAC awake—concentration required to prevent an appropriate response to command in 50% of individuals.
4. MAC amnesia—concentration required to produce amnesia in 50% of pts. Memory loss typically occurs at concentrations just below MAC awake, although this can be variable depending on the potency of the agent.
5. MAC_{BAR}—MAC concentration required to suppress the sympathetic surge associated with supramaximal stimulation in 50% of individuals; typically $1.5 \times$ MAC.

B. PHYSICAL PROPERTIES

1. Early VA (chloroform) used chlorine for halogenation.
2. Modern VAs (isoflurane, halothane) are halogenated with fluorine and chlorine, creating less flammability and toxicity.
3. The newest VAs (desflurane and sevoflurane) are halogenated by fluorine alone, resulting in agents that are less soluble in blood and tissue, allowing for a more rapid recovery.

C. MECHANISM OF ACTION

1. VAs are thought to work in the CNS at the level of the brain and spinal cord to create amnesia, analgesia, and some degree of muscle relaxation, although the exact mechanism is unknown.

2. Various theories suggest that site of action is at the level of the neuronal membrane.
3. The unitary theory suggests that all VAs share a common mechanism of action.
a. This theory is supported by the Meyer-Overton hypothesis, which implies that potency of the anesthetic is directly correlated to its lipid solubility.
b. Some compounds are inconsistent with this hypothesis.
4. The five-angstrom theory states that anesthesia is produced through interaction with two sites/receptors separated by five angstroms.
a. This theory comes from experimental data that show that the potency of an agent is highest in compounds that are exactly five carbons/angstroms long.

D. PHARMACOKINETICS
1. Inspiratory and alveolar concentration.
a. VAs are delivered to the pt via a breathing circuit.
b. VA concentration that reaches the pt is the *inspiratory concentration* (Fi).
c. Owing to uptake of VA by the body, the *alveolar concentration* (Fa), is less than the Fi.
d. Expressed as *Fa/Fi*.
e. Equilibrium is reached as Fa/Fi approaches 1.
2. Uptake.
a. VAs with greater uptake by the body have a lower Fa/Fi and slower induction time.
b. Uptake of VAs is determined by:
   i.   Anesthetic's solubility in blood.
   ii. Alveolar blood flow.
   iii. Difference between alveolar and venous partial pressures.
c. Solubility.
   i.   VAs are relatively insoluble in plasma and tissue, allowing rapid accumulation in the bloodstream and CNS.
        • The less soluble the VA is, the more quickly it works and wears off.
   ii. Solubility of VA is expressed as a partition coefficient.
   iii. The coefficient is the ratio of the agent in two compartments at equilibrium.
   iv. The blood/gas partition coefficient is typically used for comparison.
   v.   Less soluble VAs (nitrous oxide, desflurane) have a lower blood gas coefficient, as less agent is absorbed by blood.
        • As a result, alveolar and blood partial pressures reach equilibrium rapidly, leading to a faster induction.
d. Alveolar blood flow.

    i.   Because alveolar blood flow in a structurally normal heart is equal to cardiac output, changes in cardiac output affect uptake.

    ii. If cardiac output is increased, increase in uptake of agent, a slower rise in alveolar partial pressure, and delayed induction will occur.

    iii. In low output states, decreased uptake, a faster rise in alveolar partial pressure, and a more rapid induction occur.

e. Partial pressure difference between alveolar gas and venous blood.

    i.   Reflects the transfer of VA from blood to tissue.

    ii. Highly perfused organs such as the brain, heart, liver, and kidney reach equilibrium rapidly because of their intermediate solubility and small percentage of body weight.

    iii. As muscle has a large volume and intermediate solubility but is not as highly perfused as the organ group, it would take several hours to reach equilibrium.

    iv. Fat is extremely soluble but not highly perfused; it would take days to reach equilibrium.

3. Elimination

a. Occurs primarily through expired alveolar gas.

b. Trivial losses include skin, open abdomen, and biotransformation.

7

GENERAL ANESTHETIC CARE

Text continued on p. 108

TABLE 7.1

INTRAVENOUS AGENTS

Agent	Mechanism of Action	Dose	Physiologic Effects	Other Features
Propofol—isopropylphenol compound solubilized in lipid emulsion; contains soybean oil and lecithin	Facilitates inhibitory action of GABA.	Induction: 2–3 mg/kg Sedation/maintenance: • 30–300 mcg/kg/min or higher dose infusion as needed. CSHT increases by 10 min every hr after first 2–3 hr of infusion. Elimination half-life 3–12 hr.	CNS Decreases CBF/CBV and intraocular pressure. Potent antiepileptic effects with EEG burst suppression at higher doses. Antipruritic and antiemetic effects at subhypnotic doses. Muscle twitching and tonic-clonic jerking (due to subcortical glycine antagonism). Effects on SSEP—latency, increased; amplitude, decreased. Respiratory Depresses upper airway reflexes. Inhibits hypoxic and hypercapnic respiratory drive; apnea at induction doses. CV Dose-dependent hypotension due to inhibition of sympathetic vasoconstrictor activity with decreased SVR, cardiac contractility, and preload. Blunted baroreceptor response, leading to minimal change in HR. Exaggerated hypotension may be seen in the elderly and in hypovolemic pts.	Venous irritation causes pain on injection, particularly of small peripheral veins. May administer 0.5 mg/kg lidocaine IV with tourniquet 1–2 min prior to propofol administration to blunt painful effect. Lipid emulsion is a medium for bacterial growth; must be accessed with sterile technique and discarded after 6 hr to avoid possibility of bacteremia. High lipid content—has been reported to precipitate pancreatitis. Propofol infusion syndrome—life-threatening syndrome associated with continuous infusion, particularly in neurosurgical and pediatric pt populations. Characterized by metabolic acidosis, hyperlipidemia, renal failure, cardiac failure, and rhabdomyolysis. Hepatic metabolism. Renal excretion (90%).

| Thiopental—barbiturate | Enhances action of GABA, thereby depressing reticular activating system. | Induction: 3–5 mg/kg CSHT increases dramatically even after short infusions. | **CNS** Decreases CBF/CBV, producing decreases in ICP. Lowers $CMRO_2$ and induces burst suppression, which may be protective during focal brain ischemia. Potent antiepileptic effects at relatively low doses. Anti-analgesic effect of barbiturates results in a lowering of the pain threshold. Effect on SSEP—latency, increased; amplitude, decreased. **Respiratory** Depresses medullary ventilatory center, leading to dose-dependent decrease in RR/tidal volume; apnea at induction doses. May induce bronchospasm secondary to cholinergic activation, histamine release, or bronchial smooth muscle stimulation. **CV** Inhibits medullary vasomotor center, leading to venous pooling and decreased preload. Unlike propofol, barbiturates do not affect baroreceptor reflexes; often an associated rise in HR is seen. | Tissue necrosis upon infiltration or intra-arterial injection. Barbiturates induce aminolevulinic acid synthetase and therefore may precipitate porphyric crisis in inducible forms of porphyria (acute intermittent porphyria and variegate porphyria). Rapid offset related to redistribution from vessel-rich tissues to vessel-poor tissues. Reduce dosage in elderly and pts with renal failure. |

Continued

TABLE 7.1

INTRAVENOUS AGENTS—cont'd

Agent	Mechanism of Action	Dose	Physiologic Effects	Other Features
Etomidate— carboxylated imidazole (dissolved in propylene glycol)	Mimics effects of GABA and depresses reticular activating system.	Induction: 0.3 mg/kg	**CNS** Decreases CBF/CBV, producing decreases in ICP. Lowers $CMRO_2$. Causes disinhibition of the extrapyramidal motor center, resulting in myoclonus (this effect may be minimized by opioids). High association with postoperative N/V. Effects on SSEP—latency, increased; amplitude, increased. **Respiratory** Dose-dependent reductions in tidal volume and RR (markedly less pronounced than with propofol or barbiturates). **CV** Minimal effect on cardiac output and contractility. Mild decrease in SVR, resulting in a slight decrement in arterial BP and increase in HR. Effects may be accentuated with large doses, rapid administration, or in the hemodynamically compromised pt.	Pain on injection is common owing to venous irritation from the propylene glycol carrier. Adrenal suppression occurs, even after single dose of etomidate, limiting its use as infusion or for daily administrations.

| Ketamine—an arylcyclo-hexylamine | Dissociates the thalamus from the limbic system. Ketamine is an NMDA-receptor antagonist, which confers its analgesic effects. | Induction: 1–2 mg/kg IV • 3–5 mg/kg IM Dilute to 10 mg/mL prior to IV injection. Elimination half-life: α phase, 10–15 min; β phase, 2.5 hr. | **CNS** Cerebral vasodilation with increased CBF/CBV and increased ICP. Increased CMRO₂. Myoclonic activity secondary to subcortical electrical activation. Dissociative amnesia. Psychotropic effects, including illusions, unpleasant dreams, and delirium with agitation, can be minimized with benzodiazepine premedication. Effects on SSEP—latency, none; amplitude, increased. **Respiratory** Airway reflexes are largely intact, and effects on ventilatory drive are minimal. Potent bronchodilator. Increased salivation can be attenuated with anticholinergic pretreatment. Mild elevations in pulmonary pressures. **CV** Direct myocardial depression is often masked by sympathetic release and inhibition of norepinephrine reuptake. Dose-dependent increase in HR, MAP, and cardiac output (in catecholamine-replete and sympathetically intact individuals). | Nystagmus, blepharospasm, diplopia, and increased intraocular pressure. Increased muscle tone with concurrent myoclonic motions can be seen. Drug interaction with St. John's Wort. Hepatic metabolism. |

Continued

GENERAL ANESTHETIC CARE

7

TABLE 7.1
INTRAVENOUS AGENTS—cont'd

Agent	Mechanism of Action	Dose	Physiologic Effects	Other Features
Midazolam—short-acting benzodiazepine	Binds to benzodiazepine receptors, thereby facilitating GABA receptor binding and chloride membrane conductance.	Induction: 0.1–0.4 mg/kg IV Sedation: 0.01–0.1 mg/kg IV	CNS Reduces $CMRO_2$ with concurrent reductions in CBF/CBV and ICP. Antianxiolytic, anterograde amnesia. Anticonvulsant activity. Effects on SSEP—latency, no effect; amplitude, decreased. Respiratory Depresses the ventilatory response to hypercarbia. Respiratory depression is significantly less than that seen with barbiturates. CV Slight decrease in MAP, SVR, and cardiac output. Drug-induced vagolysis results in a slight rise in HR.	Can cross the placenta and induce neonatal depression. Muscle relaxant property is mediated at the spinal cord level. Flumazenil (0.3 mg IV q min up to 5 mg) is a competitive antagonist.
Opioids	Bind to opioid-specific receptors (mu, kappa, delta, sigma) located throughout the CNS.		CNS Stimulation of mu receptors results in supraspinal analgesia, respiratory depression, muscle rigidity, pruritus, and physical dependence. Kappa-receptor binding results in miosis, sedation, and spinal analgesia.	Histamine release—seen with meperidine and morphine and can cause profound hypotension; can be prevented by pretreatment with H_1 and H_2 antagonists. Centrally mediated muscle rigidity can be seen, particularly at high doses of

Delta-receptor binding provides analgesia behavioral changes and CNS stimulation, leading to seizure activity.

Sigma receptors are responsible for hallucinations, dysphoria, hypertension, tachycardia, and respiratory stimulation.

Opioids as a class also reduce $CMRO_2$, with mild concurrent decreases in CBF/CBV and ICP (if normocarbia is preserved).

Respiratory

Depress hypoxic and hypercapnic respiratory drive.

Carbon dioxide response curve is shifted down and to the right.

RR is diminished.

CV

Myocardial contractility is preserved.

Vagal-mediated bradycardia.

Dose-dependent decreases in MAP can occur, particularly with more potent members of this class of drugs (i.e., remifentanil, alfentanil).

potent opioids such as fentanyl, sufentanil, and remifentanil. Treatment includes muscle relaxants or naloxone.

Sphincter of Oddi spasm may lead to increased common bile duct pressure; can be treated with glucagon, naloxone, or nitroglycerin.

N/V may occur due to direct stimulation of the chemoreceptor trigger zone in the medulla.

Bladder sphincter stimulation may result in urinary retention.

Meperidine is structurally related to atropine and can therefore result in tachycardia. Meperidine is the only opioid that demonstrates intrinsic local anesthetic activity and negative inotropic effects. Normeperidine metabolite can induce seizures.

GENERAL ANESTHETIC CARE

7

BP, blood pressure; CBF, cerebral blood flow; CBV, cerebral blood volume; CNS, central nervous system; $CMRO_2$, cerebral metabolic rate; CSHT, context-sensitive half time; CV, cardiovascular; EEG, electroencephalogram; GABA, gamma amino butyric acid; HR, heart rate; ICP, intracranial pressure; MAP, mean arterial pressure; N/V, nausea and vomiting; RR, respiratory rate; SSEP, somatosensory-evoked potentials; SVR, systemic vascular resistance.

BOX 7.1

GUEDEL'S FOUR STAGES OF ETHER ANESTHESIA

STAGE 1—ANALGESIA

Characterized by slow, regular respirations, using diaphragm and intercostal muscles and presence of the lid reflex. The pt experiences complete amnesia, analgesia, and sedation.

STAGE 2—DELIRIUM

The pt experiences an unconscious, excitatory state associated with disinhibited activity. Physical signs include irregular respiratory pattern, pupillary dilation, and presence of the lid reflex. The risk of reflex vomiting, laryngospasm, and dysrhythmias is increased.

STAGE 3—SURGICAL ANESTHESIA

Consists of four planes:

Plane 1—mild somatic muscle relaxation, regular respiratory rate, and presence of ocular movement.

Plane 2—characterized by loss of ocular movement and respiratory changes, consisting of shortened inspiratory time and brief pauses between inhalation and exhalation.

Plane 3—complete relaxation of the abdominal musculature and prominence of diaphragmatic breathing.

Plane 4—complete paralysis of intercostal muscles, irregular respiratory pattern, paradoxical chest wall movement, and pupillary dilation.

STAGE 4—RESPIRATORY PARALYSIS

Muscles become completely relaxed, pupils are widely dilated. Cardiovascular and respiratory arrest occur during this stage.

III. STAGES OF GENERAL ANESTHESIA

A. CLASSIC DESCRIPTION PUBLISHED IN THE 1930s BY ARTHUR GUEDEL, WHO USED MUSCLE TONE, RESPIRATORY PATTERN, AND OCULAR SIGNS TO DEFINE FOUR STAGES OF ETHER ANESTHESIA (Box 7.1)

CHARACTERISTICS OF VAs (see Tables 7.2 and 7.3)

IV. NEUROMUSCULAR BLOCKADE

A. OVERVIEW

1. NMB was introduced into clinical practice more than 60 yr ago.
2. The need for muscle relaxation is governed by:
a. Type of surgical procedure.
b. Surgeon preference.
c. Pt condition.
3. Though it is useful to have a paralyzed pt in many situations, NMB is not mandatory for GA.
4. NMB improves intubating conditions and mechanical ventilation and may improve surgical conditions.

TABLE 7.2

VOLATILE ANESTHETICS

Agent	Dose (%)	Agent-Specific Effects	Effects Common to All Agents
Nitrous oxide (N_2O)	MAC, 105 MAC awake, 64	Odorless, colorless inorganic gas. Nonexplosive/nonflammable but capable of supporting combustion. Regarded as a poor amnestic when used as a sole anesthetic. When used at >65%, concentrations can decrease the MAC requirements of potent VA agents by 50%. Low blood solubility allows more rapid induction and emergence. Diffuses along the concentration gradient faster than nitrogen, leaving other gases in a smaller, more concentrated space (**concentration effect**), increasing the effective concentration of other VAs (**second gas effect**). N_2O is 20–30 times more soluble than nitrogen; therefore it will displace air, particularly in closed spaces. Because N_2O diffuses in and out of spaces more rapidly than nitrogen does, **expansion of air-filled spaces** occurs. 70% N_2O can increase the size of an air bubble by an average of 63% in 10 min. This is relevant in a number of clinical scenarios, including air emboli, pneumothoraces, middle ear surgery, bowel surgery, eye surgery (particularly with the use of trihexyl fluoride), and air-filled balloon tips, including the ETT balloon. Does not provide muscle relaxation or potentiate NMB agents. When N_2O is turned off at end of anesthesia, concentration in the alveoli is lower than that in the body. N_2O floods in, displacing nitrogen and oxygen, leaving a hypoxic mixture for the pt to breathe (**diffusion hypoxia**). Thus pt should receive 100% oxygen until N_2O washes out.	

Continued

GENERAL ANESTHETIC CARE

7

TABLE 7.2

VOLATILE ANESTHETICS—cont'd

Agent	Dose (%)	Agent-Specific Effects	Effects Common to All Agents
		Thought to be a significant cause of postoperative N/V, although this theory is not supported by all studies. **CV** Stimulation of sympathetic nervous system allows for unchanged-to-increased BP and cardiac output. N_2O-induced catecholamine release confers a potential risk of epinephrine-induced dysrhythmias. Pulmonary vasoconstriction with exacerbation of pulmonary hypertension should be avoided in pts with pulmonary hypertension.	**CNS** Dose-dependent increase in CBF/CBV and a subsequent increase in ICP. This effect can be attenuated by hypocapnia, as volatile anesthetics apparently enhance carbon dioxide reactivity in cerebral vessels and reduce $CMRO_2$, thereby affecting EEG and SSEP measurements. **Respiratory** Dose-dependent increase in RR, decrease in tidal volume, and overall decrease in minute ventilation, leading to rapid shallow breathing and, ultimately, apnea. All halogenated agents are bronchodilators. Central depression of hypoxic ventilatory response at levels as low as 0.1 MAC.
HALOGENATED VOLATILE ANESTHETICS			
Isoflurane	MAC, 1.15 MAC awake, 0.38	Isoflurane's odor limits its use as a mask induction agent. Coronary vasodilation creates a potential for coronary steal in which blood is diverted from fixed diseased vessels toward healthy dilated vessels; however, the clinical relevance of this effect is questionable.	
Sevoflurane	MAC, 2.1 MAC awake, 0.34	Sevoflurane is nonpungent; this, together with its low blood solubility, makes sevoflurane ideal for mask inductions. Of all VAs, sevoflurane exerts the most profound effect on reducing airway resistance. Sevoflurane is degraded by carbon dioxide absorbents (baralyme > soda lime) to form compound A (fluoromethyl-2,2-difluoro-1-vinyl ether), which has been shown to cause renal toxicity in animal models; risk of accumulation is increased when using low flow rates (<2 L/min). Carbon monoxide is also produced in the presence of desiccated soda lime. Hepatic metabolism causes an increase in serum fluoride, a potential nephrotoxin; however, the clinical significance is likely minimal.	

| Desflurane | MAC, 6.1
MAC awake, 0.34 | Low solubility allows for rapid wash-in and wash-out; wake-up times have been observed to be up to 50% less than with isoflurane.
Not to be used for inhalational induction; pungency causes upper airway irritation and can lead to coughing, breath holding, and laryngospasm, particularly at lower MAC levels.
Rapid increases in concentration can lead to transient but significant increases in sympathetic activity with concurrent rises in HR and BP.
Can be degraded by baralyme and desiccated soda lime to form carbon monoxide. | Inhibition of hypoxic pulmonary vasoconstriction in a dose-dependent fashion; concurrent bronchodilation may lead to V/Q mismatching.
Depression of mucociliary clearance that may contribute to postoperative hypoxia and atelectasis.
CV
Dose-dependent decrease in MAP. Substitution of N_2O for a portion of VA at equivalent MAC doses attenuates drop in MAP.
With the exception of halothane, HR is increased with all VAs because of a decrease in SVR and a functional carotid sinus baroreceptor reflex. Owing to rises in HR, cardiac output (HR × MAP) is largely maintained with sevoflurane, isoflurane, and desflurane, despite decreases in MAP. |
| Halothane | MAC, 0.75
MAC awake, 0.55 | Ideal for mask inductions because of its (relatively) pleasant smell. Use has been limited over the years with the advent of sevoflurane.
Halothane lowers the arrhythmogenic threshold in response to epinephrine
Halothane decreases cardiac output in a dose-dependent fashion.
Potential for rare (1 : 35,000) halothane-induced hepatitis. Mechanism is unknown but is thought to be due to an autoimmune response. | Halothane expectedly exhibits a dose-dependent decrease in cardiac output and may be associated with bradycardia, particularly in young children. |

BP, blood pressure; *CBF*, cerebral blood flow; *CBV*, cerebral blood volume; *CNS*, central nervous system; *CV*, cardiovascular; *EEG*, electroencephalogram; *ETT*, endotracheal tube; *HR*, heart rate; *ICP*, intracraneal pressure; *MAC*, minimum alveolar concentration; *MAP*, mean arterial pressure; *NMB*, neuromuscular blockade; *N/V*, nausea and vomiting; *RR*, respiratory rate; *SSEP*, somatosensory evoked potential; *VA*, volatile anesthetic; *V/Q*, ventilation/perfusion.

GENERAL ANESTHETIC CARE 7

TABLE 7.3

EFFECTS OF INHALATIONAL AGENTS

	Desflurane	Halothane	Isoflurane	Sevoflurane	Nitrous Oxide
BP	↓↓	↓↓	↓↓	↓	—
HR	↑	↓	↑	—	—
CO	—/↓	↓	—	↓	—
CBF	↑	↑↑	↑	↑	↑
ICP	↑	↑↑	↑	↑	↑
NMB	↑↑	↑↑	↑↑	↑↑	↑

BP, blood pressure; *HR*, heart rate; *CO*, cardiac output; *CBF*, cerebral blood flow, *ICP*, intracranial pressure; *NMB*, potentiation of nondepolarizing neuromuscular blockade; —, no change.

B. MECHANISM

1. Currently utilized NMBs are competitive or noncompetitive antagonists of the nicotinic (motor end plate) acetylcholine receptor.

C. DEFINITIONS

1. The ED_{95} of an NMB agent is the amount of drug needed to achieve 95% block of a single stimulus in 50% of pts.
2. The higher the ED_{95}, the less potent the NMB.
3. The more potent the agent, the lower the ED_{95}.
4. More potent drugs typically have a longer time to onset because more time is needed to block the same number of receptors.

D. MONITORING

1. Because of pt variation in sensitivity to NMB, it is important to monitor neuromuscular function when utilizing intermediate- to long-acting agents.
a. Monitoring can also be helpful in the titration of short-acting agents.
2. Typically, peripheral nerve stimulation of the ulnar nerve (measured at the adductor pollicis muscle) or the facial nerve (measured at the orbicularis oculi muscle) is performed using a pair of standard ECG pads.
a. Direct muscle stimulation (a false-positive test) should be avoided by placing the electrodes over the course of the nerve and not over the muscle itself.
3. The degree of NMB is monitored by applying various patterns of electrical stimulation. Most commonly used are:
a. The twitch—a single square-wave pulse of 0.2 msec, which may be repeated every 1 to 10 sec.
   i. Increasing blockade results in diminished muscle contraction response to each successive stimulus.
b. The train of four (TOF)—a series of four twitch stimuli in 2 sec.
   i. The muscle contraction responses to a TOF pattern (also called "twitches") progressively fade as receptor occupancy increases.

ii. The ratio of the first to the final twitch is a sensitive measure of relaxation.

iii. Because responses may be difficult to quantify in the clinical environment, it is acceptable to monitor the sequential disappearance of muscle contractions, where disappearance of the fourth twitch approximates a block of 75% of the receptors of the end plate; the third twitch, an 80% block; and the second twitch, a 90% block.

c. Tetany—a 50 Hz or 100 Hz maximal stimulus.

i. Sustained contraction (at least 5 sec) represents clinically adequate recovery from NMB.

ii. Because such a stimulus increases the concentration of acetylcholine at the motor end plate, a successive TOF stimulus may result in greater response than if no tetany had occurred.

iii. This phenomenon is called *post-tetanic facilitation*.

E. CLASSES OF NMB AGENTS

1. Depolarizing agents.

a. Succinylcholine (SCH) is the only commercially available depolarizing NMB agent.

b. Acts at presynaptic, postsynaptic, and extrajunctional receptors of the motor end plate.

c. Although the exact mechanism is unknown, it is thought that SCH binds to the acetylcholine receptors, causing depolarization of the motor end plate with muscle contraction, followed by inactivation of the terminal and flaccid paralysis.

d. The ED_{95} is 0.05 mg/kg in the absence of other drugs.

i. When used for intubation, a 1 to 1.5 mg/kg dose is used.

e. The exact dose depends on whether a defasciculating dose of a nondepolarizing NMB is used (see below.)

f. Phase I blockade.

i. Normal blockade that occurs after SCH administration.

ii. Characteristics of phase I block.
- Decreased muscle contraction in response to a single stimulus.
- Decreased amplitude, but sustained response, to continuous stimulus.
- >70% decrease in TOF.
- No post-tetanic facilitation.

g. Phase II blockade.

i. Occurs after multiple doses of SCH or after prolonged use of SCH infusion.

ii. Elicits a pattern of nerve stimulation similar to that of nondepolarizing NMBs.

iii. Characteristics of phase II blockade.
- Decreased muscle contraction in response to a single stimulus.
- Presence of tetanic fade.

- TOF <40%.
- Presence of post-tetanic facilitation.

h. The side effects of SCH include sinus bradycardia with escape beats, anaphylaxis (1 in 10,000 doses), fasciculations, myalgias, increased gastric pressure, increased intraocular pressure (increases by 5–15 mm Hg), increased ICP, and elevation in serum potassium by 0.5 to 1.0 meq/L.

i. Contraindications for SCH.

  i. Pts with malignant hyperthermia.

  ii. Pts who may be susceptible to malignant hyperthermia, including those with Duchenne muscular dystrophy and central core disease.

  iii. Conditions secondary to the increased risk of hyperkalemia.

  - Major denervation injuries, stroke, trauma, extensive burns, prolonged immobility, spinal cord transection, and muscular dystrophies.

  iv. Open globe injuries (concern over extrusion of intraocular contents).

  v. Relatively contraindicated in pts with evisceration injury or suspicion of increased ICP because of concerns over increasing abdominal or intracranial pressures, respectively.

  vi. Use in pts with history of atypical plasma cholinesterase or plasma cholinesterase deficiency should be avoided because of the tendency for prolonged NMB.

  vii. Many practitioners avoid the use of SCH in children <10 yr old, owing to reports of hyperkalemic arrests in children with occult musculoskeletal disorders, for example, Becker muscular dystrophy.

2. Nondepolarizing agents (Tables 7.4 and 7.5).

a. Nondepolarizing NMB agents act by competitively binding to the α subunits of the acetylcholine receptors and blocking stimulus transmission, resulting in paralysis.

b. Two classes of nondepolarizing NMBs.

  i. Aminosteroids (e.g., rocuronium, vecuronium, pancuronium).

  ii. Benzylisoquinoliniums (e.g., atracurium, cis-atracurium).

TABLE 7.4

PROPERTIES OF COMMONLY USED NEUROMUSCULAR BLOCKERS

Drug	Intubating Dose (mg/kg)	Infusion Rate (mcg/kg/min)	Onset (sec)	Duration	Type of Elimination
Atracurium	0.05	3–12	90–150	Intermediate	Hofmann degradation
Cisatracurium	0.15–0.2	1–3	90–120	Intermediate	Hofmann degradation
Pancuronium	0.08–0.12	—	120–240	Long	Kidney, liver
Rocuronium	0.9–1.2	9–12	60–90	Intermediate	Kidney, liver
Succinylcholine	1.5	—	30–90	Very short	Pseudocholinesterases
Vecuronium	0.08–0.12	1–2	90–150	Intermediate	Kidney, liver

TABLE 7.5

MAIN SIDE EFFECTS OF NONDEPOLARIZING NMBS

Drug	Histamine Release	Vagolysis	Other Side Effects
Atracurium	+	—	
Cisatracurium	—	—	Anaphylaxis
Pancuronium	—	+++	
Rocuronium	—	—	Anaphylaxis; precipitate may form when injected with thiopental.
Vecuronium	—	—	Precipitate may form when injected with thiopental.

c. The time to onset and the duration of nondepolarizing NMB can be increased by increasing the dose of the agent, with more potent agents typically having a longer time to onset.
d. When a rapid and profound NMB is required (e.g., rapid control of the airway) but muscle fasciculations are undesirable, a defasciculating dose of a nondepolarizing NMB may be given prior to use of SCH.

F. ANTAGONISM OF NMB
1. Depolarizing NMB agents.
a. Intrinsically reversed by plasma pseudocholinesterases.
b. No commercial reversal agent is available for SCH.
   i. Typically, none is needed because SCH is rapidly degraded by plasma cholinesterases.
c. In pts homozygous for disorders of plasma cholinesterases (1 in 2000 people), prolonged paralysis, up to 3 to 6 hr, can occur if SCH is used.
   i. Treatment is supportive care.
   ii. Because FFP has plasma cholinesterase, its use can speed recovery from depolarizing blockade in those with the deficiency.
   iii. However, because the use of FFP is not without risk, this method is not recommended.
2. Nondepolarizing NMB agents.
a. Anticholinesterases are the only drugs used currently to antagonize the effects of nondepolarizing NMB.
   i. These drugs act by inhibiting the enzyme acetylcholinesterase, which degrades acetylcholine.
   ii. The end result is more acetylcholine at the motor end plates to compete with molecules of nondepolarizing NMBs.
b. Edrophonium, neostigmine, and pyridostigmine are currently in use.
   i. All of the above have similar half lives, but their times to peak effect are different.
   ii. Pyridostigmine (15–20 min) > neostigmine (7–12 min) > edrophonium (1–2 min).
   iii. Numerous studies have deemed neostigmine more effective in antagonizing intense blockade.

7

GENERAL ANESTHETIC CARE

c. The side effects of anticholinesterases include bradycardia, increased salivation, and increased gastric motility.
d. Because profound bradycardia can be caused by the increased availability of acetylcholine at nicotinic receptors in the heart, their use should be preceded by an anticholinergic agent—atropine or glycopyrrolate.
e. No benefit is derived from using supratherapeutic doses of anticholinesterases.
   i.   For instance, the therapeutic dose of neostigmine is 0.07 mg/kg.
   ii. Using a higher dose does not increase time to peak effect or duration of the drug.
f. Sugammadex.
   i.   Rocuronium and vecuronium encapsulating reversal agent.
   ii. Rapidly reverses NMB without autonomic side effects.
   iii. Currently in phase 3 trials; therefore, not yet approved by the FDA.

G. FACTORS THAT INFLUENCE NMB
1. Myasthenia gravis.
a. Autoimmune disease with antibodies against acetylcholine receptors, resulting in pharyngeal/ocular weakness.
b. Treatment often consists of chronic anticholinesterase agents.
c. Often resistant to depolarizing NMBs and extremely sensitive to nondepolarizing agents.
d. Both prolonged blockade and refractoriness to reversal agents may be seen, resulting in profound postoperative weakness.
e. NMBs are best avoided if possible.
2. Renal and/or hepatic dysfunction.
a. Aminosteroid agents are metabolized with varying degrees of kidney versus liver metabolism.
b. In such pts, dosing and redosing should be titrated to effect, or a benzylisoquinolinium should be selected instead.
c. Hypermagnesemia, hyperthermia, and aminoglycoside antibiotics all contribute to prolonged duration of action of nondepolarizing agents.

V. INTRAVASCULAR CATHETERS
A. CATHETER-RELATED BLOODSTREAM INFECTION (CRBSI)—GENERAL
1. Statistics.
a. 90% of all CRBSIs are associated with CVCs.
b. 400,000 CRBSIs per year occur in the USA.
c. CRBSI is associated with a 10% to 20% mortality.
2. Increased risk for CRBSI.
a. In adults, femoral vein site has increased risk for infection
   i.   Subclavian vein has least risk.
b. Multi-lumen catheters.
c. Catheters with TPN or lipids.

d. Infection elsewhere in/on the body.
e. Catheter indwelling for >72 hr.
f. Inexperience of provider inserting the catheter.
g. Use of stopcocks.
h. Insertion of catheters through cutdown or open techniques.
i. Failure to clean hubs before entering the catheter tubing.

3. Steps to prevent CRBSI.

a. Remove vascular catheters as soon as possible.
   i. Ask daily on rounds whether the line is necessary.
b. Hand hygiene prior to insertion and prior to entering CVC.
   i. Wash hands with alcohol-based solution or soap and water.
c. Chlorhexidine for skin antisepsis.
   i. Press ChloraPrep sponge against skin.
   ii. Apply chlorhexidine solution using a back and forth friction scrub for at least 30 sec.
   iii. Do not wipe or blot.
   iv. Allow antiseptic solution time to dry completely before puncturing the site (may take 2 min).
d. Maximal barrier precautions for insertion of CVC.
   i. Provider wears sterile gloves and gown, hat, and mask with strings tied.
   ii. Prep and drape pt in sterile fashion surrounding insertion site as completely as possible.
   iii. Use large sterile drape to cover pt and area surrounding insertion site as completely as possible.
   iv. Instruct everyone involved in care to wear the same barriers.
   v. Ensure adequate room to perform procedure without risk of contamination.
e. Use subclavian insertion site when possible.
f. Decrease complexity by making certain that all required equipment is readily available for the provider.
g. Create redundancy by using a checklist to confirm that all best practices are being followed by all participants in the procedure.
h. Dressing
   i. Apply sterile dressing to insertion site before the sterile barriers are removed.
   ii. Transparent dressings are preferred to allow visualization of the site.
   iii. If insertion site is oozing, apply a gauze dressing instead of a transparent dressing.
   iv. Replace central-vascular access device (C-VAD) dressings when the dressing becomes damp, loosened, or soiled or after lifting the dressing to inspect the site.

4. Not recommended to reduce CRBSI.

a. IV antimicrobial prophylaxis.
b. Routine guidewire exchange or site rotation.
c. Use of antimicrobial ointment.

B. CVC INSERTION SAFETY TIPS

1. Speak up if you are uncomfortable with any part of the catheter insertion; get help early.
2. Always have qualified assistant in room.
a. NEVER work alone.
3. Do not cut the catheter or the lumens to rewire a line.
4. Always hold onto the wire and never let go!
5. Never make a skin nick with more than just the tip of the blade.
6. Pts must be supine for any catheter insertion.
7. Pts must be in Trendelenburg position for neck lines—**even for line removal**.
8. After three unsuccessful attempts turn over to a more experienced operator.

C. OBTAINING CULTURES OF CVC—METHOD

1. Remove all dressings and remove cap off of all hubs/ports.
2. Paint site with antiseptic solution, including within the sterile field.
3. Remove CVC en-bloc.
a. Under no circumstance should catheters be cut prior to removal.
4. Remove the catheter aseptically, avoiding contact with the pt's skin and catheter tray.
5. Use **sterile scissors** (not the scalpel used to cut the catheter sutures) to cut a 5 cm segment, including the tip.
6. Place it into a culture container.

VI. PREVENTION OF SURGICAL SITE INFECTION

A. ADMINISTER PROPHYLACTIC ANTIBIOTICS WITHIN 1 HR PRIOR TO SURGICAL INCISION (WITHIN 120 MIN FOR VANCOMYCIN OR FLUOROQUINOLONES)

B. USE THE APPROPRIATE ANTIBIOTIC BASED ON THE PROCEDURE PERFORMED

C. DISCONTINUE ANTIBIOTICS WITHIN 24 HR POSTOPERATIVELY (48 HR FOR CARDIAC SURGERY)

D. DO NOT USE RAZORS TO REMOVE HAIR
1. Use electric clippers if hair is to be removed.

E. AVOID HYPOTHERMIA (<36°C)

F. CONTROL POSTOPERATIVE GLUCOSE LEVELS

VII. TEMPERATURE CONTROL

A. GENERAL CONSIDERATIONS

1. Body temperature is tightly controlled in the hypothalamus.
2. Increases in body temperature result in rapid heat loss via vasodilation and sweating.

3. Decreased body temperature results in peripheral vasoconstriction and shivering responses.

B. HYPOTHERMIA

1. Definition.
a. Core body temperature less than 36°C.

2. Causes.
a. Inhibition of central thermoregulation (GA).
b. Redistribution of heat from core to peripheral tissue due to anesthetic-induced vasodilation (general and regional anesthesia).
   i. Pt experiences rapid 1° to 2° C drop in core temperature during the first hour of anesthesia.
c. Heat transfer to the environment through radiation, conduction, convection, and evaporation results in further decline in temperature until equilibrium is reached after 3 to 4 hr.

3. Risk factors.
a. Cold OR environment.
b. Extremes of age.
c. Abdominal surgery.
d. Large surgical incision.
e. Long operative duration.
f. Resuscitation with large volume of fluids or blood products.

4. Consequences.
a. Mild-to-moderate hypothermia.
   i. Increased PVR.
   ii. Cardiac dysrhythmias.
   iii. Coagulopathy and platelet dysfunction, leading to increased surgical blood loss and need for transfusion.
   iv. Shivering and impaired postoperative thermal comfort.
      • Significant increase in oxygen consumption correlates with increased risk of myocardial ischemia.
   v. Decreased drug metabolism, for example, prolonged duration of muscle relaxant.
   vi. Altered mental status.
   vii. Threefold increase in cardiac morbidity.
   viii. Threefold increase in surgical site infection rates.
   ix. Impaired wound healing.
   x. Prolonged hospitalization.
b. Severe hypothermia.
   i. Ventricular dysfunction and conduction disturbance.
   ii. Decreased renal blood flow due to increased vascular resistance.
   iii. Decreased sodium and potassium reabsorption leads to "cold diuresis."
   iv. As temperature decreases, blood becomes more alkalotic.

5. Controlled hypothermia.
a. Often utilized in cases in which coronary or cerebral perfusion insult is anticipated, for example, cardiac bypass, aneurysm clipping, circulatory arrest.

   b. Decreased tissue metabolic rate from hypothermia decreases tissue oxygen demand, providing protection against ischemia.
      i. Hypothermia slows whole body metabolism by 8% for every degree (Centigrade) decrease.
      ii. CBF decreases in proportion to metabolic rate.
   c. Can be achieved by:
      i. Forced cool-air blankets, lowering environmental temperature.
      ii. Cold IV and irrigation solutions.
      iii. Extracorporeal circulation (full or partial bypass circuit).
      iv. Ice packs to vascular areas, head/neck.

6. Prevention of hypothermia.
a. Minimize cutaneous heat loss.
b. Prevent redistribution of heat.
      i. Keep OR temperatures as warm as tolerable.
      ii. Protect pt from cold air circulation (vents) or drafts; minimize exposed skin.
      iii. Warm IV fluids and blood products, surgical irrigation.
      iv. Provide cutaneous warming with heated blankets, forced air, or warm-water circulation blankets.
         • Prewarming for 30 min prior to general or regional anesthetic may attenuate initial redistribution heat loss.
      v. Heat lamps or warming tables should be considered for pediatric pts.
      vi. Airway heating and humidification when appropriate.
      vii. If severe hypothermia, consider warm gastric/bladder lavage.

C. HYPERTHERMIA
1. Definition.
a. Core body temperature >38.5°C.
2. Causes.
a. Passive/iatrogenic hyperthermia—excessive pt heating.
b. Environmental exposure—"heat stroke."
c. Systemic inflammation.
d. Infection.
e. Central dysregulation—head trauma, stroke.
f. Neuroleptic malignant syndrome.
g. Malignant hyperthermia.
3. Prevention/treatment.
a. Development of fever is often inhibited by anesthetics, opioids.
b. Fever due to infection should not be suppressed unless deleterious physiologic effects occur.
c. Common antipyretic agents include NSAIDs and acetaminophen.
d. Remove external heat sources (if iatrogenic cause).
e. Avoid use of ice packs and cutaneous cooling methods, as these methods typically result in peripheral vasoconstriction, leading to poor efficacy and significant pt discomfort.
4. Consequences.

a. Pt discomfort.
b. Chills/rigors—usually during rapid rise or fall of temperature.
c. Tachycardia—may result in ischemia or dysrhythmias.
d. Vasodilation—may result in hypotension and/or hypoperfusion.
e. Increased metabolic rate and oxygen consumption.

D. GUIDELINES FOR INTRAOPERATIVE TEMPERATURE MONITORING

1. Core body temperature should be monitored in pts given GA.
a. Very brief procedures (e.g., <15 min) may be excluded, although postprocedure temperature should be recorded.
b. Core thermal compartment is composed of highly perfused tissues, that is, central bloodstream (pulmonary artery catheter), distal esophagus, tympanic membrane, or nasopharynx.
c. Rectal and skin temperature should be used with caution, as they fail to increase appropriately during malignant hyperthermia.
2. Temperature should be monitored during regional anesthesia, when changes in body temperature are intended, anticipated, or suspected.
3. Unless hypothermia is specifically indicated, efforts should be made to keep intraoperative core temperature higher than 36° C.

VIII. PATIENT POSITIONING

A. OPTIMAL PT POSITIONING DECREASES LIKELIHOOD OF NERVE AND SOFT TISSUE INJURIES

B. NERVE INJURIES WERE RESPONSIBLE FOR 16% OF ALL CLAIMS AGAINST ANESTHESIOLOGISTS BETWEEN 1970 AND 1995 (SECOND LEADING CAUSE)

1. Ulnar neuropathies—28%.
2. Brachial plexus—20%.
3. Lumbosacral nerve root—16%.
4. Spinal cord—13%.
5. Sciatic—5%.

C. MOST COMMON EXTREMITY NERVE INJURIES

1. Brachial plexus
a. Thought to occur most often during median sternotomy secondary to stretch of the nerve plexus during sternal separation.
b. Use of shoulder braces also implicated.
2. Ulnar neuropathy.
a. Ulnar nerve is vulnerable because of its position between the medial epicondyle of the humerus and the retinaculum of the cubital tunnel.
b. More common in men than women because women have more fat between the medial epicondyle and the retinaculum of the cubital tunnel.
   i. Men have a thicker cubital tunnel retinaculum, and the coronoid process is larger in males than females.

c. Ulnar neuropathy has also been known to occur postoperatively for unknown causes.

D. INTRAOPERATIVE POSITIONS

1. Supine position.

a. Most common surgical position.

b. Most frequently associated with ulnar neuropathy because of pressure on the ulnar groove of the elbow in the supine position.

c. It is recommended that arms be kept at <90° abduction and supinated or kept in neutral position if an arm board is used.

d. Padding of the arms is recommended; no data exist to prove that this reduces risk of neuropathy.

2. Lithotomy position (Fig 7.1).

a. Frequent position in gynecologic and urologic surgeries.

b. Common injuries are associated with lithotomy position.

   i. Peroneal nerve neuropathy if the nerve is compressed between the fibula and the leg supports.

   ii. Lower extremity compartment syndrome in long cases.

   iii. Crush injuries to the hands and fingers can occur when the foot of the bed is brought into neutral position.

3. Lateral position (Fig. 7.2).

a. Common position in thoracotomies, laparoscopic renal surgery, and hip surgeries.

b. Common injuries associated with lateral position.

   i. Brachial plexus injuries.

   ii. Crush injuries to the lower extremities because of the pressure generated by one leg resting on the other.

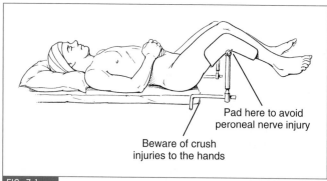

Pad here to avoid peroneal nerve injury

Beware of crush injuries to the hands

FIG. 7.1

Lithotomy position. *(Adapted from Martin JT: Lithotomy positions. In Martin JT, Warner MA [eds]: Positioning in Anesthesia and Surgery, 3rd ed. Philadelphia: WB Saunders, 1997, p 50.)*

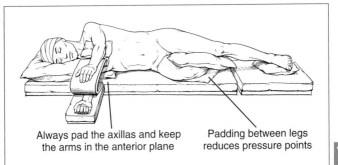

Always pad the axillas and keep
the arms in the anterior plane

Padding between legs
reduces pressure points

FIG. 7.2

Lateral position. *(Adapted from Day LJ: Unusual positions: Orthopedics: Surgical aspects. In Martin JT [ed]: Positioning in Anesthesia and Surgery, 2nd ed. Philadelphia: WB Saunders, 1987, p 226.)*

7

GENERAL ANESTHETIC CARE

    iii. Eye abrasions to the dependent eye.
    iv. Ear contusions to the dependent ear.
c. Lateral positioning pointers.
    i. If table is flexed in lateral position, avoid cervical neck injury by ensuring that neck is adequately supported to maintain alignment with thoracic spine.
    ii. If arms are placed in an anterior plane with the body, tension on the brachial plexus can be avoided.
    iii. An axillary roll should be placed to avoid stretch of the dependent brachial plexus.
    iv. Padding should be applied between the knees, ankles, and any other pressure points.
    v. Safety and positioning of the dependent eye and ear should be checked routinely throughout the case.

4. Prone position.
a. Common position for posterior spine surgeries, lower extremity, or posterior fossa surgery.
b. Chest rolls should be used to support the chest and to improve the ability of the diaphragmatic excursion.
c. Arms can be tucked to the sides in older, less flexible people.
    i. In younger people, keeping the arms at 90° and flexed at the elbows is preferred.
d. Injuries associated with prone position.
    i. Compression of the breasts.
       • Breasts should be placed in medial or lateral position and padded.
    ii. Corneal abrasions and vision loss.
       • Can occur as the result of pressure on the eyes.

- A foam pillow with slots for eyes, nose, and mouth or a horseshoe head device is often used to avoid eye compression.
- Eyes should be checked q 15 min during case and whenever the pt's head is moved.

iii. Scrotal necrosis from scrotal pressure.

5. **Sitting position** (Fig. 7.3).

a. Common position for shoulder, posterior fossa craniotomy, and surgeries of the posterior cervical spine.

b. When neck is flexed, at least two fingerbreadths of space should be between the sternum and the chin.

c. Knees should be bent to avoid sciatic nerve stretch.

d. Consider padding the area under the sciatic notch to decrease the likelihood of nerve ischemia.

e. Common problems associated with sitting position.

   i. Venous air emboli and paradoxical air emboli.

   ii. Overflexion of the neck, leading to spinal cord ischemia and compression of the vertebral and carotid arteries.

   iii. Brachial plexus injury can occur if arms are left hanging at the side.

   iv. Sciatic nerve injury due to nerve stretch can occur if the legs are kept straight.

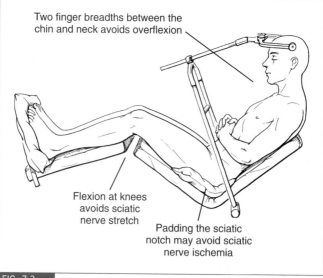

Two finger breadths between the chin and neck avoids overflexion

Flexion at knees avoids sciatic nerve stretch

Padding the sciatic notch may avoid sciatic nerve ischemia

FIG. 7.3

Sitting position. *(Adapted from Martin JT: The head-elevated positions: Anesthesiologic considerations. In Martin JT [ed]: Positioning in Anesthesia and Surgery, 2nd ed. Philadelphia: WB Saunders, 1987, p 81.)*

IX. BLOOD PRODUCT TRANSFUSION

A. INDICATIONS FOR TRANSFUSION THERAPY

1. Red blood cells (RBC) for Hb <6 g/dL in otherwise healthy pt.
2. Platelets and FFP after replacement of one blood volume of RBC or per coagulation studies.

B. TYPES OF COMPONENT THERAPY

1. **RBC.**
a. Most effective way of increasing O_2-carrying capacity
   $CaO_2 = [(1.34 \times Hb \times SaO_2) + (0.003 \times PaO_2)]$.
b. One unit contains ~200 mL of RBC and 50 mL of plasma, for a total volume of 250 mL.
c. One unit should increase Hb by 1 g/dL.
d. ABO compatibility is essential, ideally with crossmatch, except in cases of emergency product administration.
e. Rh-positive units should be avoided in Rh-negative females to avoid risk of alloimmunization.

2. **Platelet.**
a. Responsible for primary hemostasis.
b. Pooled concentrates are obtained from whole blood.
c. One equivalent (unit) of platelet contains 50 mL of volume, consisting of 3×10^{11} platelets, 80 mg of fibrinogen, and 50 mL of plasma.
d. One unit of platelets should increase platelet count by 5000 to 10,000/μL.
e. ABO compatibility is NOT required; however, may prolong the lifespan of administered platelets.
f. Rh-positive units should be avoided in Rh-negative females to avoid risk of alloimmunization.

3. **FFP.**
a. Responsible for secondary hemostasis.
b. Each unit contains 200 mL of volume, 400 mg of fibrinogen, and small quantities of WBC, RBC, platelets, and antithrombin III.
c. One unit should increase factor levels by 20% to 30%.
d. Product must be ABO compatible, and ideally, Rh-positive units should be avoided in Rh-negative females to avoid risk of alloimmunization.

4. **Cryoprecipitate.**
a. Precipitate obtained from a single unit of FFP.
b. One unit contains 15 mL of volume, consisting of 150 to 250 mg of fibrinogen, 80 to 120 units of Von Willebrand factor, 40 to 60 units of factor VIII, and fibrinogen.
c. Typically dispensed as 10-unit bag.
d. ABO compatibility is not required.

5. **Recombinant activated factor VII (rVIIa).**
a. Marketed as NovoSeven.
b. FDA-approved for treatment of pts with hemophilia A and B with inhibitors to factor VIII or IX, as well as pts with congenital factor VII deficiency.

c. Off-label use has been limited by cost of administration.

d. Cochrane review evaluating NovoSeven use in non-hemophiliac cases concluded that its off-label use should be limited.

e. Must have normal temperature and platelets for rVIIa to work.

C. SCREENING OF BLOOD PRODUCTS

1. Microbial and viral screening.

a. Standard health assessment questionnaire is used to screen potentially high-risk individuals.

b. In addition, laboratory testing of donor blood for HIV, HTLV, hepatitis B and C, and syphilis represents common practice.

2. Compatibility screening.

a. Type and screen (ABO/Rhesus [Rh] typing).

   i. Assessment of ABO/Rh status and an antibody screen is performed.

   ii. The antibody screen is an indirect Coombs test, which uses commercially available RBCs with a standard panel of antigens.

   iii. This is mixed with both donor and recipient serum to detect the presence of unexpected antibodies.

   iv. The risk of missing a potentially harmful antibody with proper antibody screening is estimated to be 1/10,000 cases.

   v. The risk of type-specific uncrossmatched blood resulting in a hemolytic reaction is ~1/50,000 units.

b. Type and cross—three phases.

   i. Immediate phase (1–5 min).

      • Ensures accurate assessment of ABO-Rh typing and MN, P, and Lewis blood group systems by mixing donor RBC with recipient serum.

   ii. Incubation phase (30–45 min).

      • Donor RBC is incubated with recipient serum, allowing detection of antibodies primarily in the Rh system.

   iii. Antiglobulin phase (60–90 min).

      • Performed only if antibody screening renders positive result.

      • Antiglobulin sera is added at the end of the incubation phase, which effectively identifies antibodies attached to the surface of the donor RBC.

      • Identifies antibodies from all blood group systems, including Rh, Kell, Kidd, and Duffy.

D. PROCESSING

1. Washed RBCs.

a. Reduces plasma protein content.

b. Indicated when there is a history of previous allergic reaction to unwashed product transfusion.

2. Leukocyte depletion.

a. Reduces the risk of CMV.

3. Irradiation.

a. Gamma radiation inactivates donor lymphocytes, thereby reducing the risk of graft-versus-host disease (GVHD). Mortality from transfusion-related GVHD is 90%.

   i. All directed donation products from pt relatives must be irradiated
   ii. Blood products for immunocompromised pts and young children should also be irradiated.

4. Preservatives.

a. CPD (citrate phosphate dextrose)—shelf life, 21 days.
b. CPDA (citrate phosphate dextrose adenine)—shelf life 35 days.
c. Adsol (additive solution)—residual plasma is removed and replaced with 100 mL of Adsol, extending the shelf life of the product to 42 days.
d. The requirement for satisfactory blood storage requires that at least 75% of erythrocytes remain in circulation for 24 hr after transfusion.

E. TEMPERATURE REQUIREMENTS

1. Frozen RBCs at −80° C can be stored for 10 yr.
2. Thawed RBCs should be used within 24 hr.
a. If stored in a blood cooler, RBCs should remain under ice packs.
3. FFP can be kept at −20° C for 1 yr.
4. Thawed cryoprecipitate should be used within 6 hr.
a. Cryoprecipitate is stored at −20° C and thawed immediately before use.
5. Platelets are stored at 20° to 24° C.
a. The risk of bacterial contamination is high and related to time in storage.
b. Ideally, platelets should be ordered just prior to administration to minimize the risk of platelet-induced sepsis.

F. ADMINISTRATION

1. Standard 170-micron filter can be used to remove debris from all component blood products.
2. RBC and FFP should be administered through a warmer, as they are administered in high volume and can potentially induce hypothermia.
3. In cases of pts with history of immunocompromise, febrile transfusion reactions, and nonhemolytic transfusion reactions, microaggregate filters (20–40 micron) can be considered to further reduce leukocyte counts.
a. Other considerations include exposure to CMV and alloimmunization to foreign antigens.
4. Platelets.
a. Microaggregate filters should not be used.
b. Platelets should be administered at room temperature.

G. TRANSFUSION RISKS

1. Infectious risk.
a. Hepatitis B—1/350,000.

b. Hepatitis C—1/2,000,000.

c. HIV—1/2,000,000.

d. Human T-cell lymphotrophic virus (HTLV)—1/2,900,000.

e. Bacterial sepsis from RBC—1/30,000 (*Yersinia*, *Serratia*, and *Pseudomonas* can potentially survive at RBC storage temperatures).

f. Bacterial sepsis from platelets—1/2000 (*Staphylococcus aureus*, *Klebsiella*, and *Serratia* are the three most common culprits).

g. CMV.

   i. Generally benign; however, may cause potentially life-threatening disease in immunocompromised pts.

   ii. Leukocyte reduction diminishes the risk of CMV transmission, but seronegative CMV donor blood is ideal.

h. Parasitic diseases.

i. Malaria and Chagas disease are endemic in some third-world nations, but their incidence is relatively small in the USA.

   i. Prion-related diseases, including Creutzfeldt-Jakob disease, have been reported but are extremely rare.

2. **Immunologically mediated transfusion reactions.**

a. Reactions to RBC antigens.

   i. Acute hemolytic transfusion reactions (1/12,000).

      - Hemolysis of donor cells can lead to acute renal failure, disseminated intravascular coagulopathy (DIC), and death.
      - Implicated antibodies, such as anti-A, anti-B, anti-Kell, anti-Kidd, anti-Lewis, and anti-Duffy, bind with donor RBC antigens, resulting in antigen-antibody complexes that activate factor XII and, subsequently, the bradykinin system.
      - Complexes also activate the complement system, which results in histamine and serotonin release from mast cells.
      - These reactions mostly involve the ABO system.
      - Treatment involves immediate discontinuation of transfusion, supportive care, fluid resuscitation, and urine alkalinization.
      - Laboratory evaluation should include a repeat crossmatch, a direct antiglobulin test, coagulation status evaluation, and DIC labs.

   ii. Delayed hemolytic transfusion reactions (1/800–2500).

      - Occurs when donor RBCs bear an antigen to which the recipient has been previously sensitized; however, over time, a decline in antibody count results in a false-negative antibody screen.
      - Upon re-exposure to the donor RBC antigen, the recipient mounts an anamnestic response, resulting in a rise in antibody level, which eventually results in extravascular RBC lyses.
      - These reactions commonly involve the Rh, Kell, Duffy, and Kidd antigens, rather than the ABO systems.
      - Reactions are typically self-limited and include low-grade fever, bilirubinemia, and drop in Hb.
      - A positive direct antiglobulin test is confirmatory.

b. Reactions to donor proteins.
  i.   Minor allergic reactions (1/200).
       • Urticarial reactions are most commonly seen with FFP.
       • Other components generally consist of small volumes of donor plasma and therefore are less likely to precipitate reactions.
       • These reactions are generally self-limiting and respond to diphenhydramine.
       • Pts with history of severe urticarial reactions should be transfused with washed RBCs.
c. Anaphylactic/anaphylactoid reactions (1/25,000–50,000).
  i.   Occur when pts with hereditary IgA deficiency sensitized with previous transfusions or pregnancy are exposed to blood with antigenic IgA protein.
  ii. These pts should be transfused with washed RBCs, frozen deglycerolized RBCs, or RBCs from IgA-deficient donors.
  iii. Treatment for anaphylaxis includes supportive therapy, epinephrine (which acts to stabilize mast cells), and discontinuation of transfusion.
d. WBC-related transfusion reactions.
  i.   Febrile reactions (1/200).
       • Increase in temperature by more than 1°C within 4 hr of transfusion.
       • Other manifestations include chills, respiratory distress, myalgia, headaches, nausea, and nonproductive coughing.
       • Secondary to recipient antibodies attacking donor leukocytes.
       • Treatment involves administration of acetaminophen and discontinuation of transfusion (depending on the severity of symptoms).
       • Use of leukocyte-depleted products can minimize severity and occurrence of these reactions.
  ii. Transfusion-related acute lung injury (TRALI).
       • Incidence is 1/2000–5000, with a reported mortality rate of 5% to 8%.
       • Manifests as fever, chills, dyspnea, and noncardiogenic pulmonary edema with bilateral pulmonary infiltrates on CXR.
       • Usually presents within 6 hr of transfusion.
       • May be associated with any blood product.
       • Pulmonary edema from TRALI is mediated by increased vascular permeability, not by increased hydrostatic pressure.
       • Diagnosed by ratio of protein in edema fluid to plasma ≥0.6; improves in 48 to 96 hr.
       • Pathogenesis is not completely clear, but two mechanisms are proposed.
       • Antibody-mediated reaction between host granulocytes and antigranulocyte antibodies in the donor serum (presumably due to sensitization from previous transfusions or pregnancy) form

7

GENERAL ANESTHETIC CARE

complexes, which ultimately leads to increased pulmonary capillary permeability.
- Donor unit components undergo spontaneous lipid breakdown, resulting in the formation of proinflammatory lipopolysaccharides that cause increased pulmonary capillary permeability.

iii. GVHD (rare occurrence).
- Transplanted donor lymphocytes become engrafted in the recipient and reject host tissue.
- Has only been associated with cellular blood components.
- No cases of occurrence with FFP or cryoprecipitate have been reported.
- Pts at high risk for developing this complication include the immunocompromised, transplant pts, and neonates.
- Irradiated leukocyte-depleted RBCs are recommended for this pt population.

iv. Immunomodulation.
- Transfused WBCs that accompany allogenic transfusions are thought to impair recipient immunity, leading to impaired wound healing and increased postoperative infections.
- Leukocyte reduction methods can potentially attenuate this effect.

e. Side effects of massive transfusion.
i. Hypothermia.
- Manifests in numerous physiologic changes, including coagulopathy, decreases in cardiac output, cardiac dysrhythmias, leftward shift of the Hb-O_2 dissociation curve, increased postoperative infection rates, and increased oxygen consumption secondary to shivering.

ii. Volume overload.
- Precipitates secondary to rapid administration of components.

iii. Dilutional coagulopathy.
- Large-volume resuscitation deficient in platelets and clotting factors can result in significant coagulopathy.
- Repletion of clotting factors with FFP and platelets should be based on clinical or laboratory assessments.

iv. Decreases in 2,3-diphosphoglycerate.
- Storage results in a progressive decline in adenosine triphosphate (ATP) and 2,3-DPG, which can cause a leftward shift of the Hb-O_2 dissociation curve, resulting in less efficient O_2-carrying capacity.
- This effect typically resolves after 12 to 24 hr.

v. Hyperkalemia.
- During storage, potassium moves out of RBCs.
- At 21 days, [K+] in a unit of RBCs in Adsol can reach 24 mEq/L.
- A unit of RBCs contains 50 to 80 mL of plasma; therefore the total [K+] in the average unit at 21 days is 1 to 2 mEq.

- During large-volume blood resuscitation, hyperkalemia can result in dysrhythmias and cardiac arrest.
- Measures should be taken to treat hyperkalemia in this situation.

vi. Citrate intoxication.
  - Citrate acts as an anticoagulant by chelating factor IV during storage.
  - Citrate is normally metabolized by the liver; however, if infusion rates exceed 1 mL/kg/min, significant hypocalcemia can occur.
  - Manifestations include hypotension, narrow pulse pressure, QRS complex widening, flattened T waves, and elevation in CVP and EDVP.
  - Washed and low-shelf-life RBCs may reduce the incidence of this complication.

vii. Acid-base changes.
  - Adding CPD (citrate phosphate dextrose) to the RBC unit results in a pH of 7.0 to 7.1.
  - After 21 days of storage, the pH can drop below 7.0, owing mostly to carbon dioxide production.
  - Bicarbonate can be administered to counteract acidosis, but overshoot should be avoided, considering that donor unit citrate will eventually be converted to bicarbonate.

viii. Microaggregate delivery.
  - Has been implicated in the pathogenesis of ARDS and pulmonary insufficiency.
  - Some advocate for periodic use of 40 micron filters when large volumes of blood are being administered.

f. Volume expanders.
  i. Dextran.
    - Water-soluble glucose polymers available in two formulations.
    - Dextran 40 is used predominantly in vascular surgery to improve rheology and prevent thrombosis.
    - Dextran 70 is used to enhance vascular oncotic pressure.
    - Potential side effects include anaphylactic/anaphylactoid reactions (1/3300), diminished platelet adhesiveness (at doses exceeding 20 mL/kg/day), and noncardiogenic pulmonary edema.
  ii. Hetastarch.
    - Hydroxyethyl starch is a commonly used synthetic colloid.
    - It is available at a pH of 5.5, with an osmolarity of 310.
    - At volumes that exceed 20 mL/kg, dilutional coagulopathy can develop.
    - Hemostasis can be altered by hetastarch movement into fibrin clots.
    - Allergic reactions can be problematic but are rare.
  iii. Albumin.
    - Available in 5% and 25%.
    - Used to increase oncotic pressure and, subsequently, plasma volume, thereby theoretically limiting third spacing.

- Evidence is lacking to support its efficacy when used in this manner.
  iv. Hypertonic saline.
  - Available as 2% or 3%.
  - Hypertonic saline 3% should only be given via a central line to limit localized RBC lyses.
  - These solutions commonly come buffered with acetate to limit the chloride content and, therefore, the incidence of hyperchloremic metabolic acidosis.
  - Some evidence has been reported that hypertonic saline can attenuate cytokine release and potentially abate the SIRS response commonly seen in surgery.
g. Blood conservation strategies.
  i. Autologous donation.
  - Limited by cost and the pt's preoperative morbidities.
  - In addition, marrow response to iatrogenically induced anemia is unpredictable, and pts may simply be rendered anemic preoperatively.
  - Autologous units do not negate the risk of clerical errors, which should be a key consideration.
  ii. Erythropoietin.
  - Use has been considered in conjunction with autologous donation; however, no benefit has been reported in this population.
  - Some benefit has been reported in the Jehovah's Witness population.
  - Without convincing evidence of clear benefit and with the high cost of administration, erythropoietin has not reached widespread use.
  iii. Acute normovolemic hemodilution.
  - Involves early intraoperative withdrawal of blood, with concurrent repletion of volume with crystalloids or colloids, resulting in a goal Hct of 27% to 33%.
  - Because whole blood is drawn off, micropore filters (40 micron) should be avoided, as they would filter out platelets.
  - No clear benefit to this strategy of blood conservation has been reported.
  iv. Intraoperative blood salvage (IBS).
  - Blood suctioned from the field is centrifuged to separate RBCs from other cellular elements and plasma.
  - Typically, IBS can salvage 50% of recovered RBCs.
  - The RBCs are washed extensively with saline and suspended in saline aliquots.
  - Common contraindications to cell saver include surgical field contamination with infection, malignant cells, urine, bowel contents, or amniotic fluid.

- Potential hazards of IBS include dilutional coagulopathy and DIC-like coagulopathy.
- Poor processing can result in fat, microaggregate, air, free Hb, heparin, debris, and bacteria from the operative field.

REFERENCES

Barash PG, Cullen BF, Stoelting RK, eds: Clinical Anesthesia, 5th ed. Philadelphia: Lippincott, Williams & Wilkins, 2005.

Bhananker SM, O'Donnell JT, Salemi JR, et al: The risk of anaphylactic reactions to rocuronium in the United States is comparable to that of vecuronium: An analysis of food and drug administration reporting of adverse events. Anesth Analg 2005;101(3):819–822.

Cheney FW, Domino KB, Caplan RA, et al: Nerve injury associated with anesthesia: A closed-claims analysis. Anesthesiology 1999;90(4): 1062–1069.

Gild WM, Posner KL, Caplan RA, et al: Eye injuries associated with anesthesia: A closed-claims analysis. Anesthesiology 1992;76(2): 204–208.

Goudsouzian NG: Recent changes in the package insert for succinylcholine chloride: Should this drug be contraindicated for routine use in children and adolescents? Anesth Analg 1995;80(1):207–208.

Kroll DA, Caplan RA, Posner K, et al: Nerve injury associated with anesthesia. Anesthesiology 1990;73(2):202–207.

Miller RD (ed): Miller's Anesthesia, 6th ed. New York: Churchill Livingstone, 2005.

Morgan GE, Mikhail MS, Murray MJ: Clinical Anesthesiology, 4th ed. New York: Lange Medical Books, 2006.

Prielipp RC, Morell RC, Butterworth J: Ulnar nerve injury and perioperative arm positioning. Anesthesiol Clin North Am 2002;20(3):589–603.

Vachon CA, Warner DO, Bacon DR: Succinylcholine and the open globe: Tracing the teaching. Anesthesiology 2003;99(1):220–223.

7

GENERAL ANESTHETIC CARE

Regional Anesthesia

Meredith Adams, MD, Mathew Belan, MD, and Benjamin Kong, MD
Edited by Jeffrey M. Richman, MD

Regional anesthesia is a safe and effective method for providing intraoperative anesthesia and postoperative pain control. The essence of performing a regional anesthesia technique is correctly placing a needle or catheter adjacent to a nerve or plexus that innervates the region of the body where surgery is to be performed, which requires that the anesthesiologist be knowledgeable in surface and internal anatomy to allow for peripheral nerves to be localized and to avoid injury to adjacent structures.

8

I. INDICATIONS

A. THE DECISION TO PERFORM A REGIONAL ANESTHESIA TECHNIQUE DEPENDS ON CLEAR COMMUNICATION AMONG ALL PARTIES INVOLVED—THE PT, THE ANESTHESIOLOGIST, AND THE SURGEON.

B. PTS MUST BE ADVISED OF THE RISKS AND BENEFITS OF REGIONAL AND GA AND BE ALLOWED TO MAKE AN INFORMED DECISION.

C. THE ADVANTAGES AND DISADVANTAGES OF A REGIONAL ANESTHESIA TECHNIQUE ARE SUMMARIZED IN Table 8.1.

II. CONTRAINDICATIONS

A. PTS WHO DO NOT DESIRE THE PROCEDURE

B. PTS WHO ARE BACTEREMIC SHOULD GENERALLY NOT HAVE AN INDWELLING CATHETER PLACED OR A NEURAXIAL TECHNIQUE OWING TO THE POTENTIAL FOR LOCALIZED INFECTION AND ABSCESS.
1. In general, a neuraxial technique should not be performed through an area that may be infected.

C. PERIPHERAL NERVE BLOCKS PERFORMED ON PTS WHO HAVE A COAGULOPATHY MAY BE ASSOCIATED WITH AN INCREASED RISK OF HEMATOMA AND NERVE INJURY OR ISCHEMIA FROM A PERINEURAL HEMATOMA.
1. In general, neuraxial techniques are contraindicated in the presence of a coagulopathy.

III. EQUIPMENT

A. NEEDLES
1. With needles that are longer, greater changes in trajectory of the tip occur with movement of the hub when compared with shorter needles.

TABLE 8.1

ADVANTAGES AND DISADVANTAGES OF REGIONAL ANESTHESIA

Advantages	Disadvantages
Delivers analgesia to the region of the body where surgery is to be performed.	Risk of discomfort during nerve localization.
Reduces side effects of GA and opioids.	Risk of inadequate or incomplete nerve blockade and the need for GA.
Potentially faster discharge from PACU and hospital.	Risk of complications directly related to regional technique, including nerve damage.
Superior postoperative analgesia.	
Safe for pts with a history of malignant hyperthermia.	Side effects and risks of LAs.
Possibly decreases morbidity and mortality.	

TABLE 8.2

RECOMMENDED NEEDLE LENGTHS FOR NERVE BLOCKS

Type of Block	Recommended Needle Length (in)
Cervical plexus block	2
Interscalene brachial plexus block	1–2
Supraclavicular brachial plexus block	1–2
Infraclavicular brachial plexus block	2–4
Axillary brachial plexus block	1–2
Thoracic paravertebral block	4
Lumbar paravertebral	4
Lumbar plexus block	4–6
Sciatic block, posterior approach	4
Sciatic block, anterior approach	6
Femoral block	1–2
Popliteal block, posterior approach	2–4
Popliteal block, lateral approach	4

2. Needles that are longer than necessary increase the risk of injuring adjacent structures if they are inadvertently advanced too deeply.
3. If a needle is too short, it will not reach its intended target and may lead to multiple attempts at localization without success.
4. Refer to Table 8.2 for recommended needle lengths for various techniques.

B. NERVE STIMULATOR

1. The nerve stimulator is connected to an insulated needle or catheter and generates an electrical impulse from the noninsulated tip of the needle.
2. When the tip of the needle is in close proximity to the intended nerve, twitches of the muscle groups innervated by that nerve will be observed.
3. It is often useful to have an assistant during the use of a nerve stimulator, as the settings will have to be adjusted during the procedure.

4. The nerve stimulator should initially be set at 1 to 1.5 mA and should be decreased when the nerve is stimulated.
5. Continued nerve stimulation in the range of 0.3 to 0.5 mA will generally provide a successful block.
6. An assistant should aspirate for blood; if blood is not present, assistant should begin injecting the LA.
7. Typically, after a small amount of LA has been injected, muscle contractions will cease.
8. It is essential to inject slowly and to discontinue injecting if the pt complains of sudden severe pain, as this may indicate an intraneural injection.
9. High initial injection pressures also have been linked with intraneural injection.
10. It is important to aspirate intermittently during the injection of LA to increase the likelihood of identifying intravascular injection.

C. ULTRASOUND
1. Ultrasound allows the anesthesiologist to visualize the needle in close proximity to the targeted nerve and the deposition of LA perineurally.
2. Advocates of ultrasound report a decreased incidence of complications and a greater success rate when ultrasound is used compared with other methods, although further data are necessary to determine if this is clinically significant.
3. The drawbacks of ultrasound include the high cost of the machines and the need for extensive training to become familiar with ultrasonography.

IV. MEDICATIONS FOR REGIONAL BLOCKS
A. LAs
1. LAs are weakly basic hydrophilic amines linked via either an ester or an amide intermediate chain to a lipophilic aromatic ring.
2. LAs are poorly water soluble and thus are manufactured as water-soluble salts.
3. Once placed in aqueous solutions, they ionize, forming a charged quaternary amine that is in equilibrium with an uncharged tertiary amine.
a. The pH at which this equilibrium occurs is called the *pKa*.
4. To achieve their effect of sensory blockade, LAs must be able to cross the neuronal axon membrane.
a. Neuronal axon membranes are penetrated by the non-ionized free base form of the medication. The degree of dissociation between the cation form and non-ionized form is determined by the drug's pKa and the solution pH.
5. The cation form binds to the receptor site within the Na channel, thereby blocking the depolarization-induced influx of Na and propagation of the nerve impulse.
a. The speed of onset is affected by the drug's pKa.

TABLE 8.3		
LOCAL ANESTHETIC PROPERTIES		
Characteristics	Esters	Amides
pKa	>8 (more basic)	<8 (less basic)
Metabolism	Pseudocholinesterase	Hepatic degradation
Significant metabolites	PABA	NONE
Allergenicity	Yes	Very rare
Agents/pKa	Tetracaine—8.4	Mepivacaine—7.7
	Procaine—8.9	Lidocaine—7.8
	2-Chlorprocaine—9.1	Etidocaine—7.9
		Prilocaine—8.0
		Bupivacaine—8.1

PABA, Para-aminobenzoic acid.

b. Because the non-ionized form is more readily able to cross the membrane, drugs with a lower pKa (closer to physiologic pH) will have a faster onset, with the exception being 2-chloroprocaine, which displays a rapid onset despite a high pKa secondary to high concentrations and total doses in clinical use.
6. Adding HCO_3^- to a solution will raise the local pH and thus promote the non-ionized (permeable) form and a faster onset of the block.
7. Blockade of functions is progressive, with sympathetic blockade first, then sensory, then motor.
a. Some agents produce more intense blockade of one over the other.
8. The pKa and additional characteristics for the most commonly used LAs are listed in Table 8.3.
9. Duration of action of LA is primarily determined by protein binding and vascular absorption.
10. All LAs except cocaine are vasodilators.
11. Increased perfusion to the site of LA injection speeds removal of the drug and shortens the duration of action.
a. Adding a vasoconstrictor such as epinephrine prolongs the duration.
b. Increasing vascularity of the site results in higher systemic absorption.
    i. Intercostal (most vascular) > Caudal > Lumbar Epidural = Brachial Plexus > Sciatic-Femoral.
12. Numerous comorbidities will affect the dosing and pharmacokinetics of LAs, as listed in Table 8.4.

B. CHOICE OF LA, DOSING, AND TOXICITY
1. Mepivacaine is relatively contraindicated in pregnant pts because it accumulates in the placenta.
2. Bupivacaine and etidocaine are associated with a higher incidence of cardiotoxicity at equivalent doses to other LAs.
a. Etidocaine produces a motor block greater than a sensory block.
3. Levo-bupivacaine is dosed the same as bupivacaine, with less cardiotoxicity.

TABLE 8.4

MEDICAL CONDITIONS AND THEIR EFFECT ON LOCAL ANESTHETICS

Condition	Effect on Dosing and/or Metabolism
Renal failure	Increased volume of distribution and accumulation of metabolic by-products
Hepatic failure	Increased amide volume of distribution and decreased amide clearance
Heart failure, β blockers, H2 blockers	Decreased hepatic blood flow and decreased amide clearance
Cholinesterase deficiency or inhibition	Decreased ester clearance
Pregnancy	Increased hepatic blood flow, increased amide clearance, decreased protein binding

TABLE 8.5

RECOMMENDED CONCENTRATIONS OF LOCAL ANESTHETICS

Drug	Concentration for Nerve Block (%)	Concentration for Epidural (%)	Concentration for Spinal (%)
Lidocaine	1–1.5	1–2	1.5–5
Bupivacaine	0.25–0.5	0.25–0.5	0.25–0.75
Ropivacaine	0.25–0.5	0.25–0.5	0.5–1
Mepivacaine	1–1.5	1–2	1–4
Chloroprocaine	2–3	2–3	2–3
Tetracaine			0.25–1

4. Ropivacaine is thought to have a sensory block greater than motor block relative to bupivacaine at equal concentrations.
5. Prilocaine in large doses may result in methemoglobinemia.
6. Chloroprocaine is rapidly hydrolyzed by plasma cholinesterase.
7. Tetracaine may result in a greater sensory block than motor subarachnoid **block**.
8. Procaine is metabolized to para-aminobenzoic acid (PABA), which may cause an allergic reaction.

C. **RECOMMENDED CONCENTRATIONS TO BE USED FOR PERIPHERAL, EPIDURAL, AND SPINAL TECHNIQUES ARE LISTED IN Table 8.5.**
1. To reduce the risk of LA toxicity, maximum dosing guidelines have been established.
a. The maximum dose recommendations for LAs and properties related to the speed of onset and duration of action are listed in Table 8.6.
2. It is important to remember that the pt's comorbidities must be taken into consideration when calculating the maximum total dose.
3. In addition, little scientific evidence supports these guidelines, and they apply only to SQ dosing, as absorption and safety vary widely by regional technique.

TABLE 8.6

PROPERTIES OF LOCAL ANESTHETICS

Name	Class	Onset of Action	Duration of Action	Maximum Dose with Epinephrine (mg/kg)
Lidocaine	Amide	Moderate	Moderate	7
Mepivacaine	Amide	Moderate	Moderate	7
Bupivacaine	Amide	Slow	Long	3
Ropivacaine	Amide	Slow	Long	3
Etidocaine	Amide	Moderate	Long	4
Prilocaine	Amide	Moderate	Moderate	8
Chloroprocaine	Ester	Rapid	Short	12
Tetracaine	Ester	Slowest	Long	3
Procaine	Ester	Slow	Short	12

4. Bolus IV dosing at these maximum doses would routinely result in toxicity.

D. LA TOXICITY

1. Symptoms and signs.
a. Will initially present with some form of CNS excitation, often in the form of tinnitus, circumoral numbness, or a metallic taste.
b. With increasing blood levels, this will progress to motor twitching and, eventually, grand mal seizures due to selective blockade of inhibitory neurons.
c. At extremely high levels, excitatory neurons are also inhibited, resulting in unconsciousness.
d. Cardiac dysrhythmias and cardiovascular collapse may occur.
e. Unintentional toxic levels are possible after intravascular or peripheral tissue injections of LA.

2. Risk factors for LA toxicity.
a. Increased total dose.
b. Increased vasculature in the area of LA injection.
c. Increasing number of injection sites (irrespective of total dose used).
d. Absence of vasoconstrictors in the solution.
e. Certain LAs such as bupivacaine and etidocaine are more likely to result in cardiovascular toxicity at clinically used doses.
f. The S-isomers (levo-bupivacaine and ropivacaine) are less likely to cause cardiovascular toxicity than the R+ isomers or racemic mixtures.

3. Management of LA toxicity
a. Requires immediate supportive care, including instituting supportive measures specific to LA toxicity.
b. Treatment should be aimed at correcting contractile depression and dysrhythmias.
c. Hypercapnia, hypoxia, and acidosis all exacerbate bupivacaine-induced toxicity and should be avoided.

d. Seizure activity can cause acidosis and thus should be treated immediately.

e. LA toxicity creates a low output state, and sympathomimetics are the principal pharmacologic agents to augment the hemodynamic compromise (epinephrine and norepinephrine).

f. Epinephrine can exacerbate dysrhythmias induced by LA; therefore alternative therapies such as vasopressin should be considered.

g. Lipid infusions are a novel mode of therapy.

   i. In animal studies, lipid pretreatment increased the toxic dose of bupivacaine.

   ii. Animals not resuscitated using American Cardiac Life Support (ACLS) guidelines recovered when given lipid emulsions.

   iii. Mechanism is thought to be related to binding of the LA by the lipid in the plasma, removing it from binding sites within the heart.

h. Consideration should be given to instituting CPB if standard drug therapies fail.

i. It may be necessary to continue CPB for many hours, given the long half-life of certain LAs.

V. PERIPHERAL NERVE BLOCKS

A. IMPORTANT POINTS

1. Best block + wrong distribution = failure.
2. Right distribution + wrong expectation = failure.
3. Side effects + no expectation = failure.
4. Complications + blame = failure.
5. Success requires an understanding of anatomy, physiology, complications, side effects, and the surgical procedure.
6. Complications common to all peripheral nerve blocks include pain, bleeding, intravascular absorption of LA, infection, and failure.
7. Known advantages of peripheral nerve blocks are an ~50% reduction in pain and 50% reduction in opioid-related side effects compared with opioids.
8. Use of continuous peripheral nerve blocks via catheters extends these benefits for days.
9. Although serious risks are minimal, inexperience or carelessness can lead to dangerous complications and high failure rates.

B. BRACHIAL PLEXUS ANATOMY AND NERVE BLOCKS
(Figs. 8.1 and 8.2)

1. Blockade at the roots is best for shoulder surgery (interscalene or posterior cervical paravertebral block).
2. Blockade at the trunks (supraclavicular) is best for any surgery below the shoulder.
3. Blockade at the cords (infraclavicular) is effective for surgery at or below the elbow.

8

REGIONAL ANESTHESIA

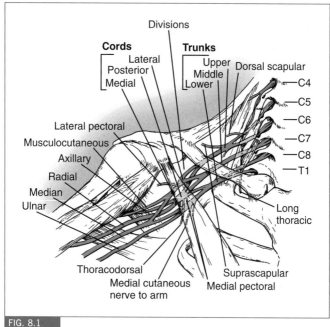

Divisions

Cords   **Trunks**

Lateral   Upper Dorsal scapular
Posterior   Middle
Medial   Lower

C4
C5
C6
C7
C8
T1

Lateral pectoral
Musculocutaneous
Axillary
Radial
Median
Ulnar

Long
thoracic

Thoracodorsal
Medial cutaneous
nerve to arm

Suprascapular
Medial pectoral

FIG. 8.1

Brachial plexus anatomy and nerve blocks. *(From Canale TC, Beatty JH: Campbell's Operative Orthopaedics, 11th ed. Philadelphia: Mosby, 2008.)*

4. Blockade at the branches (axillary) can be used for rescue blocks or with a multiple injection technique for hand and wrist surgery.

C. INTERSCALENE BLOCK
1. Indications.
a. Shoulder and upper arm surgery.
b. C8-T1 usually spared (ulnar and brachiocutaneous nerve).
2. Pt positioning.
a. Turn pt's head 45° toward nonoperative side. Palpate groove between the anterior and middle scalene muscles.
3. Needle placement.
a. Insert 1- or 2-in regional block needle 2 to 3 cm above clavicle in groove perpendicular to planes of the skin with slight caudal direction.
b. Never insert to more than 2 to 3 cm depth without experienced supervision.
c. Redirection involves shifting skin and needle in 2 to 3 mm increments either anteriorly or posteriorly.

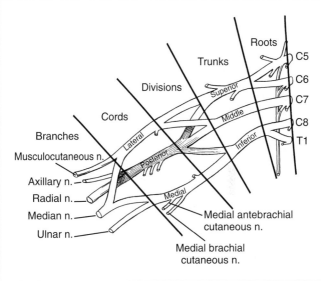

FIG. 8.2

Upper extremity peripheral nerves.

4. Position confirmation.

a. Definitive deltoid twitches or, preferably, biceps or triceps stimulation with nerve stimulation.

5. Dosing.

a. 30 to 40 mL LA in divided doses.

6. Important points.

a. The brachial plexus is usually only 1 to 2 cm deep.

b. Diaphragmatic stimulation (phrenic nerve)—reposition needle posteriorly.

c. Scapula movement (nerve to levator scapulae or dorsal scapular nerve)—reposition needle anteriorly.

D. SUPRACLAVICULAR BLOCK

1. Indications.

a. Any surgery below the shoulder.

2. Pt positioning.

a. Supine, with head turned slightly toward nonoperative side.

3. Needle placement.

a. Insert 2-in needle perpendicular to horizontal plane 1.5 cm lateral and 1.5 cm cephalad from point where lateral border of sternocleidomastoid muscle meets the clavicle.

b. Walk needle caudal in 5° increments until superior trunk stimulation occurs.

c. Flatten angle with constant stimulation until needle is parallel to floor and advance slightly until distal twitch elicited.

d. Never advance deeper than 2 to 3 cm without experienced supervision or continue to advance after blood is aspirated or after elicited twitch ceases.

4. Position confirmation.

a. Motor response in hand.

5. Dosing.

a. 30 mL LA in divided doses.

6. Important points.

a. Very challenging technique but provides fastest and best block.

b. Needle should never be directed medial or caudal to clavicle.

E. POSTERIOR CERVICAL PARAVERTEBRAL BLOCK

1. Indications.

a. Surgery on an upper extremity.

2. Pt positioning.

a. Lateral or sitting.

b. Identify point where medial border of levator scapulae passes under trapezius.

3. Needle placement.

a. Insert 17-G stimulating Tuohy needle, aiming toward sternal notch until contact with transverse process.

b. Walk needle laterally and slightly caudally off bone and advance until loss of resistance and stimulation of brachial plexus.

4. Position confirmation.

a. Stimulation of deltoids, triceps, or pectoralis for shoulder surgery, or distal stimulation for more distal surgery.

5. Dosing.

a. 20 to 30 mL LA.

6. Important points.

a. Used primarily for catheter placement owing to secure location and ease of placement.

b. Inexperience could make this an extremely risky block owing to location of spinal cord relative to initial needle insertion.

c. Beginners should not perform this block without appropriate supervision.

7. Unique side effects and complications from above-the-clavicle approaches.

a. Sympathetic ganglion blockade resulting in Horner syndrome (ptosis, miosis, anhidrosis unilateral) reported in 20% to 90% of cases.

b. Phrenic nerve (C3-C5) block results in unilateral diaphragmatic paralysis (100% with interscalene), resulting in 20% to 40% decrease in forced expiratory volume (FEV_1) and forced vital capacity (FVC).

c. Recurrent laryngeal nerve is blocked in 10% to 30%.
   i.   Results in hoarseness.
d. Epidural or intrathecal injection (even with correct needle placement).
e. Vascular injection, including vertebral, subclavian, or carotid artery.
f. Risk of pneumothorax (1 : 100–1 : 1000), depending on approach.

F.   INFRACLAVICULAR BLOCK
1. Indications.
a. Elbow, forearm, and hand surgery.
2. Pt positioning.
a. Supine with no movement of injured arm required.
3. Needle placement.
a. Insert 2- or 4-in insulated needle 2 cm medial and 2 cm caudal to the coracoid process.
b. With pt in supine position, place needle perpendicular to the floor and advance through pectoralis muscle.
4. Position confirmation.
a. Distal twitches in hand (extension best choice).
5. Dosing.
a. 40 mL LA in divided doses.
6. Unique side effects/complications.
a. Pneumothorax.
7. Important points.
a. Needle should never be directed medially (risk of pneumothorax) or laterally but should be redirected caudally or cephalad to locate the plexus.
b. Will often block musculocutaneous and brachiocutaneous nerves.
c. Abduction of the arm may make contact with artery less likely.

G.   AXILLARY BLOCK
1. Indications.
a. Hand and forearm surgery.
b. Rescue block.
2. Pt positioning.
a. The arm is placed at a right angle to the body and flexed 90° at the elbow.
3. Needle placement.
a. Insert 2-in insulated needle at a 45° angle to the skin several millimeters to either side of the artery and advance until a nerve stimulator elicits twitches distal to the elbow.
4. Position confirmation.
a. Confirm muscle stimulation of the desired nerve distribution prior to injection.
5. Dosing.
a. 30 to 50 mL LA in divided doses, preferably divided among all three distal branches.

6. Unique side effects/complications.

a. None.

7. Important points.

a. Relative to the artery, the median nerve is superior, the ulnar nerve is inferior, and the radial nerve is posterior.

b. The musculocutaneous nerve is frequently spared and is separately blocked in the body of the coracobrachialis muscle.

c. The brachiocutaneous nerve must be blocked separately.

H. LOWER EXTREMITY ANATOMY AND NERVE BLOCKS (Figs. 8.3 and 8.4, _A_)

1. Sciatic nerve block (proximal approach).

a. Indications.

    i. Major knee surgery, leg, ankle, or foot surgery.

b. Pt positioning.

    i. Classic approach.

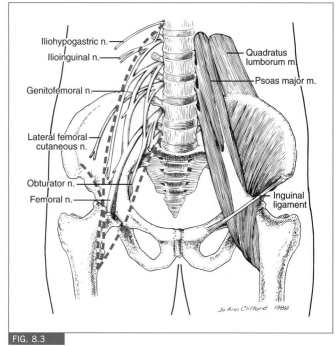

FIG. 8.3

Lower extremity anatomy. _(From Wedel DJ, Horlocker TT: Nerve blocks. In Miller RD [ed]: Miller's Anesthesia, 6th ed. Philadelphia: Churchill Livingstone, 2005.)_

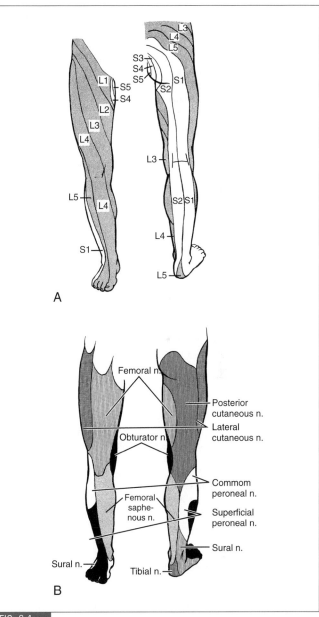

FIG. 8.4

A, Sciatic nerve sensory innervation. **B,** Lumbar plexus sensory innervation.

- Pt is positioned laterally, with operative extremity flexed at thigh and knee, and dependent extremity straight.
- Provider must be able to visualize toes.
- First line is drawn between greater trochanter of femur and posterior superior iliac spine (PSIS).
- Perpendicular line is drawn bisecting first line that extends caudally 4 cm and should bisect a second line from greater trochanter to sacral hiatus.
- Needle is inserted at intersection perpendicular to skin in all planes.
  ii. Franco approach.
    - Simpler and does not require any palpation.
    - With pt in either prone or lateral position, a point is identified 10 cm lateral from the intergluteal sulcus halfway between the upper and lower border of the buttocks.
    - Needle is inserted parallel to the floor if pt is lateral or perpendicular to the floor if pt is prone.
  c. Needle placement/position confirmation.
    i. Advance 4-in insulated needle deep to gluteal twitch until inversion or plantar flexion of foot is seen.
    ii. If eversion or dorsiflexion is seen, redirect needle medially.
  d. Dosing.
    i. Prior to injection, aspirate needle. If blood is present, reposition needle.
    ii. 20 to 30 mL LA in divided doses.
  e. Unique side effects/complications.
    i. Pts require adequate sedation due to pain from the procedure.
  f. Important points.
    i. Redirection is either lateral or medial in 5° increments for both approaches.
    ii. Posterior superior iliac spine and greater trochanter are often misidentified with classic approach.
  g. Franco approach is simpler based on the concept that the sciatic nerve exits the pelvis in the same location consistently and bones do not change size dependent on weight.
    i. Very long duration block.
    ii. This block often takes 30 min for onset.
    iii. Sciatic is largest nerve in body and is really two nerves (tibial [medial] and common peroneal [lateral]) that divide 5 to 12 cm above the knee.
    iv. Blockade at this level also involves posterior femoral cutaneous nerve, which covers skin on posterior thigh.

2. Sciatic nerve block at popliteal fossa.
  a. Indications.
    i. Surgery on the leg and foot.
    ii. Saphenous nerve block is also needed if surgery involves the medial aspect of the leg.

b. Pt positioning.
    i.   Lateral approach.
        • Pt in supine position.
        • Groove between biceps femoris and vastus lateralis is identified at a point 7 cm above knee crease.
    ii.   Posterior (intertendinous) approach.
        • Pt should be in prone position, with foot extending off edge of bed.
        • Tendons from biceps femoris and semimembranosus are identified at crease in knee and bisected.
        • Line is extended 7 cm cephalad.

c. Needle placement.
    i.   Lateral approach.
        • Insert 4-in stimulating needle parallel to floor and slightly cephalad and advance to identify femur.
        • Withdraw needle and redirect 30° posterior and no more than 2 to 3 cm deeper than femur contact.
        • Redirection is anterior or posterior in 5° increments.
    ii.   Posterior approach.
        • Insert 2-in insulated needle at 30° cephalad angle.
        • Redirection is medial or lateral in 5° increments.

d. Position confirmation.
    i.   Plantar flexion (tibial nerve) or inversion (combination of tibial and common peroneal) of foot.

e. Dosing.
    i.   Inject 30 to 40 mL LA, with careful aspiration.

f. Unique side effects/complications.
    i.   None.

g. Important points.
    i.   The nerves are just lateral and posterior to the popliteal artery.
    ii.   The common peroneal nerve may be spared and can be blocked separately with infiltration of 5 mL LA just below the head of the fibula.
    iii. Separately stimulating and injecting for common peroneal and tibial nerve increases success if the two are not very close to each other.
    iv. Tibial stimulation results in plantar flexion and inversion.
    v.   Common peroneal stimulation results in dorsiflexion and eversion and partly contributes to inversion.
    vi. Onset time is often 30 min.

3. Ankle block.
a. Multiple field blocks are performed without nerve stimulator.
b. Indications.
    i.   Foot surgery below mid-foot.
c. Pt positioning/needle placement/dosing.
    i.   Deep peroneal nerve.
        • Insert needle lateral to anterior tibial artery and inject 3 to 5 mL.

8

REGIONAL ANESTHESIA

      ii.   Superficial peroneal nerve.
- SQ injection is made from medial malleolus to lateral malleolus.

     iii.   Saphenous nerve.
- SQ injection from above medial malleolus and directed posteriorly.

     iv.   Sural nerve.
- Place needle anterior to Achilles tendon.
- Inject 10 mL with needle directed toward the malleolus.

     v.   Posterior tibial.
- Insert needle posterolaterally to posterior tibial artery.
- Inject 10 mL, fanning out at the level of the medial malleolus.

d. Position confirmation.
    i.   Nerve stimulator is not necessary but can be used for posterior tibial stimulation (plantar flexion).

e. Unique side effects/complications.
    i.   Increased pain with block placement because of necessary multiple injections.
    ii.   Intravascular injection risk is increased secondary to large area injected and prohibition of epinephrine as an intravascular marker.

f. Important points.
    i.   Injuries to the foot that cause induration, infection, or edema can decrease the effectiveness of the block.
    ii.   Epinephrine should not be used in blocks involving distal extremities.

4. Lumbar plexus block (see Fig. 8.4, _B_).
a. L1-L4 single-shot nerve block.

b. Indications.
    i.   Procedures involving hip, thigh (lateral, anterior, and medial aspects), knee, and medial leg.

c. Pt positioning.
    i.   Lateral or prone position.
    ii.   Line is drawn connecting iliac crests with midline (L4 vertebrae).

d. Needle placement.
    i.   Insert 4-in insulated needle perpendicular to the skin 4 to 5 cm lateral to the fourth lumbar spine until contact with transverse process.
    ii.   Can then redirect cephalad or caudad and advance 2 to 2.5 cm deeper.

e. Position confirmation.
    i.   Quadriceps twitches.

f. Dosing.
    i.   Prior to injection, aspirate needle. If blood is present, reposition needle.
    ii.   30 mL LA.

g. Unique side effects/complications.
    i.   Pain and hematoma formation are the most common.
    ii.   Risks also include bowel, bladder, ureter, and renal perforation.
    iii.   Epidural or intrathecal spread occurs in between 1% and 5% of cases.

h. Important points.
  i.   The pt should be well sedated prior to performing block.
  ii. Block may last 12 to 24 hr with long-acting anesthetics.
  iii. Sympathectomy is common but generally not significant.
  iv. The block often takes 30 min to work.
  v.   Blocks femoral, lateral femoral cutaneous (LFCN), and obturator nerves with single injection but is one of the highest-risk blocks.

5. Femoral nerve block.

a. Indications.
  i.   Knee arthroscopies, patellar fractures, anterior thigh procedures.
  ii. Used with other blocks for more extensive thigh and leg surgeries.
  iii. Useful adjunct for postoperative pain associated with femur fracture.

b. Pt positioning.
  i.   With pt in supine position, palpate femoral artery at the inguinal crease.

c. Needle placement.
  i.   Advance 2-in insulated needle 1 cm lateral to femoral artery.

d. Position confirmation.
  i.   Stimulation of the quadriceps muscle with patella ascension.

e. Dosing.
  i.   Prior to injection, aspirate needle. If blood is present, reposition needle.
  ii. 20 mL LA.

f. Unique side effects/complications.
  i.   None.

g. Important points.
  i.   Femoral nerve is superficial in all pts.
  ii. Most common failure is accepting sartorius stimulation (medial thigh with no patellar twitch).
    • Needle is redirected deep and slightly lateral.

6. Lateral femoral cutaneous nerve (LFCN) block.

a. Indications.
  i.   Lateral thigh procedures.

b. Pt positioning.
  i.   Supine.

c. Needle placement.
  i.   Insert 2-in needle 2 cm medial and inferior to anterior superior iliac spine.
  ii. Advance needle until it passes through fascia.

d. Position confirmation.
  i.   May stimulate for lateral thigh sensory paresthesias.

e. Dosing.
  i.   Prior to injection, aspirate needle. If blood is present, reposition needle.
  ii. Inject 10 to 15 mL LA above and below fascia, fanning in the direction of the anterior superior iliac spine.

f. Important point.
   i. Nerve has no motor component.

7. **Testing block function.**
a. Lumbar plexus 4Ps.
   i. *Pinch* mid-lateral thigh—LFCN.
   ii. *Pinch* medial thigh at midpoint—anterior femoral.
   iii. *Push* against extension at knee—posterior femoral.
   iv. *Push* against adduction of thigh—obturator.
b. Sacral plexus 4Ps.
   i. *Pinch* mid-posterior thigh—posterior femoral cutaneous.
   ii. *Pinch* dorsum mid-foot—anterior branch of common peroneal.
   iii. *Push* against dorsiflexion—deep branch of common peroneal.
   iv. *Push* against plantar flexion—tibial.
c. Brachial plexus 4Ps.
   i. *Push* the arm against force by extension at the elbow—radial nerve.
   ii. *Pull* decreased strength with flexion at the elbow—musculocutaneous.
   iii. *Pinch* palmar base of the index finger—median nerve.
   iv. *Pinch* palmar base of the fifth digit—ulnar nerve.

VI. NEURAXIAL ANESTHESIA

A. **ANATOMY (Figs. 8.5, 8.6, and 8.7)**
1. 7 cervical, 12 thoracic, 5 lumbar vertebrae.

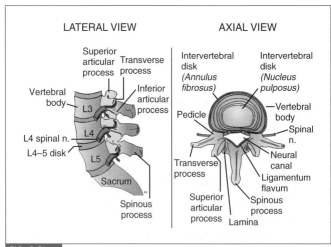

FIG. 8.5

Lumbar vertebral anatomy. *(From Lin M: Musculoskeletal back pain. In Marx JA [ed]: Rosen's Emergency Medicine: Concepts and Clinical Practice, 6th ed. Philadelphia: Mosby, 2006.)*

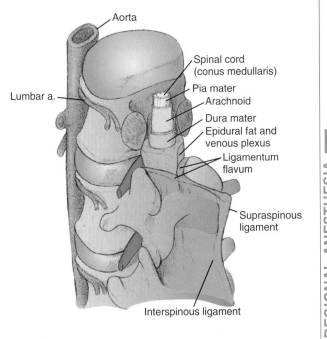

FIG. 8.6

Anatomy of the spinal canal.

2. Spinal cord ends at L1-L2; dural sac ends at S2.
3. To reach spinal canal by **midline approach**, needle must pass through skin, SQ fat, supraspinous ligament, interspinous ligament, and ligamentum flavum.
4. To reach spinal canal by **paramedian approach**, needle must pass through skin, SQ fat, and ligamentum flavum.
5. Epidural space surrounds spinal dura.
a. It contains valveless veins, fat, and exiting vertebral nerve roots.
b. It is separated from CSF by spinal meninges (dura, arachnoid, pia).
6. Subdural space is potential space between dura and arachnoid.
a. May get excessively high-level or patchy block if LA accidentally enters this space during intended epidural injection.
7. Intrathecal space extends along spinal nerve roots.
a. Accidental puncture (e.g., during paravertebral block or interscalene block) may cause spinal block or postdural puncture headache (PDPH).

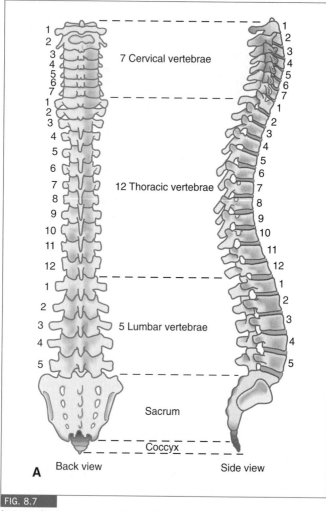

1 2 3 4 5 6 7   7 Cervical vertebrae

1 2 3 4 5 6 7 8 9 10 11 12   12 Thoracic vertebrae

1 2 3 4 5   5 Lumbar vertebrae

Sacrum

Coccyx

A   Back view   Side view

FIG. 8.7

Anatomy of the spinal canal. **A,** Vertebral column. *Continued.*

B. INDICATIONS FOR NEURAXIAL ANESTHESIA

1. Pt preference.
2. Pt's underlying disease places pt at high risk for GA.
3. Benefits.
a. Superior postoperative analgesia with epidural.

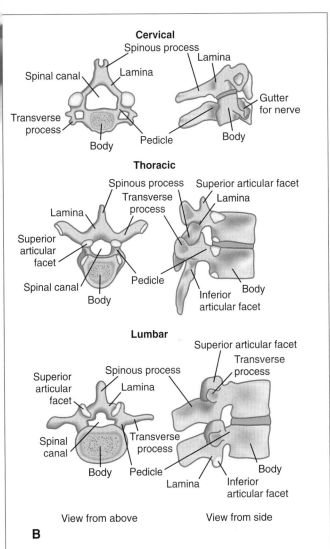

Cervical

Spinal canal

Spinous process

Lamina

Transverse process

Body

Pedicle

Lamina

Gutter for nerve

Body

Thoracic

Spinous process

Transverse process

Lamina

Superior articular facet

Lamina

Superior articular facet

Spinal canal

Pedicle

Body

Inferior articular facet

Body

Lumbar

Superior articular facet

Spinous process

Lamina

Superior articular facet

Transverse process

Spinal canal

Transverse process

Body

Pedicle

Lamina

Inferior articular facet

Body

View from above

View from side

B

FIG. 8.7—cont'd

B, Typical vertebrae. *(From Hockberger RS, Kaji AH, Newton EJ: Spinal injuries. In Marx JA [ed]: Rosen's Emergency Medicine: Concepts and Clinical Practice, 6th ed. Philadelphia: Mosby, 2006.)*

8

REGIONAL ANESTHESIA

b. May decrease intraoperative blood loss and transfusion requirements.
   i.   This benefit is lost when combined with positive-pressure ventilation.
c. Several large meta-analyses indicate decreased mortality, pulmonary, CV, GI, and coagulation-related morbidity with epidural anesthesia.
   i.   These results are controversial.

C. CONTRAINDICATIONS TO NEURAXIAL ANESTHESIA
1. Absolute.
a. Pt refusal.
b. Active infection at site of needle insertion, septicemia, meningitis.
c. Therapeutic anticoagulation.
d. True allergy to LAs.
e. Uncorrected hypovolemia.
2. Relative.
a. Peripheral neuropathy, demyelinating CNS disease.
b. Partial anticoagulation.
c. Uncooperative pts.
d. Although it is almost always possible to "talk" pts into regional anesthesia, it is not appropriate to force the issue for reluctant pts.

D. INTRAOPERATIVE COMPLICATIONS ASSOCIATED WITH NEURAXIAL ANESTHESIA
1. Hypotension.
a. Secondary to peripheral vasodilation from preganglionic sympathetic block.
b. Related to extent of sympathetic block.
c. Hypotension results from arterial dilation and resultant decrease in vascular tone.
   i.   Severe hypotension may also be related to decreased preload (due to decreased HR and stroke volume).
d. May manifest initially as nausea (central medullary ischemia).
2. Inadvertent total spinal.
a. Usually occurs with accidental intrathecal administration of epidural LA dose.
b. May also occur with accidental intrathecal injection during brachial plexus or stellate blocks.
c. Ventilation and CV support is required.
d. Block usually recedes in 1 to 2 hr.
e. Will see dilated pupils.
f. Generally, pt has no recall of the event.
   i.   Verbal reassurance is encouraged.
g. Apnea is secondary to cerebral hypotension, not C3-C5 blockade.
3. Asystole—bradycardia.
a. Abrupt onset of bradycardia or asystole without evidence of hemodynamic instability or hypoxemia.

b. May occur at any time during anesthesia.
c. Early treatment with epinephrine is associated with improved outcomes.
d. Early administration of vagolytic drugs such as atropine or glycopyrrolate decrease risk of asystole.
e. Etiology is most likely Bezold-Jarisch reflex (BJR) (intracardiac vasodepressor reflex).
   i. The BJR reflex originates in cardiac sensory receptors with nonmyelinated vagal afferent pathways.
   ii. The LV, particularly the inferoposterior wall, is a principal location for these sensory receptors.
   iii. Stimulation of these inhibitory cardiac receptors by stretch, chemical substances, or drugs increases parasympathetic activity and inhibits sympathetic activity.
   iv. These effects promote reflex bradycardia, vasodilation, and hypotension (BJR) and modulate renin release and vasopressin secretion.
f. Normally, hypovolemia causes decrease in inhibitory activity of BJR, which results in subsequent increase in sympathetic tone.
   i. A sudden decrease in central venous return associated with neuraxial blockade causes paradoxical activation of BJR.
   ii. The empty LV vigorously contracts and activates BJR receptors, resulting in abrupt withdrawal of sympathetic tone, bradycardia, and hypotension.
   iii. Stretch receptors in right atrium, SA node, and vena cava respond to decreased volume by slowing HR to improve stroke volume.

E. POSTOPERATIVE COMPLICATIONS
1. PDPH.
a. Pathophysiology of PDPH.
   i. CSF leakage.
     • PDPH occurs when CSF leakage > CSF production.
   ii. Cerebrovasodilation.
     • Body attempts to maintain homeostasis within cranium.
   iii. CSF leads to compensatory cerebrovasodilation and headache.
   iv. Meningeal irritation.
   v. Pneumocephalus.
     • Accidental intrathecal injection of air during epidural may cause relatively sudden onset of headache.
b. Risk factors of PDPH.
   i. Pt factors.
     • Gender—females at higher risk.
     • Age—younger pts at higher risk.
     • History of headache—positive history at higher risk.
   ii. Needle characteristics.
     • Size—larger needle size increases loss of CSF and incidence of PDPH.

8

REGIONAL ANESTHESIA

- Shape—sharp, cutting-edge beveled needle has increased incidence of PDPH when compared with pencil-point needles.
  iii. Procedural factors.
  - Needle should be inserted "parallel" to dural fibers. Usually, dural fibers run longitudinally.
  - Paramedian versus midline approach: paramedian may have decreased incidence of PDPH ("flap" rather than a "tin-lid" opening).
  - Multiple punctures increase risk of PDPH because of increased loss of CSF.
- c. Clinical assessment of PDPH.
  i. PDPH is a diagnosis of exclusion.
  ii. Usually, diagnosis is straightforward owing to the temporal nature and absence of other reasons for headache.
  iii. Presence of other etiologies for headache may cloud clinical picture.
  - Migraine and tension headache may be present (and initiated by concurrent PDPH).
  - Cortical venous thrombosis in parturients is also possible.
  - LP may have been performed as part of headache or meningitis workup.
  - Neurology team should be consulted if there is any doubt.
  iv. Pathognomonic sign: postural component to headache.
  v. PDPH usually appears 1 to 2 days after dural puncture and lasts (if untreated) for up to 7 days in most cases.
  vi. Other associated symptoms (not reliable).
  - Photophobia, nausea, vomiting, auditory disturbances.
  - Cranial nerve involvement (diplopia).
  - 6th cranial nerve involvement (longest cranial nerve).
- d. Treatment of PDPH.
  i. Conservative.
  - Symptomatic treatment until dural puncture heals.
  - Hydration, oral analgesics, caffeine (IV or oral).
  - Cannot increase CSF production with overhydration.
  - Caffeine provides transient relief via vasoconstriction.
  ii. Invasive.
  - Epidural blood patch (gold standard).
  - Success rate is quoted at 70% to 90%.
  - Injection of 15 to 20 mL of autologous blood (collected at the time the blood patch is performed) via epidural needle inserted in interspace below original puncture.
  - Inject slowly.
  - Pt may note severe back pain, neck stiffness, transient paresthesias in legs.
  - Pt should note headache relief within 10 to 15 min (because of displacement of CSF cephalad).

- Prolonged relief of headache is a result of sealant effect of blood over dural puncture.
- May require a second epidural blood patch.
- Reevaluate etiology of headache (with neurology consultation) if >2 epidural blood patches are required.

2. Transient neurologic syndrome.

a. Primarily associated with use of lidocaine anesthesia.
b. Not clearly associated with concentration, baricity, osmolarity, or addition of glucose.
c. Risk factors include use of lidocaine spinal, lithotomy, and outpatient surgery.
d. Incidence.
   i.   15% to 40% with lidocaine.
   ii. <5% with other agents.
e. Symptoms.
   i.   Cramping or burning in thighs.
   ii. Low back pain.
   iii. Radiation to lower extremities.
   iv. Onset 12 to 24 hr after surgery.
   v.   May last hours to days.
f. Treatment.
   i.   Supportive with opioids, NSAIDS, and muscle relaxants.

3. Epidural hematoma.

a. Incidence of traumatic epidural placement, 1% to 18% (highest in OB).
b. Risks include multiple attempts and large-gauge needles.
c. Almost all cases are related to a coagulopathy.
d. Incidence.
   i.   1:150,000 epidural and 1:200,000 spinal prior to LMWH.
   ii. Increased to 1:6600 epidural and 1:40,000 spinal in the late 1990s.
e. Presentation, diagnosis, and treatment.
   i.   Often painless with progressive neurologic deterioration.
   ii. Diagnosis and treatment must be swift to prevent permanent injury
   iii. Diagnosis confirmed with MRI.
   iv. Treatment is immediate surgical decompression.

4. Neuropathy.

a. Risk factors.
   i.   Severe pain on injection.
   ii. High initial injection pressure.
   iii. Paresthesia technique.
   iv. Multiple injection techniques.
   v.   Repeated block on an anesthetized extremity.
   vi. No increased risk demonstrated with continuous catheter techniques.

> vii. Needle type.
>> • Cutting needle with higher transient neuropathy versus B-bevel needle with higher permanent neuropathy.

b. Incidence.
>> i. 0.038%—spinal.
>> ii. 0.022%—epidural.
>> iii. 0.019%—peripheral nerve block.
>> iv. Incidence of postoperative transient dysesthesias from peripheral nerve block is ~3%.

c. Anesthetic causes.
>> i. Direct transection/crush.
>> ii. Pressure induced (e.g., intraneural injection).
>> iii. Hematoma.
>> iv. Intraneural edema.
>> v. Direct LA toxicity.
>> vi. Prolonged vasoconstriction/vascular compromise.
>> vii. Herniation of nerve fibers.

F. DURATION OF ACTION OF NEURAXIAL ANESTHESIA

1. Factors most important in influencing duration of action.

a. Degree of protein binding.
>> i. Highly bound drugs (tetracaine, bupivacaine) have a longer duration of action.

b. Use of vasoconstrictors (epinephrine, phenylephrine).
>> i. Decrease blood flow and vascular absorption of LA.
>> ii. May also improve quality of block by increased neuronal uptake of LA.

c. Dosage.
>> i. ↑ dose = ↑ duration of action.

d. Isobaric solutions produce a longer block than the same dose of hyperbaric LA for spinal anesthesia.
>> i. Less spread of isobaric solution results in a higher concentration of LA per segment.

G. NEEDLES AND CATHETERS

1. Spinal needles (22- to 29-G).

a. Cutting bevel needles.
>> i. Quincke.

b. Higher-gauge needles (smaller diameter) decrease risk of PDPH.

c. Pencil-point needles.
>> i. Greene, Whitacre, Sprotte.
>> ii. Low incidence of PDPH when compared with same caliber Quincke.

2. Epidural needles (17- to 20-G).

a. Thin-walled needles to allow passage of catheter.

b. Tuohy—directional tip.
>> i. No guarantee of the direction a catheter will take once inside the epidural space.

c. Crawford.
   i.   45° bevel.
3. Epidural catheters.
a. Open-tip, single-orifice versus bullet-tip, multi-orifice.
b. Wire supported (Arrow) versus polyamide (Braun).
c. Arrow catheter is more flexible, with the advantage of minimizing intrathecal or intravascular catheterization.

H. NEEDLE INSERTION
1. Anatomic considerations.
2. Intercrest line (drawn from superior aspect iliac crest) = L4 vertebrae.
3. Line between the most caudad points of the scapula = T7.
4. Midline approach.
a. Landmarks may be easier to identify when pt is sitting.
b. May be easier for beginners.
   i.   Assuming that needle is midline, if bone is encountered the needle is either too cephalad or too caudad.
5. Paramedian approach.
a. May be used when inserting needle between the spinous processes is expected to be difficult.
b. Pt unable to flex the back or with calcified ligaments.
c. Thoracic epidural (overlapping spinous processes).
d. Provides larger target area for needle insertion.

I. NEURAXIAL LAS (Table 8.7)

J. EPIDURAL ADJUVANT AGENTS
1. Epinephrine.
a. Used in test dose.
b. Decreases peak plasma LA concentrations by 20% to 50%.
c. Improves quality of motor block.
d. Contraindications to use of epinephrine.
   i.   Uncontrolled hypertension, known cerebrovascular aneurysm.
   ii. Severe preeclampsia.

REGIONAL ANESTHESIA   **8**

TABLE 8.7						
NEURAXIAL LOCAL ANESTHETICS						
Drug	**Class**	**Onset**	**Epidural Bolus Dose (mg)**	**Epidural Duration (min)**	**Spinal Dose (mg)**	**Spinal Duration (min)**
Lidocaine	Amide	Moderate	60–400	45–120	20–80	45–120
Bupivacaine	Amide	Slow	15–75	60–180	2.5–21	60–210
Ropivacaine	Amide	Slow	15–75	60–180	2.5–21	60–180
Mepivacaine	Amide	Moderate	60–400	45–120	20–80	45–120
Chloroprocaine	Ester	Fast	100–500	30–60	30–70	30–60
Tetracaine	Ester	Slowest			15–25	100–240

iii. Untreated thyrotoxicosis, monoamine oxidase inhibitor therapy, or malignant hyperthermia.

2. Bicarbonate (data is equivocal on use for epidural anesthesia).

a. More rapid onset of block and improved quality of block.

b. Increases relative amount of LA in non-ionized form (pKa).

c. Dose.

i. 1 mEq $NaHCO_3$/10 mL lidocaine.

ii. Should not be used with bupivacaine.

K. EPIDURAL TEST DOSE

1. What does the "test dose" test?

a. Test dose = 3 mg of 1.5% to 2% lidocaine with 1:200,000 epinephrine.

b. Intravascular placement (15 mcg of epinephrine).

i. Increase in HR by 20 to 30 bpm or 10% to 15%.

ii. Time of onset, ~30 sec.

iii. Duration, 30 to 60 sec.

c. Intrathecal placement (45–60 mg of lidocaine).

i. Motor blockade in lower extremity within 2 min.

d. Correct placement of catheter.

i. Sensory level of 1 to 8 dermatomes should be present bilaterally 10 to 15 min after test dose if catheter is correctly placed.

2. Clinical situations when a test dose may not be valid.

a. Parturients during contraction.

b. Pts taking β blockers.

c. Elderly pts.

d. Pts under GA.

L. DOSING OF EPIDURAL CATHETERS

1. Volume is most important factor for number of dermatomes.

2. Density of block is directly related to concentration of LA.

3. Catheter tip should be placed in the middle of the postoperative dermatomes needed for pain control.

a. T7-T8 epidural for Whipple procedure (incision is T5-T10).

b. T11-T12 for hysterectomy with Pfannenstiel incision (T11-T12).

c. L3-L4 for knee replacement (L2-L4 incision and pain from L2-S3).

4. Factors that affect spread of injection.

a. Greater spread in thoracic (versus lumbar) area due to decreased area of thoracic epidural space (leads to greater spread of solutions).

b. Increased age increases spread of injectate, possibly due to increased calcification of neural foramina (decreased leakage of LA from epidural space).

c. Term pregnancy and morbid obesity may cause increased spread, and reduction in volume up to 30% may be necessary.

d. Continuous infusion results in decreased spread compared with bolus infusion.

M. GENERAL GUIDELINES FOR INITIAL BOLUS

1. Base dose if possible on spread observed from test dose.
2. Thoracic epidural.
a. 1.2 mg per dermatome intended to block.
   i. T10 epidural and need for T4 block intraoperatively requires 15 mg LA, which would cover 13 dermatomes.
3. Lumbar epidural.
a. 1.5 mg per dermatome intended to block.
4. Doses should be reduced by 5% to 10% for every decade over 30 yr of age.
5. Doses should be reduced by 0% to 30% for obesity or term pregnancy (5% for mild obesity to 30% for morbid obesity).

N. GENERAL GUIDELINES FOR REDOSING

1. If continuous infusion is used, it should be run at same rate as initial bolus.
2. If intermittent bolus is used, 1/2 to 2/3 of initial bolus should be used approximately every 90 min for bupivacaine or approximately every 60 min for lidocaine.
3. Continuous infusion is simpler and more hemodynamically stable but uses higher doses of LA and may not work if operative site is nondependent.

O. INTRAOPERATIVE MANAGEMENT: GENERAL EPIDURAL ANESTHESIA

1. Epidural anesthesia may be difficult as sole anesthetic agent in upper abdominal or thoracic procedures.
2. Use intraoperative epidural anesthesia-analgesia with "light" GA.
3. Advantages.
a. Potentially faster emergence.
b. Physiologic benefits from regional anesthesia-analgesia.
c. Superior postoperative analgesia.
d. *Key*: Confirmation that the epidural catheter is functioning *prior* to induction of GA.
e. Enough LA is administered prior to incision to obtain appropriate sensory level.
f. LA is continued intraoperatively either as a bolus or continuous infusion

P. POSTOPERATIVE EPIDURAL PCA ORDERS (Table 8.8)

Q. TECHNICAL PROBLEMS: EPIDURAL ANESTHESIA

1. Aspiration of blood via catheter.
a. Most likely accidental placement into epidural vein.
   i. Aspiration of no blood does not guarantee that catheter is in the epidural space.
b. May pull back until no blood is aspirated.

8

REGIONAL ANESTHESIA

TABLE 8.8

POSTOPERATIVE EPIDURAL PCA ORDERS (STARTING DOSES UNLESS CHANGE IS INDICATED BY INTRAOPERATIVE RESPONSE)

Surgical Site	Drug and Concentration	Basal Rate (mL/hr)	Demand (mL)	Lockout (min)
Lower abdomen, lower extremity (lumbar epidural)	Bupivacaine 0.0625% and fentanyl, 5 mcg/mL	4	4	10
Lower abdomen (thoracic epidural)	Bupivacaine 0.125% and fentanyl, 5 mcg/mL	4	2	10
Upper abdomen and thoracic surgery	Bupivacaine 0.125% and fentanyl, 5 mcg/mL	5	3	10
Hip surgery—lumbar epidural	Bupivacaine 0.0625% and fentanyl, 5 mcg/mL	6	3	10

   i. May or may not be inside epidural space.
   ii. Some advocate removing catheter and inserting in another location.
2. Aspiration of clear fluid via catheter.
a. May be CSF or LA.
   i. Consider testing for presence of glucose (+CSF).
b. Consider using catheter for continuous spinal anesthesia.
   i. Lower concentration such as hyperbaric lidocaine (2%) should be used.
   ii. Continuous spinal catheter should not be left in postoperatively.
3. Difficulty in inserting catheter through needle.
a. Use of a nylon catheter (more support) may be better than use of an Arrow catheter.
b. Consider advancing Tuohy 1 to 2 mm or turning Tuohy 90°.
   i. Caution—may result in accidental dural puncture.
4. Difficulty with catheter removal.
a. Having pt flex back may open space between spinous processes.
5. Sheared epidural catheter.
a. Catheter should be left in place.
   i. It will be walled off by fibrosis.
b. Risks of surgical exploration likely higher than leaving catheter in epidural space.
c. Sheared intrathecal catheter requires neurosurgery consult.
d. Catheter may migrate (no fibrosis).

VII. SPINAL ANESTHESIA
A. ADVANTAGES (VERSUS EPIDURAL)
1. Faster onset.
2. "Denser" block.
3. Technically easier.
4. Less pt discomfort during placement.
5. Lower failure rate.

B. DISADVANTAGES
1. Faster onset.
2. Level of anesthesia not as easily titrated.
3. Limited postoperative analgesia.
4. Limited duration.
5. Greater risk of bradycardia (asystole).
6. Slightly greater risk of permanent neuropathy.
7. Transient neurologic syndrome.

C. SPINAL ADJUVANT AGENTS
1. Vasoconstrictors.
a. Increase duration of action of LA.
   i.   Lidocaine from <1 to 1.5 hr and tetracaine from <2 hr to ~3 hr.
b. Spinal dose.
   i.   Epinephrine—0.2 to 0.3 mg.
   ii. Phenylephrine—5 mg.
2. Bicarbonate is *not* used as spinal adjuvant agent.

D. FACTORS THAT AFFECT SPREAD OF SPINAL ANESTHESIA
1. Baricity and position of pt.
a. Must account for the natural curvatures of the spine.
b. Hyperbaric solutions injected at L3-L4 will spread cephalad and caudad owing to lumbar lordosis.
2. Dose of drug most important for spread.
a. Mass = concentration × volume.
3. Age of pt.
a. Greater spread with increasing age.
4. Factors that do **not** influence spread of spinal anesthesia.
a. Gender, volume of injected solution, needle direction, barbotage.

E. INTRAOPERATIVE: SPINAL ANESTHESIA
1. Increase preload prior to spinal.
a. Typically, 1 to 1.5 L crystalloid is given before injection.
b. More effective in decreasing risk of bradycardia than in preventing hypotension.
2. Sedation (applies to other regional anesthetic techniques).
a. Many spinal and epidural anesthetics fail because of inadequate IV sedation, rather than because of technically flawed blocks.
b. May increase customer (pt, surgeon) satisfaction and acceptability of regional anesthesia.

F. COMBINED SPINAL-EPIDURAL ANESTHESIA
1. Procedure.
a. Enter epidural space as usual.
b. Insert a 4–11/16-in, 27-G spinal needle or 26-G Gertie Marx needle through the Tuohy.

8

REGIONAL ANESTHESIA

   i. Administer spinal anesthetic and thread epidural catheter.
   ii. Advantage.
      • Faster onset of anesthesia.
   iii. Disadvantage.
      • Does not guarantee that epidural catheter will function postoperatively.
2. Consider use of isobaric solutions.
a. Use of hyperbaric solutions results in a saddle block when trouble is encountered threading the epidural catheter.
3. Dural puncture does not allow passage of catheter or exaggerated spread of subsequently administered LA or opioids.
a. Increased lumbar pressure of epidural injectate (if given immediately following spinal anesthetic) may increase spread of spinal anesthetic.

REFERENCES CONSULTED

Enneking KF, Chan VC, Greger A, et al: Lower extremity peripheral nerve blockade: Essentials of our current understanding. Reg Anesth Pain Med 2005;30:6.

Neal JM, Hebl JR, Gerancher JC, et al: Brachial plexus anesthesia: Essentials of our current understanding. Reg Anesth Pain Med 2002;27(4):403.

Richman JM, Rowlingson AJ, Maine DN, et al: Does neuraxial anesthesia reduce intraoperative blood loss? A meta-analysis. J Clin Anesth 2006;18:427–435.

Wu CL, Cohen SR, Richman JM, et al: Efficacy of postoperative patient-controlled and continuous infusion epidural analgesia versus intravenous patient-controlled analgesia with opioids: A meta-analysis. Anesthesiology 2005;103:1079–1088.

Cardiovascular and Thoracic Anesthesia

M. Hassan Ahmad, MD, Rahul Baijal, MD,
Ana Fernandez-Bustamante, MD, Brenda M. McKnight, MD,
and Polly-Anna Silver, MD
Edited by Joshua D. Stearns, MD, and Kelly L. Grogan, MD

I. CORONARY ARTERY BYPASS GRAFTING (CABG)

A. OVERVIEW
1. CABG is one of the most frequently performed cardiac surgeries in the US.
2. Location and severity of lesion are critical features for determining need for revascularization.
a. >75% stenosis is considered significant.

B. TREATMENTS TO REDUCE CARDIAC ISCHEMIA
1. Decrease myocardial oxygen demand.
a. Decrease HR.
b. Decrease myocardial wall tension.
2. Increase myocardial oxygen supply.
a. Higher FiO_2.
b. Increase oxygen-carrying capacity by increasing Hb if pt is anemic.
3. Improve coronary blood flow with decrease in HR.
a. Decreased HR leads to greater diastolic filling of the coronaries and greater diastolic subendocardial oxygenation.

C. MONITORING FOR CABG WITH CPB
1. ECG.
a. 12-lead ECG.
b. Continuous monitoring of leads II and V5.
c. Continuous ST-segment monitoring.
2. Arterial line for beat-to-beat BP monitoring.
3. Pulmonary artery catheter (PAC) (Swan-Ganz catheter).
a. Much debate surrounds routine use in pts with ischemic disease.
b. May be of limited value in detecting ischemia.
c. May provide valuable information in regard to cardiac output (CO) and overall volume status.
4. TEE.
a. Able to detect segmental or regional wall motion abnormalities.
b. Provides both a qualitative and quantitative evaluation of LV and RV function.
c. Transvenous or epicardial pacing may make the interpretation of regional wall motion abnormalities more difficult.

9

D. OFF-PUMP CORONARY ARTERY BYPASS
1. Advantages.
a. Decreased inflammatory response as elicited by CPB.
b. Increased platelet salvage or decreased platelet destruction by CPB.
c. Maintains pulsatile blood flow to end organs (e.g., brain, kidneys).
d. Decreased aortic manipulation in pts with advanced aortic disease.
e. Reduced requirement of blood transfusion.

2. Disadvantages.
a. Very surgeon dependent.
b. Graft patency may be impaired.
c. Induced ischemia with or without intracoronary shunting.
   i. Right coronary artery occlusion/ischemia can lead to dysrhythmias and mitral regurgitation (MR) from posteromedial papillary dysfunction.

3. Monitoring.
a. CVP monitoring is particularly important.
   i. Positioning of the heart with retractors and/or stabilizers may impair venous return, thus affecting ventricular filling.
   ii. Adjustments in preload may be achieved with volume, cessation of vasodilators (nitroglycerin, nitroprusside, calcium-channel blockers), pt positioning (Trendelenburg), and inotropic support (e.g., epinephrine or dobutamine infusions).

E. SURGICAL APPROACH (Fig. 9.1)
1. First graft—most immediately available artery with significant lesion.
a. Often, a left internal mammary artery is grafted to the left anterior descending artery.
b. Left internal mammary artery-to-left anterior descending artery graft is preferred owing to the limited amount of cardiac manipulation and the immediate reperfusion of left anterior descending artery territory by virtue of being a native arterial conduit.

2. Subsequent grafts.
a. Typically involve saphenous vein, radial artery, or right internal mammary grafts.
b. Distal anastomosis is performed for saphenous vein grafts and radial artery grafts.
   i. Distal anastomoses require an increase in BP often higher than baseline BP.
   ii. The increased BP ensures adequate coronary perfusion pressure to non-grafted coronary vessels and increases collateral flow critical to reduction of ischemia.
   iii. May require inotrope or volume.
c. Proximal anastomosis is achieved using a side-biting aortic clamp.
   i. The clamp may impair blood flow to reduce systemic BP. Typically, surgeons prefer a reduction in BP—often less than baseline BP—during proximal anastomosis.

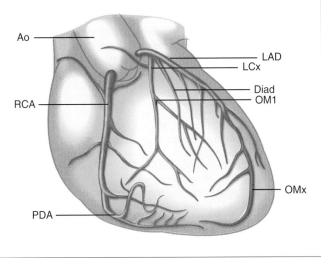

FIG. 9.1

Coronary artery anatomy. *Ao*, Aorta; *RCA*, right coronary artery; *PDA*, posterior descending artery; *OM1*, obtuse marginal 1; *LCx*, left circumflex artery; *Diad*, first diagonal branch of LAD; *LAD*, left anterior descending artery; *OMx*, obtuse marginal.

F. ANTICOAGULATION

1. Amount of anticoagulation differs by procedure (and institution).
a. Reasonable range of activated clotting time can be 250 sec for off-pump procedures to >480 sec for CPB.

II. VALVULAR DISEASES

A. GENERAL EVALUATION OF THE PT WITH VALVULAR HEART DISEASE

1. Complete and full detailed medical history.
2. Determine severity of the lesion.
a. Determine hemodynamic significance.
b. Determine LV and RV function.
c. Evaluate for presence of concomitant CAD.
3. Evaluate for secondary liver, kidney, or pulmonary dysfunction.
4. History should focus on symptoms, including exercise tolerance, fatigability, lower extremity edema, orthopnea, paroxysmal nocturnal dyspnea, chest pain or pressure, dysrhythmias, syncope, or lightheadedness.

5. Physical exam should focus on clinical signs of heart failure (HF), neurologic deficits, cardiac murmurs, carotid bruits, and dental exam.
6. Laboratory evaluation should include Hb, WBC, platelets, coagulation studies, renal function, liver function, ECG, and CXR.
a. Should consider carotid ultrasound in the elderly and echocardiographic studies and cardiac catheterization if clinically indicated.

B. AORTIC STENOSIS
1. Definitions.
a. Normal valve area is 2.5 to 3.5 cm^2.
b. Mild stenosis—valve area exceeds 1.5 cm^2; peak gradient is <30 mm Hg.
c. Moderate stenosis—valve area is 1.0 to 1.4 cm^2; peak gradient is 30 to 50 mm Hg.
d. Severe stenosis—valve area is <0.8 to 1.0 cm^2, peak gradient is >50 mm Hg, or mean gradient is >30 mm Hg.

2. Etiology.
a. Leaflet disease.
   i. Congenital—unicuspid or bicuspid aortic valve.
      • Present at birth, but clinical problems do not appear until fifth or sixth decade of life.
      • Bicuspid aortic valve is most common congenital heart lesion.
   ii. Rheumatic fever.
   iii. Degenerative or senile calcification.
   iv. Atherosclerosis and inflammation.
b. Subvalvular disease.
   i. Thin membrane, thick fibromuscular ridge, accessory endocardial cushion tissue.
   ii. Hypertrophic cardiomyopathy.
c. Supravalvular disease.
   i. "Hourglass deformity."
   ii. Homozygous familial hypercholesterolemia.

3. Pathophysiology.
a. Occurs gradually, causing an obstruction to LV outflow.
b. Gradual onset and progression allows the LV to accommodate to increased pressure.
c. LV myocardium develops concentric hypertrophy.
d. Allows generation of higher pressure during systole.
e. Hypertrophy in the presence of elevated LV pressure maintains LV wall tension; (wall tension = [pressure × radius]/[wall thickness × 2]).
f. LV becomes less compliant, and LV end-diastolic pressure (LVEDP) becomes elevated, with ventricular size initially remaining normal.
g. LV becomes very dependent on atrial contraction for filling (40%).
h. LV output may be maintained for many years before clinical symptoms appear.

. Without surgical intervention, LV develops incoordinate contraction, resulting from regional wall motion abnormalities, fibrosis, and subendocardial ischemia.

. Reduction in myocardial function develops.

k. LV eventually fails, resulting in reduction in stroke volume and CO and eventual HF.

4. Clinical presentation.

a. Often asymptomatic until fifth decade of life.

b. Symptoms usually occur when valve area is <1.0 cm^2 or peak transvalvular gradient is >50 mm Hg.

c. Three cardinal symptoms.

   i.   Angina (from myocardial ischemia).

      ● ~50% have underlying CAD as well.

      ● Imbalance in myocardial oxygen supply and demand.

      ● Increased LV oxygen supply from:

        - Increased LV mass.

        - Increased LV systolic pressure.

        - Increased LV ejection time.

      ● Decreased LV supply from:

        - Compression of intramyocardial coronary arteries from prolonged contraction and impaired myocardial relaxation.

        - Decreased aortic pressure.

        - Increased LVEDP (decreased CPP).

        - Decreased diastolic time.

   ii.   Dyspnea (from pulmonary congestion).

      ● Combined diastolic and systolic dysfunction.

   iii.   Syncope (from inadequate cerebral perfusion).

      ● Exercise-induced vasodilation in the presence of an obstruction and fixed CO can result in hypotension.

      ● Abnormalities in baroreceptor response.

      ● Dysrhythmias.

5. Clinical course.

a. Survival is excellent during asymptomatic phase.

b. 5-yr survival rate for pts in whom angina develops is 50%.

c. Syncope and dyspnea are associated with a worse prognosis, with 50% survival rates at 3 and 2 yr, respectively.

d. Symptomatic pts should undergo aortic valve replacement.

   i.   Mortality exceeds 90% within a few years of symptom development.

6. Hemodynamic goals.

a. Maintenance of normal sinus rhythm, HR, and intravascular volume is critical in pts with aortic stenosis.

b. Avoid systemic hypotension.

   i.   Coronary perfusion = AoDP − LVEDP.

c. Maintain sinus rhythm.

   i.   Need atrial kick for filling noncompliant LV.

d. Maintain slow rate.
  i. More time in diastole for filling noncompliant LV.
  ii. Increased coronary perfusion time.
  iii. Decreased myocardial demand.
e. Maintain adequate intravascular volume.
f. Avoid myocardial ischemia.

7. Anesthetic considerations for pts with aortic stenosis undergoing noncardiac surgery.
a. Severe aortic stenosis is risk factor for perioperative morbidity and mortality.
b. Elective noncardiac surgery should be postponed until valve has been replaced.
c. Pts with moderate-to-severe aortic stenosis have a bleeding tendency due to acquired von Willebrand syndrome—mechanical disruption of von Willebrand multimers during turbulent flow through narrowed valve.
  i. GI angiodysplasia.
d. Asymptomatic pts with good exercise tolerance do not present excessive risk.
e. Regional anesthesia.
  i. Pts with mild-to-moderate aortic stenosis may tolerate spinal or epidural anesthesia, with epidural anesthesia preferable because of its slower onset of hypotension.
  ii. Epidural and spinal anesthesia are contraindicated in pts with severe aortic stenosis.

C. IDIOPATHIC HYPERTROPHIC SUBAORTIC STENOSIS
1. Epidemiology.
a. Ventricular hypertrophy without an obvious cause such as HTN or aortic stenosis.
b. Incidence is $1:500$.
c. Inherited as an autosomal-dominant lesion and is the most common genetic cardiac disease.
d. Most common cause of sudden cardiac death (SCD) in children and adolescents.

2. Pathophysiology.
a. LV outflow obstruction leads to more hypertrophy.
b. Oxygen consumption increases.
c. LV filling pressures increase.
d. Diastolic dysfunction.
e. Systolic dynamic obstruction is unique.
  i. Occurs between hypertrophied septum and anterior leaflet of mitral valve, and the mitral valve apparatus is pulled forward during mid- to late-systole, known as systolic anterior motion, resulting in acute MR.

3. Clinical course.

a. Most pts have benign course.

b. Risk of SCD and obstruction of the LV outflow tract.

c. History of syncope, ventricular tachycardia (VT), flat or hypotensive response to exercise, and echo results should be used to identify pts at high risk of SCD.

    i. Automatic implantable cardioverter-defibrillator (AICD) may be indicated.

d. Maximum LV wall thickness <15 mm is not associated with SCD.

    i. If >30 mm, SCD occurs at rate of 2%/yr.

e. Eventually, the LV fails.

4. Hemodynamic goals.

a. Avoid worsening dynamic obstruction.

b. Decrease contractility to decrease obstruction.

c. Keep pt "slow, tight, and full."

    i. Avoid sympathetic stimulation and increase HR.

    ii. Increase afterload; use phenylephrine to maintain BP.

    iii. Maintain preload.

D. AORTIC REGURGITATION

1. Etiology.

a. Acute aortic regurgitation.

    i. Traumatic rupture of aortic leaflets.

    ii. Acute endocarditis with leaflet deterioration.

    iii. Aortic root dissection.

    iv. Acute dysfunction of a prosthetic or tissue valve.

    v. Acute perivalvular leak for suture rupture.

    vi. Aortic balloon valvuloplasty.

b. Chronic aortic regurgitation.

    i. Leaflet abnormalities.
  - Rheumatic fever.
  - Endocarditis.
  - Trauma.
  - Bicuspid aortic valve.
  - Myxomatous degeneration.
  - Marfan syndrome.
  - Ankylosing spondylitis.
  - Acromegaly.

    ii. Aortic root or ascending aorta abnormalities.
  - Systemic HTN.
  - Marfan syndrome.
  - Trauma.
  - Dissection.
  - Ehlers-Danlos syndrome.

2. Pathophysiology.

a. Acute regurgitation.

9

CARDIOVASCULAR AND THORACIC ANESTHESIA

    i.   Acute increase in end-diastolic volume (EDV) caused by regurgitant jet.

    ii.   LV cannot acutely dilate and increase stroke volume in response to increased EDV.

    iii.   Results in decreased forward stroke volume and CO—hypotension and shock.

    iv.   LV diastolic pressure sharply increases, resulting in MR if EDP remains markedly elevated.

    v.   Rising LA pressure eventually leads to pulmonary edema.

    vi.   Fall in stroke volume elicits a reflex sympathetic response—tachycardia and increased SVR.

    vii.   CPP may be depressed from acute increase in LVEDP and subnormal diastolic arterial pressure.
- May result in myocardial ischemia.

b. Chronic regurgitation.

    i.   Inability of aortic valve to coapt during diastole.

    ii.   Portion of LV stroke volume regurgitates from aorta into LV.

    iii.   Increased LVEDV results in elevated wall stress (Laplace law).

    iv.   Compensatory myocardial eccentric hypertrophy develops.
- Returns wall stress to normal.
- Hypertrophy and chamber enlargement raises total stroke volume.

    v.   SVR and systolic pressure drop to facilitate forward flow.
- CO is initially maintained.
- LV volume is increased, but EDP remains normal because of increased LV compliance.

    vi.   Eventually, LV dilatation and cardiomegaly with myocardial dysfunction occur.

3. Clinical presentation—chronic aortic regurgitation.

a. Pts may remain asymptomatic for many years.

b. Subsequently develop dyspnea, orthopnea, and paroxysmal nocturnal dyspnea secondary to LV volume overload.

c. Exertional fatigue reflects inadequate forward flow.

d. Angina is a manifestation of reduced forward flow and inadequate coronary blood flow.

4. Clinical course.

a. Asymptomatic pts with normal LV systolic function.

    i.   Progression to symptoms and/or LV dysfunction = 6% per yr.

    ii.   Progression to asymptomatic LV dysfunction = 3.5% per yr.

    iii.   Sudden death = <0.2% per yr.

b. Asymptomatic pts with LV systolic dysfunction.

    i.   Progression to cardiac symptoms = >25% per yr.

c. Symptomatic pts.

    i.   Mortality rate = >10% per yr.

d. Symptomatic pts should undergo aortic valve replacement, whereas asymptomatic pts may be medically treated.

5. Hemodynamic goals.

a. Regurgitant volume depends on the HR (diastolic time) and the diastolic pressure gradient across the aortic valve (diastolic aortic pressure minus LVEDP).

b. Avoid a slow HR because it will increase diastolic time and favor backward flow, increasing regurgitant volume.

c. Pts should be treated with afterload reduction, while maintaining coronary perfusion pressure.

d. Tachycardia should maximize net forward flow by preferentially compromising the diastolic time interval during which regurgitation occurs.

e. It bears noting that "asymptomatic" pts may have significant LV dysfunction.

E. MITRAL STENOSIS

1. Definition.

a. Normal = 4–6 cm^2.

b. Mild = 1.5 to 2.5 cm^2; mean gradient is <5 mm Hg.

c. Moderate = 1.1 to 1.5 cm^2; mean gradient is 5 to 10 mm Hg.

d. Severe = <1 cm^2; mean gradient is >10 mm Hg.

2. Etiology.

a. Associated with rheumatic fever.

　i. Usually presents in the third or fourth decade of life.

　ii. Mitral stenosis alone occurs in 25% of pts; remaining have combined lesions of MR and mitral stenosis, or mitral stenosis and aortic stenosis.

　iii. Women are affected twice as much as men.

　iv. Decreasing incidence of rheumatic fever-induced mitral stenosis due to widespread use of antibiotics.

b. Congenital abnormalities.

c. Infective endocarditis.

d. Mitral annular calcification.

e. Prolapse of LA myxomas into the mitral valve opening, causing functional mitral stenosis.

3. Pathophysiology.

a. Leaflet immobility—obstruction in flow of blood from LA to LV.

b. Progressive elevations in LA pressure to maintain diastolic flow into LV.

c. Progressive dilation of LA.

d. Distortion of depolarization pathways, setting stage for atrial dysrhythmias.

e. Increased pulmonary artery pressures—pulmonary HTN.

f. RV dilatation and failure.

g. With severe mitral stenosis, decrease in LV filling, and EDV (preload) may result in decreased SV and CO.

4. Clinical presentation.

a. Asymptomatic for years.

b. Dyspnea—vascular congestion; initially occurs with activity or atrial fibrillation.

c. Hemoptysis—increased pulmonary pressure and vascular congestion.

d. Thromboembolism—mostly cerebral; from LA enlargement and atrial fibrillation.

e. Chest pain—usually secondary to pulmonary HTN and RV hypertrophy.

f. Infective endocarditis.

g. Right-sided HF.

h. Hoarseness—Ortner syndrome.

i. Dysphagia.

5. Hemodynamic goals.

a. Avoid atrial fibrillation with rapid ventricular response.

b. Maintain adequate volume (increased filling volumes).

c. Avoid volume overload (RV failure).

d. Maintain normal afterload.

e. Avoid increasing PVR (hypoxia, hypercarbia, acidosis).

6. Interventions.

a. Pts with asymptomatic mitral stenosis are medically managed with diuretic therapy.

b. Pts with symptomatic critical stenosis and those with thromboembolic phenomena are managed surgically.

c. Mitral stenosis generally requires replacement with a bioprosthetic or mechanical valve.

F. MITRAL REGURGITATION

1. Etiology (Table 9.1).

2. Pathophysiology.

a. The degree of MR is directly related to the orifice size, the HR, and the pressure gradient between the LV and the LA.

   i. Dynamic process.

   ii. Increased preload, increased afterload, and decreasing contractility all worsen MR.

b. Reduction in forward stroke volume due to backward flow into the LA during systole.

c. LV compensates by dilating and increasing LVEDV.

d. By increasing LVEDV, the volume overloaded LV maintains a normal CO, even as ejection fraction decreases.

e. Eventual development of LV hypertrophy and progressive impairment in contractility, as reflected by reduced ejection fraction.

f. Atrial enlargement, dysrhythmias, pulmonary HTN, and eventual HF.

3. Natural history.

a. Symptoms are determined by underlying disorder, volume of regurgitation, and status of LV function.

   i. Pts with regurgitation fractions <30% have mild symptoms.

   ii. Regurgitant volumes of 30% to 60% cause moderate symptoms.

   iii. Fractions >60% are associated with severe symptoms.

TABLE 9.1

ETIOLOGIES OF ACUTE AND CHRONIC MITRAL REGURGITATION

Acute	Chronic
LEAFLETS	**LEAFLETS**
Traumatic rupture	Rheumatic fever
Infective endocarditis	Infective endocarditis
LA myxoma	Connective tissue disease (Marfan syndrome; Ehlers-Danlos)
	Congenital
	Myxomas
	LA myxoma
	IHSS
CHORDAE TENDINEAE	**CHORDAE TENDINEAE**
Traumatic rupture	Myxomatous
Spontaneous rupture	Infective endocarditis
Infective endocarditis	Trauma
	Rheumatic fever
	Rupture (spontaneous, MI, trauma)
PAPILLARY MUSCLES	**PAPILLARY MUSCLES**
Dysfunction or rupture due to acute myocardial or severe ischemia	Dysfunction due to ischemia, MI, dilated CM, LV aneurysm
Traumatic rupture	Papillary muscle rupture (MI, trauma)
Acute LV dilatation	
PROSTHETIC OR TISSUE VALVE DYSFUNCTION	**PROSTHETIC OR TISSUE VALVE DYSFUNCTION**
Deterioration of tissue leaflets	Perivalvular leak
Ring or strut fracture, perivalvular leak for ruptured sutures	Infective endocarditis
Infective endocarditis	Ring or strut fracture
Dysfunction or deterioration of disc, ball, or leaflet of prosthetic	Disc dysfunction or dislodge
	MITRAL ANNULUS
	Calcification (idiopathic, rheumatic, CRI)
	Dilatation from connective tissue disorder or dilated CM

CM, Cardiomyopathy; *CRI*, chronic renal insufficiency; *IHSS*, idiopathic hypertrophic subaortic stenosis; *LA*, left atrial; *LV*, left ventricular; *MI*, myocardial infarction.

b. Long latency from diagnosis until symptoms develop.

c. Generally present with fatigability, chronic weakness.

d. Massively dilated and highly compliant LA protects pulmonary circulation until LA compliance is reduced.

4. Hemodynamic goals.

a. Normal-to-fast HR—decrease diastolic regurgitation time.

b. Avoid increasing SVR—increase regurgitation.

c. Maintain adequate volume, but avoid hypervolemia.

d. Medical management of MR includes digoxin, diuretics, and vasodilators, including ACE inhibitors.

e. Afterload regurgitation may be life saving in pts with acute MR.

G. TRICUSPID REGURGITATION

1. Etiology.

a. 70% to 90% of pts have mild tricuspid regurgitation with insignificant regurgitant tricuspid volume.

b. Most common cause is functional disease (secondary to pulmonary HTN with dilated RV).

c. Trauma.

d. Carcinoid syndrome.

e. Congenital abnormalities (Ebstein anomaly).

f. Endocarditis.

g. CAD with ischemia, infarction, and/or rupture of RV papillary muscle.

2. Pathophysiology.

a. Chronic LV failure leads to sustained increases in pulmonary vascular changes and progressive dilation of the thin-walled RV and tricuspid valve annulus.

b. An increased EDV allows the RV to compensate for the regurgitant volume and maintain effective forward flow.

c. Elevations in pulmonary artery pressure increase the regurgitant volume and CVP. In addition, marked increases in RV afterload reduce RV output and result in systemic hypotension.

d. Chronic venous HTN leads to progressive congestion of the liver and hepatic dysfunction or to cardiac cirrhosis.

3. Clinical presentation.

a. Pts with isolated tricuspid regurgitation are relatively asymptomatic in absence of severe pulmonary HTN.

b. If in association with chronic MV disease and pulmonary HTN, pts may present with biventricular failure:

   i. Pulmonary congestion.

   ii. Hepatomegaly.

   iii. Peripheral edema.

   iv. Ascites.

4. Anesthetic management.

a. Should be directed at the underlying disease process.

b. Avoid hypovolemia—need adequate filling volumes.

c. Avoid hypervolemia—do not overload the struggling RV.

d. Avoid factors that increase RV afterload, such as hypoxia, acidosis, and hypercarbia.

e. During GA, N_2O may exacerbate pulmonary HTN and should be administered cautiously, if at all.

f. Avoid excessive peak airway pressures during positive-pressure ventilation to maintain adequate venous return.

g. Avoid bradycardia to increase regurgitant time.

h. Increasing CVP may imply worsening RV dysfunction.

i. Prominent "c" and "v" waves are usually present on the CVP waveform.

j. Often, PACs are avoided in tricuspid valve repairs.

III. PACEMAKERS AND IMPLANTABLE CARDIOVERTER-DEFIBRILLATORS (ICDS)

A. INDICATIONS—PACEMAKERS

1. Guidelines for implantation of cardiac pacemakers have been established by a joint task force formed by the American College of Cardiology (ACC), the American Heart Association (AHA), and the North American Society for Pacing and Electrophysiology (NASPE).
2. Some indications for permanent pacing are relatively certain, whereas others require considerable expertise and judgment.
3. The indications for pacemaker implantation can be divided into three specific categories as defined by the ACC/AHA/NASPE guidelines.
   a. Class I—Conditions in which permanent pacing is definitely beneficial, useful, and effective. Implantation of a pacemaker is considered acceptable and necessary, provided that the condition is not due to a transient cause.
   b. Class II—Conditions in which permanent pacing may be indicated but conflicting evidence and/or divergence of opinion exists.
      i. Class IIA refers to conditions in which the weight of evidence/opinion is in favor of usefulness/efficacy.
      ii. Class IIB refers to conditions in which the usefulness/efficacy is less well established by evidence/opinion.
   c. Class III—Conditions in which permanent pacing is not useful/effective and in some cases may be harmful.
4. Two major factors guide the decision to place a pacemaker.
   a. The association of symptoms with a dysrhythmia.
   b. Location of the conduction abnormality.
5. Symptoms often include dizziness, lightheadedness, syncope, fatigue, and poor exercise tolerance.
6. A direct correlation between symptoms and bradyarrhythmias will increase likelihood of recommending a pacemaker.
7. The location of an atrioventricular (AV) conduction abnormality is an important determinant of both the probability and the likely pace of progression of disease of the conduction system.
8. Disease within the AV node is suggested by the following:
   a. Significant PR prolongation.
   b. Mobitz type I or AV Wenckebach block.
   c. Normal QRS complex.
9. Disease below the AV node, in the His-Purkinje system, is suggested by:
   a. Normal or minimally prolonged PR interval.
   b. Mobitz type II.
   c. QRS complex abnormalities (bundle-branch block and/or fascicular block).

9

CARDIOVASCULAR AND THORACIC ANESTHESIA

10. Disease in the His-Purkinje system is generally considered to be less stable; therefore, permanent pacemaker placement is more likely to be recommended.

B. COMMON CONDITIONS REQUIRING PACEMAKERS

1. Sinus node dysfunction—need for pacemaker based largely upon correlation of bradycardia with symptoms (syncope, seizures, HF, dizziness and confusion).

a. Class I.
   i. Sinus bradycardia in which symptoms are clearly related to bradycardia (HR <40 bpm or frequent sinus pauses).
   ii. Symptomatic chronotropic incompetence.

b. Class II.
   i. Sinus bradycardia in a pt with symptoms but without clearly demonstrated association between bradycardia and symptoms.
   ii. Sinus node dysfunction in a pt with unexplained syncope.
   iii. Chronic HR <30 bpm in the awake and minimally symptomatic pt.

2. Acquired AV block—second most common indication for pacemaker therapy.

a. Class I.
   i. Complete (third-degree) AV block.
   ii. Advanced second-degree AV block.
   iii. Symptomatic Mobitz I or Mobitz II second-degree AV block.
   iv. Mobitz II second-degree AV block with a widened QRS or chronic bifascicular block, regardless of symptoms.

b. Class II.
   i. Asymptomatic Mobitz II second-degree AV block with a narrow QRS interval; pts with associated symptoms or a widened QRS interval have a class I indication.
   ii. First-degree AV block when a hemodynamic compromise occurs because of effective AV dissociation secondary to a very long PR interval.
   iii. Bifascicular or trifascicular block associated with syncope that can be attributed to transient complete heart block, with exclusion of other causes of syncope.

3. Post-MI.

a. Class I.
   i. Third-degree AV block within or below His-Purkinje system.
   ii. Persistent second-degree AV block in His-Purkinje system, with bilateral bundle-branch block.
   iii. Transient advanced infranodal AV block with associated bundle-branch block.

b. Class II.
   i. Persistent, asymptomatic second- or third-degree AV block at the level of the AV node.

1. Neurocardiogenic syncope.
a. Use of pacemakers in this disorder is limited to selected pts whose syncopal events are clearly associated with a cardioinhibitory or bradycardic event.
b. Class I.
   i.   Significant carotid sinus hypersensitivity, defined by syncope and >3 sec of asystole following minimal carotid sinus massage.
c. Class II.
   i.   Pts with syncope of unexplained origin in whom major abnormalities of sinus node function are discovered during electrophysiologic study.
   ii. Pts with recurrent syncope of unexplained origin and an abnormal response to carotid sinus massage but who do not have syncope caused by carotid sinus massage on examination.
   iii. Pts with recurrent neurocardiogenic syncope associated with bradycardia documented spontaneously or at the time of tilt-table testing.

5. Other.
a. Congenital complete heart block.
   i.   Significant symptoms attributable to bradycardia.
   ii. Wide QRS escape rhythm.
   iii. Complex ventricular ectopy.
   iv. Ventricular dysfunction.
   v.   In the first year of life, regardless of symptoms, ventricular rates <50 to 55 bpm or <70 bpm when associated with congenital heart disease.
b. Neuromuscular disease.
   i.   Diseases including myotonic muscular dystrophy, Kearns-Sayre syndrome, Erb syndrome, and peroneal muscular atrophy are associated with AV block and have class I indication for pacemaker with second- or third-degree heart block.

C. PACEMAKER MODE CODING
1. The North American Society of Pacing and Electrophysiology (NASPE) and the British Pacing and Electrophysiology Group (BPEG) first published a generic pacemaker code (NBG code) in 1987 and revised it in 2001 in light of developing technology (Table 9.2). In 2004, almost 95% of all newly inserted permanent pacemakers were accounted for by four different modes: VVI (16.9%), VVIR (24.8%), DDD (27.3%), and DDDR (25.4%) (see Table 9.2).
2. Pacemaker modes.
a. VOO or DOO mode.
   i.   Both are asynchronous pacing modes, most often used for temporary pacing in the perioperative setting.
   ii. Sensing is deactivated and the single (VOO) or dual (DOO) pacemaker emits stimuli at a set rate without regard for underlying rhythm.

TABLE 9.2

GENERIC PACEMAKER CODE (NBG) OF THE NORTH AMERICAN SOCIETY OF PACING AND ELECTROPHYSIOLOGY (NASPE) AND THE BRITISH PACING AND ELECTROPHYSIOLOGY GROUP (BPEG)

(I)[a] Chamber Pace	(II)[b] Chamber Sensed	(III)[c] Response to Sensing	(IV)[d] Rate Modulation	(V)[e] Multisite Pacing
O = No action	O = No action	O = No action	O = No action	O = No action
A = Atrium	A = Atrium	T = Triggered	R = Rate	A = Atrium
V = Ventricle	V = Ventricle	I = Inhibited	modulation	V = Ventricle
D = Dual	D = Dual	D = Dual		D = Dual

[a]Position I indicates the chamber in which pacing occurs and may be atrial (A), ventricular (V), or both (D).

[b]Position II indicates the chamber in which sensing occurs, and again may be assigned the letter A, V, or D. The designation O may be used if the pacemaker discharges independently without sensing.

[c]Position III indicates the effect of sensing, which may be either to trigger a pacing stimulus or to inhibit a pacing stimulate.

[d]Position IV indicates the presence (R) or absence (O) of any rate-adaptive mechanisms.

[e]Position V is used to indicate whether multisite pacing is present in none of the chambers (O), one or both atria (A), one or both ventricles (V), or a combination of both (D). For a device to have multisite pacing, the additional leads can either be placed within the same chamber (e.g., two leads pacing the RV) or within opposite chambers (e.g., one lead pacing the RV and another lead pacing the LV).

b. VVI.
   i. The pacemaker will both sense and pace the ventricle.
   ii. If no intrinsic activity is sensed within the ventricle, the pacemaker will pace at a preprogrammed rate.
   iii. If the electrical impulse generated by the SA node is able to pass through the AV node and successfully depolarize the ventricular tissue, pacing will be inhibited.

c. DDD.
   i. Both atrium and ventricle are sensed and paced.
   ii. If both the SA and AV nodes are functioning correctly, the pacemaker will do nothing more than sense this activity.
   iii. If the atrium fails to produce a native beat, the pacemaker will pace the atrium at a preprogrammed rate.
   iv. If either a native or paced atrial beat is not conveyed through the ventricles after the preprogrammed PR interval, the pacemaker will pace the ventricle.

d. VVIR and DDDR.
   i. VVIR—Same as VVI with rate-adaptive mechanism installed, which will alter the pacing rate to match the physiologic needs of the pt.
   ii. DDDR—Same as DDD with rate-adaptive mechanism that will alter the atrial pacing rate to match the physiologic needs of the pt.

iii. Most rate-adaptive sensors respond to stimuli such as movement (by using a piezoelectric crystal) and minute ventilation (by monitoring transthoracic impedance). Other sensors may include QT interval, temperature, venous oxygen saturation, and RV contractility.

- Thus rate adaptive sensors help to meet increases in oxidative requirements (i.e., exercise, illness, stress) that may not be adequately met by a fixed-rate pacemaker.
- Additional rate-adaptive sensors have been incorporated into pacemakers to detect "secondary" stimuli that may indicate the need for a faster pacing rate.

D. ICDS

1. Indications.

a. Pts with prior episode of resuscitated VT/ventricular fibrillation (VF) or sustained hemodynamically unstable VT.

b. Pts with one or more episodes of spontaneous sustained VT in the presence of structural heart disease.

c. Selected pts with a prior documented MI and impaired LV systolic dysfunction.

d. Pts with an ischemic or nonischemic cardiomyopathy, NYHA (New York Heart Association) functional class II-III, and an LVEF <35%.

e. Selected pts with syncope, structural heart disease, and inducible VT/VF during electrophysiologic study.

f. Selected pts with certain underlying disorders who are deemed to be at high risk for life-threatening VT/VF.

  i. Pts with congenital long QT syndrome who have recurrent symptoms or torsade de pointes despite β-blocker therapy.

  ii. High-risk pts with hypertrophic cardiomyopathies.

  iii. High-risk pts with arrhythmogenic RV dysplasia.

2. Tiered-therapy ICDs.

a. Modern ICDs have the capacity to perform antibradycardia pacing, antitachycardia pacing, low-energy cardioversion, high-energy defibrillation, and electrogram storage.

  i. These devices are multi-programmable and can be programmed to respond differently to tachycardias in multiple rate zones or tiers, allowing for therapy to be tailored for each tachycardia that a pt experiences.

b. Antibradycardia pacing.

  i. VVI only—protects against bradyarrhythmias that are either primary or follow a tachycardia or shock.

c. Antitachycardia pacing.

  i. Antitachycardia (overdrive) pacing diminishes the requirement for cardioversion or defibrillation in pts with VT, reverting 89% to 95% of episodes of spontaneous VT.

  ii. Atrial tachyarrhythmias are common in pts with ventricular dysrhythmias.

    iii. Inappropriate shocks occur in 20% to 25% of pts in whom ICD interprets the atrial arrhythmia incorrectly.
- Additional programming can reduce the frequency of this problem.
- Dual-chamber ICDs can discriminate between ventricular and atrial tachyarrhythmias and between atrial tachycardia/atrial flutter and atrial fibrillation.

d. Low-energy cardioversion.

    i. Defined as a DC shock of <2 J that must be synchronized to the R wave.
- Backup defibrillation is essential, as low-energy cardioversion can accelerate the rate of VT.

    ii. Antitachycardia pacing is painless and usually used first, followed by low-energy cardioversion if needed.

e. High-energy defibrillation.

    i. Modern devices will reconfirm the rhythm prior to shock delivery.

    ii. This feature avoids inappropriate shocks for nonsustained VT.

    iii. Defibrillation threshold is usually <15 J and often less than 10 J with biphasic shocks and improved lead systems.

3. Defibrillator coding conventions.

a. NASPE/BPEG devised a four-position defibrillator code in 1993 (Table 9.3).

4. Perioperative management for ICDs and pacemakers.

a. In 2005, ASA published a practice advisory that outlined management.

b. Medicines and Healthcare Products Regulatory Agency (MHRA) and Heart Rhythm UK (HRUK) released guidelines in 2006.

5. Preoperative evaluation.

a. Determine if device is an ICD, pacemaker, or biventricular pacing device, also known as cardiac resynchronization therapy (CRT), and nature of underlying condition that led to its implantation.

b. Identify device registration card with model and serial numbers, manufacturer's name, programmed mode, and set rate.

TABLE 9.3			
NASPE/BPEG FOUR-POSITION DEFIBRILLATOR CODE			
(I)[a] Chamber Shock	(II)[b] Anti-tachycardia Pacing Chamber	(III)[c] Anti-tachycardia Detection	(II)[d] Pacing Chamber
O = No action	O = No action	E = Electrocardiogram	O = No action
A = Atrium	A = Atrium	H = Hemodynamic	A = Atrium
V = Ventricle	V = Ventricle		V = Ventricle
D = Dual	D = Dual		D = Dual

[a]Position I indicates which chamber is shocked.
[b]Position II indicates the chamber in which any antitachycardia pacing is administered.
[c]Position III identifies the detection method.
[d]Position IV indicates which chamber delivers antibradycardia pacing.

i. If not available, CXR studies can be used to identify the type of device.

c. Determine the extent to which pt is device dependent. This can be determined by:

i. A verbal history or an indication in the medical record that the pt has experienced a bradyarrhythmia that caused syncope or other symptoms requiring implantation of a pacemaker or ICD.

ii. A history of successful AV nodal ablation that resulted in device placement.

iii. An evaluation that shows no evidence of spontaneous ventricular activity when the pacemaking function of the device is programmed to VVI pacing at the lowest programmable rate.

d. If device has been interrogated within the last 3 mo, there is probably no benefit in requesting repeat check preoperatively.

e. Battery depletion causes pacemakers to reprogram automatically to slower rates, single-chamber pacing, and/or nonphysiologic (fixed-rate) pacing modes.

f. Presence of more complex features such as rate-adaptive pacing or anti-tachycardia modalities should be elicited.

6. Preinduction preparation.

a. Deciding whether a device requires reprogramming or disabling before surgery will depend on the following factors:

i. Anticipated amount of electromagnetic interference (EMI) and surgical-site proximity to device.

ii. Device type (pacemaker, ICD, or CRT).

iii. Pacemaker dependency.

iv. Rate-adaptive features.

b. EMI.

i. When EMI is likely to be high or when the surgical site lies in close proximity to the device, the ICD should be reprogrammed to "monitor only" mode to prevent inappropriate defibrillation shocks.

- Defibrillator pads should be placed on the pt in the event that the pt may actually have a dysrhythmia that requires defibrillation.
- The external defibrillation pads should be placed >10 cm away from the pulse generator to avoid risk of device damage, reprogramming, or serious burn to the myocardium via high-energy currents through the device leads.

ii. Effects of EMI on a pacemaker or ICD are unpredictable and include inappropriate inhibition or triggering of pacing activity, asynchronous pacing, reprogramming or software resetting of the device, damage to the internal circuitry, and activation of antitachycardia pacing or even defibrillation shocks.

iii. Heat damage may occur in the myocardium at the point of contact with the electrodes of the device, although unlikely and only reported following exposure to high-powered radiofrequency fields.

9

CARDIOVASCULAR AND THORACIC ANESTHESIA

iv. A common consequence of electrocautery is the pacemaker incorrectly interpreting the cautery signal as cardiac activity, thus causing inappropriate pacemaker inhibition.

v. Unipolar electrocautery is more hazardous than bipolar.
- If unipolar electrocautery is necessary, the grounding pad should be placed as far away from the device as possible.
- For head and neck surgery, the recommended placement of the grounding pad is on the posterior aspect of the shoulder opposite the pulse generator.

vi. When using electrocautery, it should be used in short, infrequent, and irregular bursts, with the energy setting kept to a minimum.
- When a high level of EMI is likely to be generated, or when the intended site of surgery lies close to the pulse generator, expert advice regarding reprogramming should be sought.

c. For pts who are dependent on their pacemaker or CRT, their device should be reprogrammed to prevent inappropriate inhibition (VOO or DOO).

d. Rate-adaptive pacemakers that utilize the transthoracic-impedance sensor should ideally be switched to "off."
i. Ensure the availability of temporary pacing and defibrillation equipment.

e. Use of magnets with pacemakers and ICDs.
i. Do not assume that placing a magnet over a device will produce asynchronous pacing.
- Response will depend on how the device has been programmed. There is no universal effect.
ii. Information about the response of a device to the application of a magnet can be obtained from the pacemaker clinic responsible for the pt or the manufacturer of the device.
- With single-chamber ventricular pacemakers, the response to a magnet is always asynchronous pacing (VOO). However, rate of pacing varies depending on the device and battery life.
- For dual-chamber pacemakers, a magnet will usually result in dual-chamber asynchronous pacing (DOO) at a variable rate.
- ~99% of ICDs are programmed to have their anti-tachycardic function disabled in the presence of a magnet without affecting their bradycardia pacing.
- Some (e.g., Guidant) will be deactivated after a magnet is held over the generator for 20 to 30 sec, whereas others will be inhibited only if the battery remains over the generator.

7. Intraoperative management.
a. Electrolyte and metabolic disturbances may increase pacing threshold, which may result in failure to pace.
i. This may occur as a consequence of acidosis, alkalosis, hyperkalemia, hypoxemia, myocardial ischemia, and severe hyperglycemia.

b. If diathermy is essential:
    i.   Use a bipolar electrocautery system or an ultrasonic (harmonic) scalpel, if possible.
    ii. Use short, intermittent, and irregular bursts at the lowest feasible energy levels.
    iii. Ensure that the cautery tool and current-return pad are positioned so that the current pathway does not pass through or near the device pulse generator and leads.
    iv. Avoid proximity of the cautery's electrical field to the pulse generator or leads.
c. Emergency pacing systems should be available.
    i.   This is most readily provided by external pacing pads, although equipment for passing a transvenous pacing catheter may be necessary.
d. Risk of interference from radiofrequency ablation may be reduced by avoiding direct contact between the ablation catheter and the pulse generator and leads and by keeping the radiofrequency's current path as far away from the pulse generator and leads as possible.
e. During lithotripsy, the lithotripsy beam should not be focused near the pulse generator.
    i.   If the lithotripsy system triggers on the R wave, atrial pacing might need to be disabled before the procedure.
f. MRI is generally contraindicated for pts with pacemakers and ICDs.
g. Radiation therapy can be safely performed for pts with pacemakers and ICDs.
    i.   The device must be outside the field of radiation.
    ii. Most manufacturers recommend verification of pulse generator function during and at completion of therapy.
h. Electroconvulsive therapy can be performed in a pt who has a pacemaker or ICD.
    i.   All devices should undergo a comprehensive interrogation before the procedure(s).
    ii. ICD functions should be disabled during electroconvulsive therapy.
i. Where an ICD is to be disabled, consider connecting the pt to the external defibrillator pads prior to commencing surgery.
j. If a life-threatening dysrhythmia occurs, follow ACLS guidelines for management.
    i.   If defibrillation is necessary, attempt to minimize the current flowing through the pulse generator and lead system by:
        • Positioning the defibrillator or cardioversion pads or paddles as far as possible (at least 10 cm) from the pulse generator.
        • Positioning the pads or paddles perpendicular to the major axis of the device and placing the leads, to the extent possible, in an anterior-posterior location.

8. Postoperative management.

a. If there is any concern about device failure, malfunction, or the effects of EMI, the device should undergo complete telemetric testing.

b. Reprogramming back to the original settings should occur as soon as possible.

c. Antitachycardia and defibrillator modalities must be switched on immediately postoperatively.

   i. If this is not immediately possible, the pt should remain in a monitored setting until it is done.

IV. MECHANICAL ASSIST DEVICES
A. INTRAAORTIC BALLOON PUMP (IABP)
1. General concepts.

a. Counterpulsation balloon pump that is synchronized to the cardiac cycle to improve myocardial perfusion and optimize myocardial oxygen supply-and-demand relationship.

   i. Blood is displaced to proximal aorta by inflation during diastole.

   ii. Balloon inflation increases diastolic pressure and coronary perfusion gradient.

   iii. Aortic volume and afterload are reduced during systole through a vacuum effect created by rapid balloon deflation.

   iv. Aortic pressure, LV afterload, wall tension, and myocardial oxygen consumption are all thereby decreased.

b. IABP consists of a catheter with a helium-filled elongated balloon at the end, made of nonthrombogenic polyurethane material.

   i. Its volume varies between 50 and 80 mL. Helium's low viscosity permits rapid inflation and deflation of the balloon.

2. Hemodynamic effects.

a. Variable effects depend on volume of balloon, its position in the aorta, heart rate and rhythm, and compliance of the aorta.

b. Expected changes in hemodynamic profile.

   i. Decrease in systolic pressure by 20%.

   ii. Increase in diastolic pressure by 20%.

   iii. Decrease in HR by 20%.

   iv. Decrease in mean pulmonary wedge by 20%.

   v. Increase in CO by 20%.

   vi. Decrease in LV systolic work, tension, and myocardial oxygen consumption.

c. IABP may have beneficial effects on RV function.

   i. Directly through augmenting coronary perfusion and relieving RV ischemia.

   ii. By improving LV forward flow with resulting decreased RV afterload.

3. Indications.

a. Refractory unstable angina.

b. Impending infarction.

c. Acute MI and its complications (acute MR or ventricular septal defect, or papillary muscle rupture).
d. Refractory ventricular failure.
e. Cardiogenic shock.
f. Support for diagnostic, percutaneous revascularization, and interventional procedures.
g. Ischemia-related intractable ventricular dysrhythmias.
h. Septic shock.
i. Intraoperative pulsatile flow generation.
j. Weaning from bypass.
k. Cardiac support for noncardiac surgery.
l. Prophylactic support in preparation for cardiac surgery.
m. Postsurgical myocardial dysfunction/low cardiac output syndrome.
n. Myocardial contusion.
o. Mechanical bridge to other assist devices.
p. Cardiac support following correction of anatomical defects.

4. Contraindications.
a. Severe aortic insufficiency.
b. Abdominal or aortic aneurysm.
c. Severe calcific aortoiliac disease or peripheral vascular disease.
d. Sheathless insertion with severe obesity, scarring of the groin, or other contraindications to percutaneous insertion.

5. Placement and timing of device for effective IABP function.
a. Proper placement.
  i. The balloon is usually introduced through the femoral artery, either percutaneously or after surgical dissection.
  ii. In pts with severe peripheral vascular disease, it may be placed directly into the descending thoracic aorta.
  iii. If properly positioned, balloon's distal tip should be placed just below left subclavian artery takeoff, and its proximal end should lie above renal arteries.
b. Timing of inflation of the device.
  i. Triggering of the IABP may be based on ECG or on arterial pressure tracing, recorded at the tip of IABP catheter.
  ii. Inflation occurs at the peak of the T-wave (end systole).
  iii. Balloon is deflated in end-diastole, just prior to the R-wave.
  iv. Inflation occurs with the dicrotic notch, which indicates aortic valve closure.
  v. Deflation should occur with the upstroke in aortic pressure curve.
  vi. If radial arterial pressure tracing must be used, inflation should occur 25 to 50 msec before the dicrotic notch because of time delay in wave transmission to the periphery.
  vii. Properly synchronized cycling of the IABP results in the following beneficial hemodynamic effects (Fig. 9.2):
    • Diastolic augmentation with increased diastolic pressures and improved coronary perfusion.

CARDIOVASCULAR AND THORACIC ANESTHESIA

9

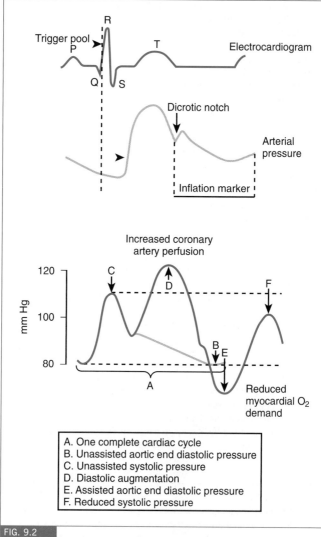

FIG. 9.2

Properly synchronized cycling of the intra-aortic balloon pump. *(Courtesy of Datascope Corp., Montvale, NJ.)*

- Reduced aortic EDP and subsequent systolic pressures that demonstrate reduced LV afterload.

viii. Inflating the balloon too soon or deflating it too late leads to an increase in LV afterload and decrease in forward flow (Figs. 9.3, 9.4, 9.5, and 9.6).

- Late inflation decreases the time of diastolic augmentation.

6. Weaning from device.

a. Device can be withdrawn when CO is satisfactory on minimal inotropic support.

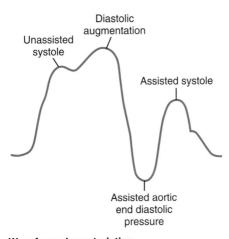

Waveform characteristics:
- Inflation of IAB prior to dicrotic notch
- Diastolic augmentation encroaches onto systole (may be unable to distinguish)

Physiologic effects:
- Potential premature closure of aortic valve
- Potential increase in LVEDV and LVEDP or PCWP
- Increased left ventricular wall stress or afterload
- Aortic regurgitation
- Increased MVO$_2$ demand

FIG. 9.3

Early inflation—inflation of the IAB prior to aortic valve closure. *(Courtesy of Datascope Corp., Montvale, NJ.)*

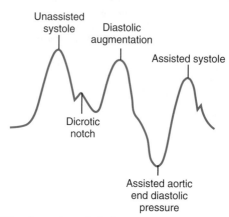

Unassisted systole

Diastolic augmentation

Assisted systole

Dicrotic notch

Assisted aortic end diastolic pressure

Waveform characteristics:
• Inflation of the IAB after the dicrotic notch
• Absence of sharp V
• Sub-optimal diastolic augmentation

Physiologic effects:
• Sub-optimal coronary artery perfusion

FIG. 9.4

Late inflation—inflation of the IAB markedly after closure of the aortic valve. *(Courtesy of Datascope Corp., Montvale, NJ.)*

b. Weaning is achieved by decreasing support from 1 : 1 (heart beat : balloon inflation) to 1 : 2 for 4 to 6 hr, and finally, 1 : 3, ensuring that hemodynamic stability remains.

c. Do not leave at 1 : 3 for extended period for risk of clot formation of balloon.

d. Contraindications.

    i. Aortic insufficiency.

    ii. Aortic aneurysm or dissection.

    iii. Uncontrolled sepsis.

    iv. Uncontrolled bleeding disorder.

    v. Severe bilateral peripheral vascular disease.

    vi. Bilateral femoral-popliteal bypass graft for severe peripheral vascular disease.

e. Complications.

    i. Limb ischemia.

    ii. Vascular laceration requiring surgical repair.

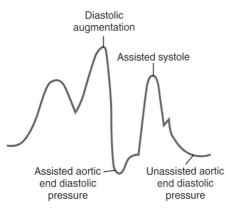

Waveform characteristics:
- Deflation of IAB is seen as a sharp drop following diastolic augmentation
- Sub-optimal diastolic augmentation
- Assisted aortic end diastolic pressure may be equal to or less than the unassisted aortic end diastolic pressure
- Assisted systolic pressure may rise

Physiologic effects:
- Sub-optimal coronary perfusion
- Potential for retrograde coronary and carotid blood flow
- Angina may occur as a result of retrograde coronary blood flow
- Sup-optimal afterload reduction
- Increased MVO_2 demand

FIG. 9.5

Early deflation—premature deflation of the IAB during the diastolic phase. *(Courtesy of Datascope Corp., Montvale, NJ.)*

   iii. Aortic dissection.
   iv. Embolism.
   v. Cerebrovascular accident (usually only if placed too high into arch of aorta).
   vi. Sepsis (usually only if placed for >7 days).
   vii. Balloon rupture.
 viii. Thrombocytopenia and hemolysis.
   ix. Spinal cord or visceral ischemia.
   x. Groin infection.
   xi. Peripheral neuropathy.

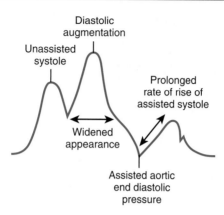

Waveform characteristics:
- Assisted aortic end-diastolic pressure may be equal to the unassisted aortic end diastolic pressure
- Rate of rise of assisted systole is prolonged
- Diastolic augmentation may appear widened

Physiologic effects:
- Afterload reduction is essentially absent
- Increased MVO$_2$ consumption due to the left ventricle ejecting against a greater resistance and a prolonged isovolumetric contraction phase
- IAB may impede left ventricular ejection and increase the afterload

FIG. 9.6

Late deflation—deflation of the IAB after opening of the aortic valve. *(Courtesy of Datascope Corp., Montvale, NJ.)*

B. **VENTRICULAR ASSIST DEVICES (VADs)**
1. Classification of devices.
a. LV assist device (LVAD).
   i.   Used for pts who face imminent death and who may need only temporary support.
   ii. Bridge-to-heart transplant.
   iii. Destination therapy.
   iv. Drains blood from LA or LV into ascending aorta.
b. RV assist device (RVAD).
   i.   Drains blood from the RA or RV into pulmonary aorta.
c. Biventricular assist device (BiVAD).

d. Cardiopulmonary assist.
  i.   Used infrequently in cardiac cath lab; limited use elsewhere.
  ii. Provides full cardiopulmonary support, analogous to that provided by intraoperative bypass machine.
  iii. Requires placement of central arterial and venous access.
  iv. Requires continuous highly technical support.
e. Total artificial heart.
  i.   Inserted orthotopically.
  ii. Requires removal of pt's ventricles.
  iii. Not widespread use due to thromboembolism, infection, and bleeding.

2. Indications for assist device placement.

a. LVAD.
  i.   SBP <80 mm Hg with either:
     • Cardiac index <2.0 L/min/m^2, **OR**
     • Pulmonary capillary wedge pressure >20 mm Hg.
  ii. SVR >2100 dynes-sec/cm^5.
  iii. Urinary output <20 mL/hr.
b. RVAD.
  i.   RA pressure >20 mm Hg.
  ii. LA pressure <15 mm Hg.
  iii. No significant tricuspid regurgitation.
c. BiVAD.
  i.   RA pressure >20 to 25 mm Hg.
  ii. LA pressure >20 mm Hg.
  iii. No significant tricuspid regurgitation.
  iv. Inability to maintain LVAD flows >2 L/min/m^2, with RA pressure >20 mm Hg.

3. Frequently used devices.

a. Abiomed BVS5000.
  i.   Considered a "short-term" device.
  ii.   Paracorporeal pump—"atrial" chamber filled by gravity drainage, flows across polyurethane valve to "ventricular" chamber, pneumatically pumped into pt.
  iii. Automatically adjusts rate of pumping to provide up to 5 L/min of outflow.
  iv.   Output depends on intravascular volume status and downstream vascular resistance.
  v.   For use as an LVAD, RVAD, or BiVAD.
  vi.   Requires anticoagulation.
  vii. Pts are generally confined to bed.
  viii. Bleeding, thromboembolism, and infection limit use to 14 days.
  ix.   Particular niche is donor heart dysfunction following transplant.
b. Abiomed AB5000.
  i.   Considered a "short-to-intermediate-term" device.
  ii. Vacuum-assisted, pneumatic compression of blood chamber.

    iii. Automatically adjusts rate of pumping to provide up to 6 L/min of outflow.

    iv. Output depends on intravascular volume status and downstream vascular resistance.

    v. For use as an LVAD, RVAD, or BiVAD.

    vi. Requires anticoagulation.

    vii. Pts are able to ambulate with device.

c. Thoratec.

    i. "Intermediate-to-long-term" support device.

    ii. Presently, the only widely available device capable of providing long-term support to the pt requiring biventricular support.

    iii. Flexible polyurethane blood sac supplied with inlet and outlet conduits and tilting-disc mechanical valves to direct blood.

    iv. Blood sac is alternately compressed and released by gas-driven diaphragm.

    v. For use as an LVAD, RVAD, or BiVAD.

    vi. Requires anticoagulation.

d. Heartmate I.

    i. Considered a "long-term" device.

    ii. Paracorporeal system.

    iii. Device rests below diaphragm in intraperitoneal or properitoneal position, depending on pt size.

    iv. For use as an LVAD only.

    v. Used for destination therapy or as a bridge to transplant.

    vi. Device is lined by "textured" surface, which promotes deposition of fibrin and circulating cells and becomes nonthrombogenic.
- Requires only aspirin for long-term anticoagulation.

    vii. Propels blood with pulsatile, pneumatic system of electrically driven motor.

    viii. Blood is drained from apex of LV, into pumping mechanism, and out to ascending aorta, with one-way valves ensuring forward flow.

    ix. Pump ejects either once chamber is full or at a set, fixed rate.

    x. Pumping mechanism is connected to external, portable console, which provides power source and control unit.

e. Heartmate II.

    i. Considered a "long-term" device.

    ii. Axial flow device; no blood chamber.

    iii. Nonpulsatile flow.

    iv. For use as an LVAD only.

    v. Requires full anticoagulation.

    vi. No back-up device; however, components are considered more durable and reliable.

    vii. Currently still investigational.

4. Anesthetic considerations for the pt with an LVAD.

a. Preload must be maintained in the face of anesthetic-induced vasodilation.

b. An unassisted ventricle may require vasoactive or inotropic support to achieve optimal hemodynamics.

c. Nonpulsatile device presents monitoring challenges, including inability to obtain noninvasive BP and pulse oximetry.

d. Maintaining relatively normal intrinsic heart rate and rhythm is important to maintaining adequate filling of LVAD devices.

5. Common complications associated with VADs.

a. Vary, depending on type of device.

b. Coagulopathic bleeding in perioperative period.

c. Infection.

d. Thromboembolic complications.

e. RV failure in the pt with only LV support.

C. EXTRACORPOREAL MEMBRANE OXYGENATION (ECMO)

1. Physiology.

a. Removes CO_2 from and adds O_2 to venous blood via an artificial membrane lung.

b. Oxygenated blood then returns to the pt via an arterial or venous route.

2. Types of ECMO.

a. Venoarterial bypass.
   i. Extracorporeal pump flow rate determines the systemic perfusion.
   ii. Pulmonary circulation is bypassed, and arterial blood gases are determined primarily by the efficiency and volume of extracorporeal gas exchange.

b. Venovenous bypass.
   i. Extracorporeally treated blood raises the O_2 content and lowers the CO_2 content in the RA.
   ii. Gas exchange is augmented by any remaining native pulmonary function, and perfusion depends upon the pt's CO.
   iii. Theoretical advantages include:
      • Maintenance of pulmonary blood flow.
      • Improved myocardial oxygenation.
      • Delivery of thrombin or platelet emboli to the pulmonary (not systemic) circulation.
      • Preservation of carotid artery.

3. Indications for ECMO.

a. Reliable predictors to identify adults who will benefit from ECMO do not exist.

b. Respiratory failure.
   i. Acute, potentially reversible, life-threatening respiratory failure that is unresponsive to optimal conventional therapy.
   ii. Provides oxygenation and ventilation so that the injured lung can "rest" at low levels of ventilatory support.
   iii. Uses venoarterial or venovenous bypass.

   c. Severe reversible myocardial dysfunction.
      i.   In addition to oxygenation/ventilation function, provides forward flow and organ perfusion.
      ii. Common indication in pediatric population—usually in pts unable to wean from CPB or HF after cardiac surgery.
      iii. LV dysfunction is less amenable to ECMO than is RV dysfunction—reserved for pts suffering from acute but reversible dysfunction (e.g., myocarditis, cardiomyopathy, postoperative cardiogenic shock).
      iv. Used as bridge to another support device—VAD or transplant.
      v.   Used to stabilize pt prior to emergent myocardial revascularization.

4. Complications.
a. Bleeding due to required systemic anticoagulation.
b. Stroke.
c. Trauma at cannulation sites.
d. Thrombosis.

5. Contraindications.
a. Pts with irreversible underlying illnesses are not appropriate candidates.
b. Pts with an absolute contraindication to systemic anticoagulation.
c. Mechanical ventilation >5 days correlates with a higher mortality.

V. SURGICAL OPTIONS FOR HEART FAILURE

An increasing number of surgical options are being created to relieve symptoms of CHF and arrest the progression of the disease. Theoretical methods of benefit include correction of abnormal myocardial depolarization, enhancement of blood supply to the myocardium, improvement in ventricular loading conditions, and restoration of more normal ventricular geometry. Options include:

- CRT with biventricular pacing.
- Revascularization.
- Mitral valve repair or replacement.
- LV remodeling or reconstruction.
- Dynamic cardiomyoplasty.
- Extrinsic compression devices (e.g., CorCap).
- Implantation of LVAD.
- Cardiac transplantation.
- New therapies in early phases—transplantation of skeletal myoblasts and stem cells, "gene" therapy, and xenotransplantation.

A. CARDIAC RESYNCHRONIZATION THERAPY

1. Pts with moderate-to-severe HF have a higher incidence of both interventricular and intraventricular asynchrony, resulting from altered conduction throughout the His-Purkinje system.
2. The effects on hemodynamic function have been well documented and include reduced diastolic filling and impaired CO.

3. CRT, also referred to as *biventricular pacing*, aims to improve diastolic filling and CO by using additional leads to pace multiple sites within the cardiac chambers.

a. Leads may be positioned within the RA and RV, and passed through the coronary sinus and veins to reach the LV.

b. Following placement of these additional leads, the pt's CO can be optimized by altering the timing of each pacing lead while observing the effects under echocardiography.

4. Mechanism of dyssynchrony.

a. Most pts with intraventricular dyssynchrony display a left bundle-branch-block pattern.

   i. Intraventricular dyssynchrony occurs in up to 25% of pts with HF and predicts a higher risk of worsened HF and SCD.

   ii. In these pts, the left lateral wall is activated well after the septum contracts.

   iii. This leads to contraction of the lateral wall during relaxation of the septum, resulting in profound mechanical dysfunction.

   iv. Results in an increase in LV volume, reduction of contractility, and worsening of MR.

5. Pt selection.

a. Advanced HF (usually NYHA class III or IV).

b. Pts should be in sinus rhythm.

c. Severe systolic dysfunction (ejection fraction < 35%).

d. Intraventricular conduction delay (QRS > 120 msec).

e. Pts who already have ICDs.

6. Mechanism of benefit.

a. Improved contractile function.

   i. In pts with HF associated with interventricular conduction delay or left bundle-branch block, causes greater coordination of global contraction.

   ii. Myocardial efficiency is increased.

      • Increased contractility is associated with no change or modest reduction in myocardial energy demands and myocardial oxygen consumption.

b. Reverse ventricular remodeling.

   i. Biventricular pacing is associated with reverse ventricular remodeling in pts with HF.

      • Reductions in LV systolic and end-diastolic dimensions, mitral regurgitant jet, and LV mass are seen.

   ii. Main mechanism of benefit is improved mechanical synchrony.

c. Other.

   i. Increase in cardiac index and a reduction in pulmonary capillary wedge pressure, when compared with normal sinus rhythm or RV pacing.

   ii. Ability to tolerate more aggressive medical therapy and neurohormonal blockade (e.g., β blockers).

   iii. Improvement in HR variability.

7. **Complications.**
a. Most common complication with transvenous CRT implantation is inability to implant the LV-pacing lead successfully.
   i. Requires placement of an epicardial lead.
   ii. Greater risk of failure to capture with chronic pacing.
   iii. Placement of an epicardial LV lead requires a limited thoracotomy, which is performed under GA and is associated with a greater operative risk.
b. Coronary sinus or coronary vein trauma.
c. Pneumothorax.
d. Diaphragmatic/phrenic nerve pacing.
e. Infection.
f. Theoretical risk that pacing from an LV lead may be proarrhythmic owing to alterations in depolarization and repolarization sequences.

8. **Further studies.**
a. Most clinical trials focus on the QRS width as the main parameter for cardiac dyssynchrony. However, little difference in QRS duration exists between responders and nonresponders.
b. Growing evidence shows that echo Doppler criteria should be used to determine mechanical dyssynchrony.
c. Other areas for further investigation include:
   i. The role and benefit of CRT in pts with atrial fibrillation.
   ii. The role and benefit in pts with mild-to-moderate HF.
   iii. The benefit in RV pacing-induced dyssynchrony.
   iv. The role in pts with narrow QRS complexes.
   v. Determining if ICD back-up is always needed.
   vi. The cost effectiveness of CRT.

B. SURGICAL LV REMODELING OR RECONSTRUCTION

1. **Indications.**
a. Used to reshape the dilated, spherical LV of pts who have had an anterior wall MI with resulting aneurysm and akinesis/dyskinesis.

2. **Mechanism of benefit.**
a. Dacron patch is placed within LV cavity to exclude the large akinetic/dyskinetic area of anterior wall.
b. Restores LV geometry to more normal elliptical shape and improved systolic function.
c. Better outcomes if performed in combination with coronary revascularization.
d. Mitral valve repair is also frequently required.

3. **Anesthetic considerations.**
a. Pts have very poor ventricular function and require careful titration of medications and fluids.
b. Invasive arterial monitoring should be placed prior to induction.
c. Recommend use of PACs (at Hopkins, we frequently use continuous SvO_2 PA catheters) and TEE.

d. Pts often have AICDs that must be disabled intraoperatively, with defibrillator pads placed prior to induction.

VI. THORACIC TRANSPLANTATION

A. HEART TRANSPLANTATION

1. **The key to successful cardiac transplantation is minimizing the time that donor's organ is ischemic.**

a. Communication with the surgical team is essential to synchronize organ arrival time with preparation of the recipient.

b. Graft function is optimized when ischemic time (from aortic crossclamp in donor to release of aortic crossclamp in recipient) is ≤4 hr; therefore delaying recipient's induction can have a negative impact on graft function.

c. Conversely, a premature induction of the recipient may prolong CPB and its associated risks.

2. **Organ-recipient matching is performed based on size, ABO typing, and cytomegalovirus serology, but not tissue crossmatching.**

a. Donors positive for hepatitis B, hepatitis C, or HIV are excluded.

3. **Preoperative evaluation of the recipient should focus on:**

a. Cause of cardiac condition (most frequently, cardiomyopathy or CAD) and current functional status (usually NYHA class IV, with an LVEF <20%).

b. Current therapeutic management, including inotropics, immunosuppressors, and devices for circulatory support (pacemaker, ICD, IABP, VAD).

c. History of pulmonary HTN and its response to oxygen and vasodilatory therapy.

   i. Pulmonary HTN >4 Woods units and unresponsive to oxygen or vasodilator therapy is usually considered a contraindication for heart transplant, but these pts may be candidates for heart-lung transplant.

d. Hepatorenal consequences of chronic hypoperfusion.

e. Previous chest surgery (longer and more complicated procedure with increased blood loss risk).

f. Electrolyte and coagulation status.

g. Fasting situation—sometimes pts are warned with very short notice; therefore NPO status must be determined.

   i. Consider premedication with sodium citrate, H_2 blocker, and/or metoclopramide.

h. Sedation is usually delayed until pt is in the OR.

4. **Monitoring.**

a. The use of the right internal jugular for central access is controversial because it is the future access for endomyocardial biopsies.

b. Placement of a PAC may be difficult owing to tricuspid regurgitation, enlarged RV with coiling of the PAC, and ventricular irritability.

   i. The PAC should be withdrawn prior to venous cannulation into its sterile sheath and refloated after CPB.

9

CARDIOVASCULAR AND THORACIC ANESTHESIA

c. TEE probe may be placed after induction.

6. Anesthetic induction.

a. Usually performed with full-stomach precautions (slight head-up position, cricoid pressure), ensuring an adequate preload (especially if a VAD is in place) and organ perfusion.

b. Consider increasing inotropic support if already being used (or adding it if not) to compensate for induction-related vasodilation.

c. Some options for anesthetic techniques include small sequential doses of 5 to 10 mcg/kg fentanyl with/without 0.1 to 0.3 mg/kg etomidate, or 1 to 2 mg/kg ketamine with 0.05 to 0.1 mg/kg midazolam.

d. 0.1 mg/kg pancuronium, 1.5 mg/kg succinylcholine, or 1 mg/kg rocuronium can be used for tracheal intubation.

7. Sternotomy and initiation of CPB are similar to other procedures in cardiac surgery.

a. Heparin is used as in other CPB procedures, followed by aggressive antifibrinolytic therapy.

b. Once pt is on CPB, the aorta and main pulmonary artery are transected and atria are incised at the level of the AV groove, so that the posterior wall of both atria with the caval and pulmonary venous connections remain in the recipient.

c. The donor ventricles and complementary portion of the atria (with the sinoatrial node) are then sutured to the donor, in order: left atrium, right atrium, great arteries.

d. The heart is flushed with saline, and intracardiac air is evacuated.

e. Finally, aortic crossclamp is removed for coronary reperfusion.

f. Methylprednisolone dose is given before unclamping.

    i. Daclizumab (Zenapax) is given after CPB.

8. The transplanted heart is denervated and lacks direct autonomic control, although the response to circulating catecholamines is normal.

a. Chronotropic support is usually performed with direct β-adrenergic agonists such as 0.5 to 10 mcg/min isoproterenol (a stronger β_1 than β_2 effect) or 0.5 to 20 mcg/kg/min dobutamine (primarily β_1 and less β_2 stimulation than isoproterenol).

b. Chronotropic support is frequently started before separation from CPB.

c. PAC is refloated and used in combination with TEE for evaluating cardiac function.

9. The most common post-CPB problems include:

a. Transient myocardial depression requiring inotropic support.

b. Slow junctional rhythms that require epicardial pacing.

c. Bleeding and HTN secondary to RV failure, usually managed with:

    i. Hyperventilation.

    ii. Nitric oxide (10–60 ppm).

    iii. Prostaglandin E1 (0.025–0.2 mcg/kg/min).

    iv. Epinephrine (0.03–0.2 mcg/kg/min).

    v. Milrinone (0.125–0.75 mcg/kg/min).

    vi. Placement of an RVAD.

10. Pts are transported to the ICU for slow arousal.
11. Postoperative complications include acute rejection, renal and hepatic dysfunction, and infections.

B. HEART-LUNG TRANSPLANTATION
1. Heart-lung transplantation is now relatively infrequent. It used to be the preferred option for Eisenmenger syndrome. Today, most Eisenmenger pts undergo isolated lung transplantation and repair of the cardiac defect; however, these pts are still the most frequent candidates for heart-lung transplantation. Pts with primary pulmonary HTN and cystic fibrosis are also candidates.
2. The surgical procedure and anesthetic management are more similar to that for cardiac transplantation than that for isolated-lung transplantation.

C. LUNG TRANSPLANTATION
1. Indications for lung transplant are end-stage pulmonary parenchymal diseases or pulmonary HTN.
a. These pts usually have dyspnea at rest or minimal activity and $PaO_2 < 50$ mm Hg at rest with increasing oxygen requirements.
b. Progressive hypercapnia is very common.
c. To be considered candidates for lung transplant, pts must have normal LV function and be free of coronary disease.
d. They may have some degree of RV dysfunction (cor pulmonale) if it is expected to improve when pulmonary artery pressure normalizes.
2. Single-lung transplantation is preferred to optimize the shortage of organ donations.
a. Double-lung transplantations are performed more frequently in pts with cystic fibrosis, bullous emphysema, and vascular diseases, and in younger pts.
3. Organ-recipient selection is based on ABO compatibility and size and, ideally, cytomegalovirus matching.
4. Team coordination is critical to minimize graft ischemia time and avoid unnecessary pretransplant anesthesia time.
5. Preoperative evaluation of the recipient should focus on:
a. Cause of pulmonary condition and current functional status (usually dyspnea at rest).
b. Current therapeutic management, including oxygen and/or ventilator requirements.
c. In cases of pulmonary HTN, response to oxygen and vasodilatory therapy.
d. Cardiac function and hepatorenal consequences of chronic hypoxemia.
e. Previous pulmonary surgery (more debridement necessary and risk of blood loss increased).

f. Electrolyte and coagulation status.

g. NPO status—as with other transplants, pts are usually warned with very short notice and may have recently eaten.

h. Sedation is delayed until the pt is monitored in the OR.

6. Monitoring and induction are very similar to that for cardiac transplant pts.

a. Invasive catheters are placed under strict asepsis.

b. Placement of a PAC may be difficult owing to tricuspid regurgitation and enlarged RV.

   i. The PAC must be withdrawn into its sterile sheath before lung resection (because of concern that it floats to the operative side) and refloated after transplantation.

c. Induction is performed with full-stomach precautions (head-up position, cricoid pressure).

d. To compensate induction vasodilation, inotropic support is preferred to large boluses of fluid.

e. Some options for anesthetic techniques include small sequential doses of 5 to 10 mcg/kg fentanyl with/without 0.1 to 0.3 mg/kg etomidate, or 1 to 2 mg/kg ketamine with 0.05 to 0.1 mg/kg midazolam.

f. 0.1 mg/kg pancuronium, 1.5 mg/kg succinylcholine, or 1 mg/kg rocuronium can be used for tracheal intubation.

g. Immunosuppressant medications are often started shortly after induction.

h. One-lung ventilation (OLV) during the procedure is obtained by placement of a double-lumen ETT or a bronchial blocker.

i. Hypoxemia and hypercapnia must be avoided to prevent further increases in pulmonary artery pressure.

j. After induction, a TEE may be placed.

7. Maintenance of anesthesia.

a. Can be performed with a volatile agent, an opioid, and an NMB agent.

b. Mechanical ventilation is usually challenging, with poor lung compliance and CO_2 retention.

c. Correct tube positioning must be checked frequently with bronchoscopy.

d. Suctioning should be performed as needed.

e. Pulmonary HTN is exacerbated by hypoxemia and hypercapnia; may be attenuated by inhaled nitric oxide, prostaglandin, β agonists, nitroglycerin, milrinone, or dobutamine.

f. IV crystalloid administration is commonly minimized to avoid postoperative lung edema.

8. Single-lung transplantation is attempted via posterior thoracotomy without CPB.

a. If CPB is finally needed, femoral cannulation is used in a left thoracotomy, and RA-to-aorta cannulation is used in a right thoracotomy.

9. Double-lung transplantation is usually performed with a "clamshell" transverse sternotomy.
a. Sequential lung transplantation is usually tried without CPB; normothermic CPB is another option.
10. After anastomosis of bronchus, artery, and vein, ventilation to the donated lung is resumed.
a. Peak inspiratory pressures and inspired oxygen fraction should be minimized to obtain adequate lung expansion and oxygenation.
b. FiO_2 should be maintained below 60%.
c. Methylprednisolone is given before the release of the vascular clamps.
d. Hyperkalemia may occur when releasing these clamps, and the preservative fluid is washed out of the donated lung.
e. TEE can be helpful in identifying RV and LV dysfunction, guiding de-airing, and evaluating blood flow in the pulmonary vessels.
f. At the end of the procedure, the double-lumen tube (DLT) is replaced by a single-lumen tube, and a bronchoscopy is carefully performed to revise the bronchial anastomoses and clear secretions and blood.
11. Ideally, pts are extubated postoperatively when warm and stable, usually within the first 24 hr. However, pts with significant pulmonary HTN who show hemodynamic instability benefit from a longer period of sedation.
12. As the cough reflex is abolished below the carina in the transplanted lung, pulmonary toilet is critical to avoid atelectasis and infection.
a. Frequent suctioning and good pain control with an epidural catheter (placed preoperatively or postoperatively) are helpful.
b. Sometimes pts demonstrate bronchial hyperreactivity.
13. Postoperative complications include early graft dysfunction, acute rejection, infections, and renal and hepatic dysfunction.
a. Frequent bronchoscopies with lavage and biopsies are necessary to differentiate infection versus rejection.

VII. DEEP HYPOTHERMIC CIRCULATORY ARREST (DHCA)

A. INDICATIONS
1. Any cardiopulmonary procedure that requires a bloodless field.
2. Repair of the distal ascending aorta or the aortic arch.
3. Atherosclerotic disease or heavy calcification of the aorta that would make clamping of the aorta hazardous.
4. Control and repair of massive hemorrhage as a result of cardiac or aortic laceration from reopening prior median sternotomy.
5. Selected extracardiac vascular procedures that otherwise would be complicated by uncontrolled bleeding (e.g., excision of renal tumors invading the IVC).

B. PROCEDURE
1. Although techniques differ from institution to institution, DHCA typically consists of systemic cooling to 18° to 20° C (core

temperature), with a period of time in which cerebral blood flow is interrupted.

2. 30 to 40 min is usually considered a safe limit of DHCA, but up to 90 min has been reported to be successful with selective cerebral perfusion (see below).

a. Brain is most sensitive organ with lowest tolerance to ischemia during DHCA.

b. Inadequate cooling can lead to cerebral rewarming during circulatory arrest period, resulting in neurologic injury.

c. Cool for at least 20 to 25 min before induction of DHCA to ensure adequate suppression of cerebral metabolic activity.

C. METHODS TO MONITOR CEREBRAL METABOLISM

1. EEG.

a. Cooling is continued for ~45 min after electrical silence is achieved on EEG.

2. Internal jugular venous saturation.

a. Saturation >95% signifies minimal cerebral oxygen extraction.

3. Near-infrared spectroscopy.

4. Currently, no correlation has been defined between any method of cerebral monitoring and eventual outcome after circulatory arrest.

5. Arterial cannula is usually placed in the femoral artery instead of the ascending aorta, but arterial access via the right subclavian/axillary artery may also be used.

a. Venous cannulation may be performed in the femoral vein, the RA, or caval veins.

b. Circulatory arrest is initiated to complete the distal aortic anastomosis.

c. The graft is then clamped, filled with blood, and cannulated, and CPB inflow is reestablished.

d. Proximal anastomoses of the aorta are completed during either hypothermic low flow or full CPB flow.

e. Rewarming is initiated.

6. Management during DHCA includes various measures to minimize the sequelae from the transient lack of CBF.

a. Application of ice around the head to reduce cerebral metabolism and oxygen consumption.

b. Administration of drugs such as sodium thiopental, magnesium, ketamine, methylprednisolone, mannitol, and additional heparin before CPB.

c. Trendelenburg position—to prevent entrainment of air in the great vessels.

d. Selective cerebral perfusion.

    i. Carried out with arterialized blood through the innominate artery (anterograde) or the internal jugular vein (retrograde) at a flow of 300 to 600 mL/min and a pressure of 25 mm Hg.

ii. Pressure is usually monitored through the sidearm of the PAC introducer.

e. Aggressive rewarming or overwarming of the body core temperature to >36° C can increase the risk of neurologic injury and should be avoided.

VIII. VASCULAR SURGERY

A. **VASCULAR SURGERIES INCLUDE THE FOLLOWING PROCEDURES:**

1. **Carotid endarterectomy.**
2. **Peripheral arterial bypass.**
a. Femoral-popliteal bypass.
b. Femoral-femoral bypass.
3. **Aortobifemoral bypass.**
4. **Abdominal aortic aneurysm (AAA) repair.**
5. **Thoracic outlet syndrome repair.**
6. **Axillary-femoral bypass.**

B. **PREOPERATIVE CONSIDERATIONS**

1. **Pts with either central or peripheral vascular disease typically have one or more comorbidities, thereby increasing their associated risks of surgery and anesthesia. Comorbidities may include:**
a. HTN.
b. Diabetes mellitus.
c. Hypercholesterolemia.
d. CAD.
e. Renal Insufficiency.
f. CHF.
2. **Preoperative considerations for pts undergoing vascular surgery must take into account the impact that these comorbidities have on surgical outcome.**
a. The so-called "cardiac workup" may prove particularly important in the setting of vascular surgery.
3. **The American College of Cardiology and the American Heart Association have published guidelines for stratifying CV risk for pts undergoing noncardiac surgery. The guidelines describe clinical predictors of increased morbidity (see Table 4.2).**
4. **The guidelines also consider the type of surgery and classify common surgeries according to mild-, moderate-, and high-risk procedures (Box 9.1).**
5. **ACC/AHA guidelines recommend the algorithm in Figure 9.7 for determining cardiac risk and the appropriate preoperative interventions to reduce perioperative risk of CV events (MI, HF, and death).**

9

CARDIOVASCULAR AND THORACIC ANESTHESIA

BOX 9.1

ACC/AHA GUIDELINES: RISK STRATIFICATION OF VASCULAR PROCEDURES

HIGH RISK

Aortic and other major vascular surgery.

Peripheral vascular surgery.

INTERMEDIATE RISK

Carotid endarterectomy.

Intrathoracic surgery (e.g., thoracic outlet syndrome repair).

LOW RISK

No vascular surgeries listed.

C. INTRAOPERATIVE ANESTHETIC TECHNIQUES AND MANAGEMENT

1. Peripheral vascular bypass.

a. Depending on location of procedure, may be amenable to use of regional or neuraxial technique (especially spinal anesthetic).

2. Thoracic outlet syndrome.

a. Generally performed under GA with a single-lumen ETT.

b. If used, arterial pressure monitoring should be via the opposite arm owing to frequent manipulation of the operative side axillary artery.

3. Carotid endarterectomy.

a. Preoperative assessment should include a thorough neurologic exam to determine any preoperative deficits.

b. Anesthetic techniques.

  i. Awake technique using local blockade (deep and superficial cervical plexus blocks).

  ii. General endotracheal anesthesia.

c. An arterial cannula is typically placed to monitor hemodynamic perturbations during induction and to assess baseline BP.

d. Short-acting agents should be chosen with special consideration for their impact on the assessment of immediately postoperative neurologic function.

  i. Avoidance of benzodiazepine use may be prudent in elderly pts.

  ii. Short-acting narcotics (fentanyl, sufentanil, remifentanil) are most often used for placement of arterial catheter and for postoperative pain relief.

  iii. Induction agents such as propofol, etomidate, and sodium thiopental are at the discretion of the anesthesiologist.

  iv. Maintenance anesthetic typically employs low-dose volatile agent, +/– N_2O, narcotic, and muscle relaxant.

e. Monitoring.

  i. Arterial catheter for beat-to-beat BP measurement.

  ii. Some surgeons routinely use EEG monitoring intraoperatively.

  iii. Some surgeons use cerebral oximetry.

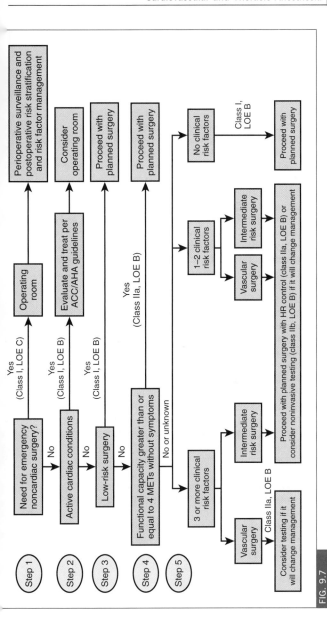

FIG. 9.7

Algorithm for cardiac evaluation for noncardiac surgery for patients >50 years of age. *(From Fleisher LA, Beckman JA, Brown KA: ACC/AHA 2007 Guidelines on Perioperative Cardiovascular Evaluation and Care for Noncardiac Surgery. JACC 2007;50:17:1707–1732, with permission.)*

    iv.   Long-arm CVCs via antecubital veins are used to deliver vasoactive medications.

f. BP management usually includes maintenance of BP within 10% of established baseline levels.

    i.   Some surgeons use intracarotid shunts that maintain flow through the operative carotid throughout the "clamp time."

    ii.   In cases where shunts are not used, an increased BP may be requested during carotid clamp time.

g. Pts should be extubated in the OR, with particular attention paid to limiting coughing or "bucking," which can cause bleeding.

h. Perioperative use of β blockers in vascular surgery.

    i.   Particular interest has been directed toward the use of β blockers in pts undergoing vascular surgery in an effort to reduce perioperative CV complications.

    ii.   In general, the literature supports routine use of β blockers in this pt population, citing numerous publications that demonstrate reduced rate of CV complications.

    iii. More recent publications have challenged the notion that β blockers are beneficial in ALL pts undergoing vascular surgery.

    iv.   Currently, recommendation is routine use of β blockers for pts undergoing vascular surgery—except in the case of direct contraindication to their use.

4. Abdominal aortic aneurysm.

a. Definitions and epidemiology.

    i.   AAA is defined as aortic diameter at least 1 1/2 times the diameter measured at the level of the renal arteries.

    ii.   Abdominal aorta is the most common site of arterial aneurysm.
       • Most occur between the renal and mesenteric arteries.

    iii. Aneurysm size is one of the strongest predictors of rupture, with risk increasing markedly at aneurysm diameters >5.5 cm.
       • Rate of expansion may also be an important determinant of risk of rupture.

b. Risk factors.

    i.   Age >60 yr.

    ii.   Male gender—4 to 5 times more common in men.

    iii. Race—twice as frequent in whites compared with blacks.

    iv.   History of smoking—risk factor most strongly associated with AAA and promotes rate of aneurysmal growth.

    v.   HTN.

    vi.   Presence of CAD.

    vii. Serum creatinine >1.2 mg/dL.

    viii. BUN >40 mg/dL.

    ix.   Emergency surgery.

c. Clinical presentation.

    i.   Typically asymptomatic, found incidentally on CT, MRI, or US.

    ii.   Aneurysms that produce symptoms are at increased risk for rupture.

- Two main findings suggestive of recent aneurysm expansion are abdominal or back pain, and an aneurysm tender to palpation.
- iii. Ruptured aneurysm presents with abdominal or back pain, hypotension, and a pulsatile abdominal mass.
- iv. Survival rate of pts who experience a ruptured AAA is <50% versus mortality of <5% for elective surgical repair.

d. Management.
- i. AAA monitoring schedule per ACC/AHA published guidelines (2005).
  - For most pts with AAA <5 cm, the annual risk of rupture is similar to, or lower than, the risk of surgery.
  - 4.0- to 5.4-cm aneurysms should be monitored by US or CT every 6 to 12 mo.
  - 3.4- to 4.0-cm aneurysms should be monitored every 2 to 3 yr.
- ii. Medical therapy.
  - Smoking cessation—continued smoking increases the rate of aneurysmal growth by 20% to 25%.
  - Treat HTN and dyslipidemia.
  - β blockers.
- iii. Surgical therapy.
  - Symptomatic AAA should undergo repair, regardless of size.
  - Asymptomatic AAA >5.5 cm should be repaired.
  - Early repair may be beneficial in selected pts whose AAA increases in diameter more than 0.5 cm in 6 mo.
  - Repair of suprarenal and/or thoracoabdominal aneurysms involves more extensive surgery and greater operative risk; repair may not be beneficial until aneurysm is >5.5 to 6.0 cm.
  - Repair in medium-sized aneurysms may be indicated with an iliac or femoral artery aneurysm, coexistent occlusive disease, or thrombotic or embolic disease.

e. Preoperative evaluation.
- i. Careful preoperative assessment to determine CV risk.
- ii. Evaluate for other common concomitant diseases, such as COPD, renal insufficiency, HTN, diabetes mellitus.
- iii. Preoperative laboratory tests.
  - CBC.
  - Complete metabolic panel.
  - Coagulation profile.
  - Urinalysis.
  - CXR.
  - ECG.

f. Surgical technique.
- i. Vertical anterior midline incision with transperitoneal approach to retroperitoneal space.
  - Advantages: less pain and pulmonary impairment postoperatively.
  - Disadvantages: major heat and fluid losses and prolonged ileus.

    ii. Retroperitoneal approach through left flank incision with pt in right lateral decubitus position.
- May have less respiratory and wound complications, less postoperative ileus, less blood loss, lower fluid requirements, and earlier hospital discharge.

    iii. Endoluminal aortic stent graft.
- Minimally invasive.
- Complications include vessel perforation, inability to seal the aneurysm (endoleak), and inability to advance the device past the iliac artery.
- When compared with conventional approach, showed decreased transfusion requirements, earlier extubation, and shorter ICU and hospital lengths of stay.
- Overall mortality is the same as conventional approach.

g. Intraoperative monitors.
    i. Routine ASA monitors, including five-lead ECG.
    ii. Arterial catheter for BP monitoring.
    iii. Central venous access.
    iv. PAC for pts with decreased LV function or anticipated supraceliac crossclamp.
    v. TEE for pts with LV dysfunction and/or high aortic crossclamping.

h. Anesthetic management.
    i. Plan for large fluid losses and possibly large blood loss.
    ii. Renal prophylaxis with mannitol should be considered for anticipated decrease in renal blood flow.
    iii. Type of anesthesia depends on surgical technique.
- Epidural anesthesia and/or GA for open repairs can be utilized; goal is to maintain stable hemodynamics.
  - Keep in mind that pts do receive heparin during clamping of the aorta.
- Endovascular repairs can be done under local anesthesia with sedation.

i. Pathophysiology of aortic crossclamp.
    i. Depending on location of lesion, the crossclamp will be applied supraceliac, suprarenal, or infrarenal.
    ii. The further from the aorta the distal clamp is applied, the less the effect on LV afterload.
    iii. Systemic hemodynamic response to application of aortic crossclamp:
- Blood flow to lower extremities halted.
- Afterload and preload suddenly increased, increasing LVED wall stress and systemic pressure.
- CO decreased.
- Possible LV failure and ischemia.
  - Ischemia can be managed with IV nitroglycerin.
- Metabolism goes from aerobic to anaerobic.
- Maximal vasodilation and lactic acid production.

iv. Systemic hemodynamic response to removal of aortic crossclamp.
  - When crossclamp is released, SVR and arterial BP decrease.
  - Peripheral vasodilation results in relative volume depletion and hypotension. This is minimized by:
    - Volume loading prior to unclamping.
    - Gradual release of clamp by surgeons to allow time for adjustment in volume, pressors, and sodium bicarbonate replacement.
    - If pressure remains low, surgeon may need to reapply clamp.
j. Complications of AAA repair.
  i. MI is the single most common cause of early morbidity in AAA resection.
  ii. Renal insufficiency.
  iii. Pulmonary infections and pulmonary failure.
  iv. Colon ischemia.
  v. Hepatic failure.
  vi. Paraplegia.

5. Thoracoabdominal aneurysm.

a. Etiology.
  i. Most thoracoabdominal aneurysms are due to degenerative atherosclerotic disease.
  ii. 20% are a result of chronic dissections.
  iii. Other less common etiologies include Marfan syndrome, giant cell arteritis, and infectious causes.
b. Crawford classification (Fig. 9.8).
c. Symptoms.
  i. Back pain.
  ii. Epigastric pain.
  iii. Hoarseness—secondary to compression of recurrent laryngeal nerve.
  iv. Symptoms related to compression.
    - Cough.
    - Shortness of breath.
d. Indications for surgical repair.
  i. Aneurysm >6 cm in diameter.
  ii. Aneurysm size increases >1 cm/yr.
  iii. Associated pain symptoms.
  iv. Marked irregularity in shape is noted.
e. Anesthetic management.
  i. Monitoring (capability to transduce five pressures).
    - Right radial arterial catheter.
    - Femoral arterial catheter.
    - CSF catheter.
    - Typically need three catheter-introducer (Cordis) sheaths.
      - One for PAC/CVP.
      - Remaining two for rapid-infusion system.
    - TEE, if available.

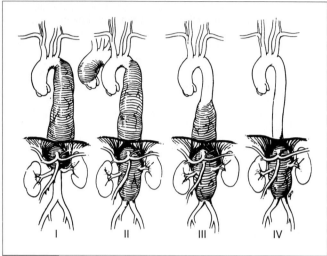

FIG. 9.8

The Crawford classification of thoracoabdominal aortic aneurysms is defined by anatomic location and the extent of involvement. Type I aneurysms involve all or most of the descending thoracic aorta and the upper abdominal aorta, type II aneurysms involve all or most of the descending thoracic aorta and all or most of the abdominal aorta, type III aneurysms involve the lower portion of the descending thoracic aorta and most of the abdominal aorta, and type IV aneurysms involve all or most of the abdominal aorta, including the visceral segment. *(Adapted from Crawford ES: Thoracoabdominal and suprarenal abdominal aortic aneurysm. In Ernst CB, Stanley JC [eds]: Current Therapy in Vascular Surgery, Philadelphia: Decker, 1987, pp 96–98.)*

    ii.   Routine infusions.
- Sodium nitroprusside.
- Nitroglycerin.
- Phenylephrine.
- Total IV anesthetic if following motor-evoked potentials.

   iii.   DLT for OLV with appropriate tube changers for end of case.

   iv.   Three temperature-monitoring sites.
- Bladder.
- Nasopharyngeal.
- Blood (from PAC thermistor).

    v.   Blood warmer.
- Sufficient blood products should be available (e.g., 15 units RBC and 15 units FFP).

   vi.   Cell saver.

TABLE 9.4

PERCENT CHANGE IN CARDIOVASCULAR VARIABLES ON INITIATION OF
AORTIC OCCLUSION

| Cardiovascular Variable | Percent Change after Occlusion | | |
	Supraceliac	Suprarenal-Infraceliac	Infrarenal
Mean arterial BP	54	5*	2*
Pulmonary capillary wedge pressure	38	10*	0*
End-diastolic area	28	2*	9*
End-systolic area	69	10*	11*
Ejection fraction	−38	−10*	−3*
Pts with wall motion abnormalities	92	33	0

*Statistically different ($p < 0.05$) from the group undergoing supraceliac aortic occlusion.
(From Roizen MF, et al: J Vasc Surg 1984;1(2):300–305, with permission.)

vii. Associated intraoperative issues.
- Renal.
  - Renal artery cold perfusion (4° C/1 L LR/mannitol/steroids).
  - Crossclamp time >100 min is only intraoperative predictor of renal failure.
  - Renal failure significantly increases risk of perioperative death.
- Cardiac hemodynamics (Table 9.4).
- Neuroprotection.
  - 5% to 15% paralysis rate, depending on location of aneurysm.
  - Goal is to maintain spinal cord blood supply.
  - Spinal drain to monitor CSF pressure; set pop-off at 10 cm H_2O.
  - Neuromonitoring.
    - Motor-evoked potentials—good correlation with neurologic outcome.
      - Intraoperative management of motor-evoked potentials changes (Fig. 9.9).
    - Somatosensory-evoked potentials—poor correlation with neurologic outcome.
  - Distal perfusion using left heart bypass.
    - Above-clamp goal MAP = 75 to 125 mm Hg.
    - Below-clamp goal MAP = 50 to 75 mm Hg.
    - Moderate heparinization (100 U/kg).
    - Intraoperative management of left heart bypass (Table 9.5).
  - Variety of adjuncts.
    - Systemic hypothermia—30° to 34° C.
    - Epidural cooling.
    - Pharmacologic interventions.
      - IV naloxone.
      - Intrathecal papaverine.

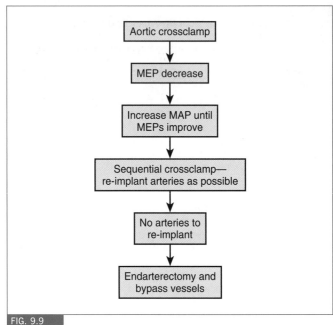

FIG. 9.9
Intraoperative management strategy for changes in motor-evoked potentials (MEPs).

TABLE 9.5

HEMODYNAMIC MANAGEMENT OF LEFT HEART BYPASS

MAP Variable	Intervention
High above and below aortic clamp	↑ Anesthesia
	↑ Vasodilators
	↓ Vasopressors
Low above and below aortic clamp	Volume resuscitate
	↓ Anesthesia
	↓ Vasodilators
	↑ Vasopressors
High above aortic clamp	↑ Flow of left-heart bypass
Low below aortic clamp	↓ Flow of left-heart bypass

IX. ANESTHESIA FOR THE THORACIC SURGICAL PATIENT

A. PREOPERATIVE EVALUATION

1. Standard detailed H&P.
2. Risk assessment of underlying cardiac disease.
3. Define nature and severity of pulmonary dysfunction.

4. Optimize clinically.
a. Attempt to have pt quit smoking 4 to 6 wk before surgery.
b. Acute and chronic infections should be aggressively treated before surgery.
c. Bronchoconstriction should be maximally treated; consider steroid administration.

5. Preoperative pulmonary function tests.
a. Considered controversial because their utility in directing management is unclear. However, the following findings are associated with greater morbidity during thoracic procedures:
    i. FEV_1 <2 L.
    ii. FEV_1/FVC <0.5.
    iii. Vital capacity <15 mL/kg.
    iv. Arterial hypoxemia or hypercarbia.

B. MONITORING

1. Standard ASA monitors, including five-lead ECG and temperature monitoring.
2. Arterial catheter.
a. Continuous monitoring of BP for potential hemodynamic instability due to cardiac manipulation, effects of anesthesia, and potential bleeding.
b. Frequent blood gas analysis to assess gas exchange and oxygenation.
3. Central venous access and/or PAC.
a. Decision to place is dependent on pt comorbidities and anticipated need for vasoactive agents or volume resuscitation.
4. TEE.
a. Determined by pt's comorbidities.
b. Mediastinal mass may be an indication for placement.

C. CHOICE OF ANESTHESIA

1. GA is generally required for most major thoracic procedures.
2. Regional anesthesia allows for postoperative pain control, minimizing sedation, and respiratory depression associated with narcotic analgesia.
3. Thoracotomy is one of the most painful incisions.
a. Thoracic incisions have immediate and intermediate lasting adverse effects on respiratory mechanics.
4. Postoperative pain control management options.
a. Thoracic epidural.
b. Intrathecal narcotics.
c. Intrapleural catheter.
d. Intercostal nerve blocks.

D. ANESTHETIC CONSIDERATIONS FOR SPECIFIC SURGICAL PROCEDURES

1. Bronchoscopy.
a. Flexible.

     i.   Often performed in remote locations.

     ii.   Performed under sedation or GA.

     iii.   Airway managed via LMA or ETT; no airway protection from aspiration with LMA.

     iv.   Topical lidocaine administered to larynx and trachea will decrease stimulation.

     v.   Small IV dose of glycopyrrolate is often useful as an antisialagogue.

b. Rigid.

     i.   GA is needed, as deep muscle relaxation is required.

     ii.   IV anesthesia may be preferable.

        • Delivery of inhaled anesthetics can be administered only intermittently during procedure.

2. Mediastinoscopy.

a. Preoperative evaluation should include a search for airway obstruction or distortion.

b. Rare but significant risk of injury to mediastinal structures.

c. Vascular structures may be compressed or injured, resulting in significant bleeding, hypotension, or dysrhythmias.

d. Recommend GA with muscle relaxation.

e. Monitoring.

     i.   Innominate artery may be compressed during the procedure, making BP monitoring in the right arm unreliable.

     ii.   BP monitoring via BP cuff or arterial line should be performed in the left arm.

     iii.   Pulse oximeter can be placed on the right arm to monitor compromised perfusion to right arm.

     iv.   Invasive BP monitoring should be considered in those pts in whom brief periods of hypotension may be poorly tolerated.

f. Positioning.

     i.   Usually, both arms are tucked at the pt's sides.

     ii.   Good peripheral IV access must be established before positioning.

3. Anterior mediastinal mass.

a. Special considerations.

     i.   Large tumors may compress the trachea, main bronchi, or both.

     ii.   Airway obstruction may not occur until induction of GA or muscle relaxation, causing reduction in distending pressure on intrathoracic airways.

     iii.   Obstruction may result in inability to ventilate or intubate pt.

b. Additional preoperative evaluation.

     i.   Detailed history to elicit symptoms of positional (supine) stridor or dyspnea or difficulty swallowing.

     ii.   Flow-volume loops showing evidence of intrathoracic variable obstruction.

     iii.   Radiographic evidence to evaluate for tracheobronchial compression.

c. Anesthetic plan, if airway compression is at risk.
  i. Ensure careful preoperative planning, including discussions with surgeons.
  ii. Place preinduction invasive arterial monitor and establish adequate IV access.
  iii. Inhaled spontaneous approach with pt in semi-sitting position (head of bed elevated 45°).
  iv. Slowly deepen anesthesia and flatten table and gradually attempt to assist ventilation.
  v. If able to assist easily, including complete exhalation, deepen anesthesia rapidly and give short-acting muscle relaxant.
  vi. If ventilation is difficult, inhaled anesthesia can be lightened in a controlled pattern.
  vii. If unable to pass ETT, a rigid bronchoscope can be placed past the compression, and ventilation can be provided through it.
  viii. Consider keeping pt intubated and sedated until definitive management (chemotherapy, radiation, or surgery) of mass is provided.

4. Thoracotomy.
a. Single-lung ventilation greatly facilitates surgical exposure but is not mandatory.
b. Consider plan for postoperative pain management (options discussed above).
c. Invasive BP monitoring recommended.
d. Pt is positioned in lateral decubitus position, with surgical side up.
  i. Caution in pt positioning and padding is necessary.
e. Recommend cautious fluid administration.
  i. Goal is to keep pt relatively "dry."

5. Thoracoscopy.
a. Involves insertion of an endoscope into the thoracic cavity and pleural space.
  i. Used for diagnosis of pleural disease, effusion, infectious disease, staging procedure, chemical pleurodesis, and lung biopsy.
b. Single-lung ventilation is required to permit operative exposure in the closed chest.
c. Can be performed under local, regional, or general anesthesia.
  i. Depends on duration of procedure and clinical status of pt.
  ii. If spontaneously awake pt does not tolerate procedure, convert to GA.
    • Intubation in lateral position may be challenging.
d. Postoperative pain control generally does not require neuraxial analgesia.

6. Thymectomy.
a. Indications.
  i. Management of myasthenia gravis.
  ii. Surgery should preferably be performed electively when pt is in remission.

CARDIOVASCULAR AND THORACIC ANESTHESIA

9

b. Special considerations.
   i. Determine significance of disease and possible need for postoperative mechanical ventilation.
   ii. Evaluate pt clinically and radiographically for evidence of airway compression.
   iii. Avoid or minimize the use of nondepolarizing muscle relaxants, as pts with myasthenia gravis may be sensitive.
      • Pts with myasthenia gravis may be resistant to NMB effects of succinylcholine.
   iv. Calculate pt's total outpatient pyridostigmine (Mestinon) dose and convert it to a neostigmine infusion in the OR if pt is particularly symptomatic.
   v. Consider using combined general-epidural anesthesia for intraoperative and postoperative pain management.

7. Lung volume reduction surgery.
a. Indications.
   i. Advanced emphysema.
      • Typical FEV_1 is 600 to 800 mL.
b. Special considerations.
   i. Pts preoperatively undergo course of pulmonary rehab, exercising with supplemental oxygen to improve their conditioning, strength, and nutritional status.
   ii. Pts must be free of any pulmonary infections and must be medically optimized.
c. Anesthetic considerations.
   i. Avoid medications that may cause postoperative respiratory depression.
   ii. High thoracic epidurals may be placed; a segmental sensory block should be confirmed prior to the induction of GA.
   iii. Additional monitors include an arterial catheter and adequate peripheral IV access (or central line if necessary).
   iv. Double lumen tube (DLT) is necessary for lung isolation.
   v. Aggressively treat bronchospasm with inhaled bronchodilators.
   vi. Pts must be awake, spontaneously ventilating, and showing adequate ventilation via serial blood gases before extubation is appropriate.
   vii. Pts should be monitored closely in the OR for adequate ventilation prior to transfer to the ICU.
d. Potential problems in the OR and ICU.
   i. Air trapping and auto-PEEP may result in hypotension.
   ii. Pts are kept "dry"—may result in hypotension.
   iii. Air leaks are common.
      • If >50% of tidal volume is being lost, may need to address surgically.
   iv. If epidural use results in hypotension, vasoactive agents should be initiated.
      • Postoperative pain control must be a priority.

X. ONE-LUNG VENTILATION

A. ABSOLUTE INDICATIONS

1. Isolation for spillage or contamination.
   a. Infection—bronchiectasis and lung abscess.
   b. Massive hemorrhage.
2. Control of the distribution of ventilation.
   a. Bronchopleural fistula.
   b. Bronchopleural cutaneous fistula.
   c. Giant unilateral lung cyst or bulla.
   d. Tracheobronchial tree disruption.
   e. Life-threatening hypoxemia resulting from unilateral lung disease.
   f. Unilateral bronchopulmonary lavage.
   g. Pulmonary alveolar proteinosis.

B. SURGICAL PROCEDURES FOR WHICH OLV IS DESIRED FOR SURGICAL EXPOSURE

1. Thoracic aortic aneurysm.
2. Pneumonectomy.
3. Upper lobectomy.
4. Mediastinal exposure.
5. Thoracoscopy.
6. Pulmonary resection via median sternotomy.
7. Esophageal resection.
8. Middle and lower lobectomies and segmental resection.
9. Procedures on the thoracic spine.

C. ISSUES RELATED TO OLV

1. For surgery-related indications, OLV provides a "quiet" surgical field, usually by collapse of the nondependent lung in the lateral decubitus position.
   a. Can greatly increase the complexity of anesthetic management.
2. The main physiologic concern is arterial hypoxemia secondary to ventilation and perfusion mismatching.
   a. CO_2 elimination is typically not altered by OLV, as long as minute ventilation remains constant.
   b. Frequent sampling of PaO_2 and $PaCO_2$ is often necessary, and arterial catheters are almost always utilized.
3. In the lateral position, the nondependent lung is preferentially ventilated because of its increased compliance.
   a. Conversely, the dependent lung receives more perfusion because of gravity (~60% of total blood flow).
   b. Hence, V/Q mismatching occurs.
4. When the nondependent lung is collapsed, as it is to accommodate thoracic surgery, all ventilation goes to the dependent lung.
   a. However, blood flow continues to the nondependent—and now nonventilated—lung, resulting in a right-to-left intrapulmonary shunt.

b. Mixing of oxygenated and deoxygenated blood in the pulmonary veins leads to hypoxemia.

5. **The primary mechanism to blunt this effect is hypoxic pulmonary vasoconstriction.**

a. Because of the low oxygen tension in the nondependent lung, PVR increases, thereby redirecting blood flow to the ventilated lung.

b. A single-lung hypoxic pulmonary vasoconstriction response should decrease the blood flow to that lung by 50%.

c. Several factors can inhibit hypoxic pulmonary vasoconstriction, including inhalation anesthetics, vasodilators such as nitroglycerin and nitroprusside, and pulmonary infection.

6. **The anesthesiologist can take some maneuvers to improve oxygenation during OLV.**

a. Increased FiO_2.

   i. Greater inspired oxygen concentration will not only increase PaO_2 but will also decrease PVR in the ventilated lung and will improve blood flow.

b. Positive end-expiratory pressure.

   i. Application of 2.5 to 10 mL H_2O PEEP to the dependent lung can help to reduce atelectasis and improve ventilation.

   ii. Caution must be taken because higher pressures can lead to increases in PVR.

c. CPAP.

   i. CPAP to the nonventilated lung will potentially lead to oxygenation of blood that does enter the collapsed lung. It also increases vascular resistance in that lung, further diverting flow to the ventilated lung.

   ii. CPAP can be provided by connecting a Mapleson circuit to the nonventilated lung.

      • Communication with the surgeon is important because this maneuver can lead to gradual reinflation of the lung, and adjustments of the oxygen flow and adjustable pressure-limiting (APL) valve should be made accordingly.

d. Should hypoxemia persist, periodically returning to two-lung ventilation may be necessary.

   i. Finally, the surgeon can be asked to temporarily clamp the pulmonary artery to the nondependent lung.

e. As always, the surgeon should be kept aware of persistent hypoxemia.

D. LUNG-ISOLATION TECHNIQUES

Single-lung isolation is usually accomplished by one of two methods: bronchial blocker or double-lumen ETT. In the pediatric pt, and rarely in the adult, lung isolation may also be accomplished by advancing a conventional ETT into a mainstem bronchus.

1. Bronchial blockers.

a. A bronchial blocker is a catheter with a balloon at its tip that is passed through or alongside a standard single-lumen ETT and inflated in the mainstem bronchus of the operative lung.

 i.   A fiberoptic bronchoscope is required to position the blocker properly. The most commonly used endobronchial blocker (Arndt Endobronchial Blocker, Cook Critical Care) can be placed through any adequately sized ETT and guided to the correct position using a small nylon loop that slips over the bronchoscope.

 ii. A special three-port ETT connector allows simultaneous ventilation, bronchoscopy, and introduction of the blocker, facilitating positioning of the blocker.

b. Advantages of the bronchial blocker over a DLT.

 i.   The outside diameters of DLTs are significantly larger than single-lumen tubes, making them challenging to place in children, small adults, and pts with difficult airways, tracheostomies, or other anatomical abnormalities.

 ii. Ability to place catheter via an existing single-lumen tube in emergent situations.

 iii. Removes the need to change ETTs for postoperative mechanical ventilation.

 iv. For pts with limited pulmonary reserve, the balloon may be advanced into a lobar bronchus for selective lobar blockade.

 v.   Can be used in long cases in which lung isolation may be required only for a short period (back surgery).

c. Disadvantages of the bronchial blocker.

 i.   Blockers may be difficult to place in the left side.

 ii. Lung deflation is slow because it relies primarily on absorption of trapped oxygen.

 iii. Suctioning and administration of CPAP to the deflated lung for hypoxemia may be difficult.

 iv. It may be impossible to achieve right-lung isolation in 5% of pts with tracheal or proximal right upper lobe bronchial takeoff.

2. DLT.

a. Technical considerations.

 i.   The most commonly used DLTs are disposable versions of the Robertshaw tube.

  • Consists of two D-shaped lumens:
    - The longer bronchial lumen has a bend designed to enter a mainstem bronchus.
    - The shorter tracheal lumen opens above the carina.

  • A bronchial cuff is at the end of the bronchial lumen, and a tracheal cuff is proximal to the opening of the tracheal lumen.

  • They are available in right- and left-sided tubes, and sizes 35F, 37F, 39F, and 41F.

9

CARDIOVASCULAR AND THORACIC ANESTHESIA

- Typically, 37F DLTs are used for average-sized female pts, and 39F DLTs are used for males.
ii. Although both right- and left-sided tubes are available, almost all cases can be performed with a left-sided tube.
iii. The proximity of the right upper lobe takeoff to the carina (~2 cm) necessitates an aperture in the bronchial cuff of the right-sided tube to ventilate the right upper lobe.
    - This can make placement more challenging.
    - Use of right-sided DLTs is limited to cases that involve large exophytic lesions on the left mainstem bronchus, tight left mainstem bronchus stenoses, or distortion of the left mainstem bronchus by an adjacent tumor.
b. Placement of the DLT.
    i. Can be more challenging than single-lumen tube intubation because the larger and stiffer DLT can be difficult to manipulate.
    ii. Laryngoscopy is usually performed with a Macintosh blade, as this creates a wider channel through which the larger tube can enter.
    iii. The more distal bronchial portion of the DLT should be introduced into the glottic opening, with the bend in an anterior orientation.
    iv. Because a very rigid stylet is used, it should be removed before advancing the DLT into the trachea to avoid trauma and rupture.
    v. Once the bronchial cuff has passed the vocal cords, the tube is rotated 90° (left for left-sided, right for right-sided) and advanced until resistance is met (usually at 29 cm).
    vi. The tracheal cuff is then inflated, and endotracheal positioning is confirmed (auscultation, E_TCO_2, etc.).
    vii. Confirmation of DLT placement consists of clinical assessment and flexible FOB.
    viii. After endotracheal placement has been confirmed, the following steps should be taken to ensure proper positioning of a left-sided tube.
        - Inflate the bronchial cuff (1 to 2 mL).
        - Clamp the tracheal lumen.
        - Auscultate both lungs.
            - Unilateral left-sided breath sounds indicate entry of the bronchial lumen into the left mainstem.
            - Persistence of bilateral breath sounds indicates that the bronchial opening is in the trachea or that the seal of the bronchial cuff is inadequate.
            - Unilateral right-sided breath sounds indicate that the bronchial lumen has entered the right (incorrect) mainstem.
        - Unclamp the tracheal lumen and clamp the bronchial lumen.
            - Absence of any breath sounds indicates that the bronchial lumen is obstructing the distal trachea or that the tracheal opening is abutting the carina.
    ix. A flexible FOB should be passed into the tracheal lumen.

x. The carina should be clearly visualized, and anterior/posterior orientation confirmed by tracheal rings (complete rings anteriorly, incomplete rings posteriorly).

xi. The endobronchial portion of the tube should be seen entering the left mainstem, with the proximal rim of the blue bronchial cuff visible.

xii. Advancing the bronchoscope into the right mainstem should reveal the right upper lobe takeoff ~2 cm distal to the carina.

xiii. Tube placement should be confirmed again after positioning the pt, as displacement is common.

c. Contraindications to DLT.

i. Pt with a lesion (e.g., airway stricture and endoluminal tumor) that is present somewhere along the pathway of the tube.

ii. Small pts for whom a 35F tube is too large to fit comfortably through the larynx.

iii. Extremely sick pt who is already intubated with a single-lumen tube and will not tolerate being taken off of mechanical ventilation and PEEP for even a short period of time.

d. Complications.

i. The tracheal cuff can be lacerated by the pt's teeth. If placement of a single-lumen tube is necessary, specially designed tube-exchanger stylets can be utilized.

ii. Hypoxemia due to malpositioning.

iii. Trauma to the trachea and larynx; tracheobronchial rupture.

iv. Inadvertent suturing of the tube to the bronchus.

XI. ANESTHESIA FOR TRACHEAL SURGERY

Tracheal surgery is usually performed for tracheal stenosis and, much less frequently, congenital malformations. Stenoses can be a result of impingement of either malignant or benign tumors, endotracheal intubation, or tracheostomy.

A. PREOPERATIVE STUDIES SHOULD FOCUS ON:

1. Causes and symptoms of tracheal stenoses.

a. Tracheal stenoses result in progressive dyspnea that may worsen in prone position, and wheezing or stridor may also be present (sometimes only with exertion).

b. Tumoral stenosis may also be associated with hemoptysis.

2. Checking airway patency, diameter, and location at preoperative CT scan.

a. Communication with the surgeon is necessary to plan airway management: whether oral intubation is possible, ETT size, need for tracheostomy, and so on.

3. Oxygenation status (check ABG and the concomitant FiO_2) and preoperative PFTs.

4. Other comorbidities.

a. The makeup of this population varies from young ASA 1 pts with no other comorbidities to elderly ASA 4 pts with other multiple associated diseases.

B. PREMEDICATION
1. Usually withheld until pt is in the OR.
2. Oxygen is usually administered.

C. INDUCTION
1. Performed in presence of the surgeon in case emergency surgical airway access is needed.
2. Spontaneous ventilation is maintained during induction, with sevoflurane or desflurane either alone (preferred in critical stenoses) or in combination with a short-acting IV anesthetic for induction.
3. If oral intubation is judged possible, direct laryngoscopy should be attempted with the pt under deep anesthesia and no muscle relaxation.
a. 1 to 2 mg/kg lidocaine can be administered to dampen the respiratory reflexes during direct laryngoscopy.
4. Once pt is intubated, plan conversion to total IV anesthetic for periods of apnea.
5. On occasion, a rigid laryngoscopy is needed to dilate a high tracheal stenosis enough to pass a small tube distal to the obstruction.
a. If this is not possible because the stenosis is too narrow, friable, or distal, spontaneous ventilation can be maintained through the rigid bronchoscope or an LMA until the trachea is incised and a distal tube is placed.
6. In low tracheal stenosis, or if other measures fail, a tracheostomy may be the best option for securing the airway.
a. Those pts with preexisting mature tracheostomies can be induced with IV agents via cannulating the tracheostomy with a cuffed, flexible, armored ETT that will be later replaced with a sterile tube by the surgeon.

D. PROCEDURE
1. FiO_2 100% should be used whenever ventilation is intermittent or at risk.
2. Invasive arterial monitoring is recommended.
a. In low tracheal stenoses, the left radial artery is preferred because of the potential risk of compression of the innominate artery.
3. High tracheal stenoses are repaired through a transverse neck incision by excising the obstructed tracheal ring and reanastomosing the remaining edges.
a. Once the trachea is incised distally to the tip of the ETT, the surgeon places a sterile armored tube into the distal trachea and passes a sterile connecting hose to the anesthesiologist for continuation of ventilation during the resection and reanastomosis of the posterior wall.
   i. This tube may often be removed and reinserted as the surgeon works around it.
b. When the anastomosis is almost complete, the tube is removed and the original tracheal tube is advanced distally past the anastomosis.

c. The distal trachea is then suctioned to clear it of blood and secretions.

4. An alternative is to use high-frequency jet ventilation (HFJV) after the incision and during the anastomosis by passing the jet cannula through the ETT.

a. This cannula is advanced by the surgeon past the distal trachea, the ETT cuff is deflated, and ventilation is then performed with HFJV.

b. Extreme caution is needed to avoid air trapping and barotrauma.

c. As administration of volatile anesthetics is difficult, total IV anesthetic is the best option with this ventilatory technique.

5. At the end of the procedure, when the return of spontaneous ventilation is achieved and the pt is awake, pt may be extubated in the OR.

a. Pts are positioned with the neck flexed for 24 to 48 hr to minimize tension on the suture line.

b. In those pts who are not likely to cooperate with this position (i.e., children) or in those with difficult anatomy or copious secretions, replacing the tube by a small tracheostomy below the anastomosis level or by a small uncuffed oral tube may be considered.

6. If reintubation is necessary, it should be performed under direct visualization with an FOB to allow inspection of the anastomosis and precise placement of the ETT.

7. Very low tracheal obstructions that involve the intrathoracic trachea or carina imply a right posterior thoracotomy or median sternotomy for surgical access.

a. Anesthetic management is similar but more frequently requires HFJV or even CPB (in complex congenital cases).

XII. ESOPHAGECTOMY

A. INDICATIONS

1. Esophageal cancer.

a. Prevalence: men (6 in 100,000), women (1.6 in 100,000).

b. Ruptured esophagus.

2. Esophageal strictures refractory to esophageal dilation.

3. Barrett esophagitis.

4. Benign obstructive tumors of the esophagus or gastroesophageal junction.

B. PREOPERATIVE CONSIDERATIONS

1. Nutritional status—because of frequent dysphagia, nutritional deficiencies can lead to metabolic and functional changes that may affect anesthesia.

a. Dehydration.

  i. Pts frequently are hypovolemic prior to surgery and may be more dramatically affected by hemodynamic effects of anesthetics.

b. Hypoalbuminemia.

  i. May lead to an increased response to anesthetic medications.

9

CARDIOVASCULAR AND THORACIC ANESTHESIA

  c. Anemia.
   i. Common because of reduced nutritional intake and/or bleeding from tumor site. Pts may be at higher risk of ischemia and blood transfusion.
  d. Electrolyte imbalance.
   i. Frequent electrolyte disturbances secondary to malnutrition include hypomagnesemia and hypokalemia.
   ii. Hypophosphatemia may lead to reduced muscle function, further compromising postoperative respiratory function.
  e. Pts are often on total peripheral nutrition (TPN), which can help offset the effects of malnutrition.
   i. TPN should be continued throughout the surgery, with the rate reduced to half of target or preoperative infusion.
   ii. Use of intraoperative TPN may lead to hypoglycemia and hypercarbia.
 2. Cardiac status.
  a. Pts undergoing esophagectomy should be evaluated in regard to cardiac status, similar to other pts undergoing surgery.
  b. The ACC/AHA Guidelines for Perioperative Evaluation of Noncardiac Surgery should be followed, with esophagectomy typically being considered a "high-risk" procedure.
 3. Airway evaluation.
  a. As with all pts undergoing anesthesia, a thorough review of pt's airway history and exam should be performed.
  b. With the frequent use of double-lumen ETT in esophagectomy, particular attention should be paid to the ability to place such an airway device.
  c. Alternative methods of intubation should be considered in advance for pts who present with history or exam findings that are suggestive of difficult intubation.

C. SURGICAL APPROACH
 1. Thoracic incision.
 2. Thoracoabdominal (three-incision approach).
 3. Transhiatal approach.

D. MONITORING
 1. Arterial catheter for BP monitoring and blood sampling—mandatory.
 2. CVC—not imperative; however, the frequent need for a large volume of fluid (IV fluids, colloid, blood products) makes the presence of CVP monitoring useful. Of course, its use in pts with limited peripheral access is standard practice.

E. ANESTHETIC CONSIDERATIONS
 1. Hemodynamic perturbations.
  a. The esophagus is positioned directly behind the heart; therefore manipulation of the heart during dissection may lead to reduced venous return, leading to reduced CO.

b. Dysrhythmias are common.
2. **OLV.**
a. Dependent on the surgical approach.
b. All anesthetic considerations attendant to OLV are applicable to an esophagectomy.
c. Double-lumen ETTs.
d. Arndt bronchial blockers.
e. FOB.
3. **Postoperative airway management.**
a. Pts are at high risk for aspiration.
b. They are also at high risk for reintubation due to major fluid resuscitation.
c. With these considerations in mind, our practice is to leave pts intubated and sedated overnight.
4. **Regional techniques.**
a. Intraoperative and postoperative use of a thoracic epidural can be helpful for pain management.
b. We routinely use thoracic epidurals in our esophagectomy pts.

XIII. HEMODYNAMIC AND RESPIRATORY FORMULAS (Tables 9.6 and 9.7)

TABLE 9.6

HEMODYNAMIC FORMULAS

Variable	Equation	Normal Values
Cardiac index (CI)	CO/BSA	2.8–4.2 L/min/m^2
Stroke volume (SV)	CO/HR × 100	60–90 mL/beat
Stroke index (SI)	SV/BSA	40–60 mL/beat/m^2
Mean arterial pressure (MAP)	Diastolic pressure + 1/3 pulse pressure	80–120 mm Hg
Systemic vascular resistance (SVR)	[(MAP − CVP) ÷ CO] × 80	900–1400 dynes/sec/cm^5
Systemic vascular resistance index (SVRI)	[(MAP − CVP) ÷ CI] × 80	1900–2400 dynes/sec/cm^5
Pulmonary vascular resistance (PVR)	[(P̄ĀP − PCWP) ÷ CO] × 80	100–250 dynes/sec/cm^5
Pulmonary vascular resistance index (PVRI)	[(P̄ĀP − PCWP) ÷ CI] × 80	45–225 dynes/sec/cm^5
Right ventricular stroke work index (RVSWI)	0.0136 (P̄ĀP − CVP) × SI	5–9 g/m/beat/m^2
Left ventricular stroke work index (LVSWI)	0.0136 (MAP − PCWP) × SI	45–60 g/m/beat/m^2

BSA, Body surface area; *CO*, cardiac output; *CVP*, central venous pressure; *HR*, heart rate; *P̄ĀP*, mean pulmonary artery pressure; *PCWP*, pulmonary capillary wedge pressure.

9

CARDIOVASCULAR AND THORACIC ANESTHESIA

TABLE 9.7	
RESPIRATORY FORMULAS	
Variable/Equation	Normal Values
Alveolar oxygen tension	110 mm Hg (FiO_2 = 0.21)
$\textbf{PaO}_2$ = FiO_2 (PB – PH_2O) – $PaCO_2$/0.8	
Alveolar-arterial oxygen gradient	<10 mm Hg (FiO_2 = 0.21)
Est. Normal = (age/4) + 6	<60 mm Hg (FiO_2 = 1.0)
$\textbf{A} - \textbf{aO}_2$ = PAO_2 – PaO_2	
Arterial-to-alveolar oxygen ratio(a/A ratio)	>0.75
$\textbf{a/A ratio}$ = PaO_2/PAO_2	
Physiologic dead space as a fraction of tidal volume	0.33
$\textbf{V}_D\textbf{/V}_T$ = ($PaCO_2$ – $P\bar{E}CO_2$)/$PaCO_2$	
Arterial oxygen content	21 mL O_2/100 mL
$\textbf{CaO}_2$ = (Hb × 1.36 × SaO_2/100) + PaO_2 (0.0031)	
Mixed venous oxygen content difference	15 mL O_2/100 mL
$\textbf{C}\bar{\textbf{v}}\textbf{O}_2$ = (Hb × 1.36 × $S\bar{v}O_2$/100) + $P\bar{v}O_2$ (0.0031)	
Ateriovenous O_2 content difference	4–5.5 mL O_2/100 mL
$\textbf{a} - \bar{\textbf{v}}\textbf{O}_2$ = CaO_2 – $C\bar{v}O_2$	
Intrapulmonary (or physiologic) shunt fraction	<5%
$\dot{\textbf{Q}}\textbf{s/}\dot{\textbf{Q}}\textbf{t}$ = (Cc'O_2 – CaO_2)/(Cc'O_2 – $C\bar{v}O_2$) *or* P(A – a)O_2 ÷ 20 *(For PaO_2 > 175 and normal CO)*	
$\textbf{Cc'O}_2$ = (Hb × 1.36) + PAO_2 (0.0031) *(use FiO_2 = 1.0)*	
O_2 consumption or Fick eq. for CO	3.5 mL O_2/kg/min (at BMR)
$\dot{\textbf{V}}\textbf{O}_2$ = CO (CaO_2 – $C\bar{v}O_2$) × 10 *or* $\textbf{CO}$ = $\dot{V}O_2$/(CaO_2 – $C\bar{v}O_2$) × 10	
$\dot{\textbf{V}}\textbf{O}_2\textbf{I}$ = CI (CaO_2 – $C\bar{v}O_2$) × 10	110–140 mL/min/m²
O_2 delivery or transport	
$\dot{\textbf{D}}\textbf{O}_2$ = CO (CaO_2) × 10	1000 mL/min
$\dot{\textbf{D}}\textbf{O}_2\textbf{I}$ = CI (CaO_2) × 10	450–550 mL/min/m²
O_2 extraction ratio	22%–30%
$\textbf{O}_2\textbf{ER}$ = ($\dot{V}O_2$/$\dot{D}O_2$) × 100 *or* [(CaO_2 – $C\bar{v}O_2$)/CaO_2] × 100	
BMR, Basal metabolic rate.	

REFERENCES

Acher CW, Wynn MM, Archibald J: Naloxone and spinal fluid drainage as adjuncts in the surgical treatment of thoracoabdominal and thoracic aneurysms. Surgery 1990;108:755–761.

Allen M: Pacemakers and implantable cardioverter defibrillators. Anesthesia, 2006;61:883–890.

Aufderheide S, Simon BA: Anesthesia for the thoracic surgical patient. In Yang SC, Cameron DE (eds): Current Therapy in Thoracic and Cardiovascular Surgery. Philadelphia: Mosby, 2004.

Barash P, Cullen BF, Stoelting RK: Clinical Anesthesia, 5th ed. Philadelphia: Lippincott Williams & Wilkins, 2006.

Benumof JL: Anesthesia for Thoracic Surgery. Philadelphia: Saunders, 1987.

Black J, Davison JK, Cambria RP: Regional hypothermia with epidural cooling for prevention of spinal cord ischemic complications after thoracoabdominal aortic surgery. Semin Thoracic Cardiovasc Surg 2003;15:345–352.

Bonow RO, Carabella BA, Chatterjee K, et al: ACC/AHA 2006 guidelines for management of pts with valvular heart disease. A report of the American College of Cardiology/American Heart Association Task Force on Practice Guidelines. J Am Coll Cardiol 2006;48:e1.

Cleland JG, Daubert JC, Erdmann E, et al: The effect of cardiac resynchronization on morbidity and mortality in heart failure. N Engl J Med 2005;352:1539–1549.

Coselli J, LeMaire SA, Miller CC III: Mortality and paraplegia after thoracoabdominal aortic aneurysm repair: A risk factor analysis. Ann Thorac Surg 2000;69:409–414.

Dardik A, Perler BA, Roseborough GS, et al: Subdural hematoma after thoracoabdominal aortic aneurysm repair: An underreported complication of spinal fluid drainage? J Vasc Surg 2002;36: 47–50.

de Haan P, Kalkman CJ, de Mol BA, et al: Efficacy of transcranial motor-evoked myogenic potentials to detect spinal cord ischemia during operations for thoracoabdominal aneurysms. J Thorac Cardiovasc Surg 1997;113:87–100.

Eagle KA, Berger PB, Calkins H, et al: ACC/AHA guideline update for perioperative cardiovascular evaluation for noncardiac surgery—executive summary a report of the American College of Cardiology/American Heart Association Task Force on Practice Guidelines (Committee to Update the 1996 Guidelines on Perioperative Cardiovascular Evaluation for Noncardiac Surgery). Circulation 2002;105:1257–1267.

Eisenkraft JB, Cohen E, Neustein SM: Anesthesia for thoracic surgery. In Barash PG, Cullen BF, Stoelting RK (eds): Clinical Anesthesia, 3rd ed. Philadelphia: Lippincott-Raven, 1997.

Ellis JE, Roizen MF, Mantha S, et al: Anesthesia for vascular surgery. In Barash PG, Cullen BF, Stoelting RK (eds): Clinical Anesthesia, 3rd ed. Philadelphia: Lippincott-Raven, 1997.

Gregoratos G, Abrams J, Epstein AE, et al: ACC/AHA/NASPE 2002 Guideline update for implantation of cardiac pacemakers and antiarrhythmia devices: Summary article. A report of the American College of Cardiology/American Heart Association Task force of practice guidelines (ACC/AHA/NASPE committee to update the 1998 pacemaker guidelines). Circulation 2002;106:2145–2161.

Heerdt PM, Triantafillou A, Yao FF: Bronchoscopy, mediastinoscopy, and thoracotomy. In Yao FF, Malhotra V, Fontes ML (eds): Yao and Artusio's Anesthesiology: Problem-Oriented Patient Management, 5th ed. Baltimore: Lippincott Williams & Wilkins, 2003.

Hurford WE, Bailin MT, Davison JK, et al: Clinical Anesthesia Procedures of the Massachusetts General Hospital, 6th ed. Philadelphia: Lippincott Williams & Wilkins, 2002.

Jacobs M, Mess WH: The role of evoked potential monitoring in operative management of type I and type II thoracoabdominal aortic aneurysms. Semin Thoracic Cardiovasc Surg 2003;15:353–364.

Juvonen T, Ergin MA, Galla JD, et al: Prospective study of the natural history of thoracic aortic aneurysms. Ann Thorac Surg 1997;63:1533–1545.

Kaplan JA, Reich DL, Lake CL, et al: Kaplan's Cardiac Anesthesia, 5th ed. Philadelphia: Saunders, 2006.

Kashap V, Cambria RP, Davison JK, et al: Renal failure after thoracoabdominal aortic surgery. J Vasc Surg 1997;26:949–955.

Levine W, Lee JJ, Black JH, et al: Thoracoabdominal aneurysm repair: Anesthetic management. Int Anesthesiol Clin 2005;43:39–60.

Meylaerts S, Jacobs MJ, van Iterson V, et al: Comparison of transcranial motor-evoked potentials and somatosensory-evoked potentials during thoracoabdominal aortic aneurysm repair. Ann Surg 1999;230: 742–749.

Miller RD: Miller's Anesthesia, 6th ed. Philadelphia: Elsevier, 2005.

Morgan GE, Mikhail MS, Murray MJ: Clinical Anesthesiology, 4th ed. New York: Lange Medical Books/McGraw-Hill, 2005.

Roizen MF, Beaupre PN, Alpert RA, et al: Monitoring with two-dimensional transesophageal echocardiography. Comparison of myocardial function in patients undergoing supraceliac, suprarenal-infraceliac, or infrarenal aortic occlusion. J Vasc Surg 1984;1(2):300–305.

Rubin LA, Rosner HL: Abdominal aortic aneurysm repair and postoperative pain management. In Yao FF, Malhotra V, Fontes ML (eds): Yao and Artusio's Anesthesiology: Problem-Oriented Patient Management, 5th ed. Baltimore: Lippincott Williams & Wilkins, 2003.

Savader S, Williams GM, Trerotola SO, et al: Preoperative spinal artery localization and its relationship to postoperative neurological complications. Radiology 1993;189:165–171.

Shanewise JS, Hug CC: Anesthesia for adult cardiac surgery. In Miller RD, Miller, ED, Reves JG, et al (eds): Anesthesia, 5th ed. New York: Churchill Livingstone, 2000.

St. John Sutton MG, Plappert T, Abraham WT, et al: Effect of cardiac resynchronization therapy on left ventricular size and function in chronic heart failure. Circulation 2003;107:1985–1990.

Sticherling C, Schaer B, Coenen M, et al: Cardiac resynchronization therapy in chronic heart failure. Swiss Med Wkly 2006;136:611–617.

Stoelting RK, Miller RD: Basics of Anesthesia, 5th ed. New York: Churchill Livingstone, 2007.

Stone ME, Fischer GW: New approaches to the surgical treatment of end-stage heart failure. In Kaplan JA, Reich DL, Lake CL, et al (eds): Kaplan's Cardiac Anesthesia, 5th ed. Philadelphia: Saunders, 2006.

Stone KR, McPherson CA: Assessment and management of patients with pacemakers and implantable cardioverter defibrillators. Crit Care Med 2004;32:S155–S165.

Svensson LG: An approach to spinal cord protection during descending or thoracoabdominal aortic repairs. Ann Thorac Surg 1999;67: 1935–1936.

Thomas SJ, Kramer JL: Manual of Cardiac Anesthesia, 2nd ed. New York: Churchill Livingstone, 1993.

Zaiden JR, Atlee JL, Belott P, et al: Practice advisory for the perioperative management of patients with cardiac rhythm management devices: Pacemakers and implantable cardioverter-defibrillators. A report by the American Society of Anesthesiologists Task Force on Perioperative Management of Patients with Cardiac Rhythm Management Devices. Anesthesiology 2005;103:186–198.

9

CARDIOVASCULAR AND THORACIC ANESTHESIA

Neuroanesthesia

*Anil Abraham, MD, PhD, Alexis Bilbow, MD, Merrie Griffin, CRNA,
and Ira Lehrer, DO
Edited by Laurel Moore, MD, Zenobia Casey MD,
and Lauren Berkow, MD*

I. NEUROPHYSIOLOGY

A. CBF

1. $CBF = (MAP - ICP)/CVP$.
2. Normal CBF = 50 mL/100 g/min.
3. EEG changes are seen when CBF < 20 mL/100 g/min.
4. Neuronal death occurs when CBF < 10 mL/100 g/min.
5. Physiologic significance.
a. Determines delivery of energy substrate.
b. Can be manipulated to optimize CPP under pathologic conditions.
6. Under normal conditions, CBF remains constant over wide range of perfusion pressures (Fig. 10.1).

B. CEREBRAL METABOLIC RATE OF OXYGEN CONSUMPTION ($CMRO_2$)

1. $CMRO_2 = CBF \times$ (arterial O_2 content—jugular venous O_2 content).
2. Normal $CMRO_2$ = 3 – 3.5 mL/100 g/min.
3. CBF is tightly coupled to local cerebral metabolism, ensuring adequate delivery of oxygen and glucose.
4. CBF and $CMRO_2$ are influenced by IV and volatile anesthetics (Table 10.1).

C. CEREBROVASCULAR RESISTANCE (CVR)

1. $CVR = CPP/CBF$.
2. Normal CVR = 1.5 to 2.1 mm Hg/100 g/min/mL.
3. Under normal circumstances, CVR adjusts to maintain constant CBF over wide range of perfusion pressures, known as *cerebral autoregulation*.

D. CPP

1. $CPP = MAP - ICP$ (or CVP if higher than ICP).
2. Normal CPP = 70 to 100 mm Hg.
a. Normal range of CPP may be higher in pts with chronic hypertension.
3. Normal ICP 8 to 12 mm Hg.

E. ELASTANCE

1. The effect of increasing volume on ICP, $\Delta P/\Delta V$.
2. The cranial vault, under normal conditions, has the capacity to tolerate large increases in volume with minimal effect on ICP (Fig. 10.2).

10

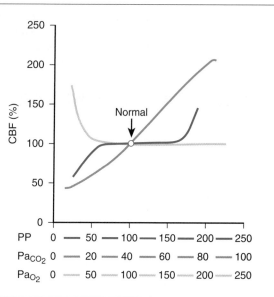

FIG. 10.1
The effect of perfusion pressure (PP), arterial carbon dioxide pressure (PaCO2), and arterial oxygen pressure (PaO2) on cerebral blood flow (CBF). *(From Bendo AA, Kass IS, Hartung J, Cottrell JE: Anesthesia for neurosurgery. In Barash PG, Cullen BF, Stoelting RK: Clinical Anesthesia, Philadelphia: Lippincott Williams & Wilkins, 2006, pp 746–752.)*

TABLE 10.1

EFFECTS OF ANESTHESIA ON CBF/CMRO$_2$

	CBF	CMRO$_2$	Direct Cerebral Vasodilation
Halothane	↑↑↑	↓	Yes
Isoflurane	↑	↓↓	Yes
Desflurane	↑	↓↓	Yes
Sevoflurane	↑	↓↓	Yes
Nitrous oxide alone	↑	↑	—
Thiopental	↓↓↓	↓↓↓	No
Etomidate	↓↓	↓↓	No
Propofol	↓↓	↓↓	No
Midazolam	↓	↓	No
Ketamine	↑↑	↑	No
Fentanyl	↓ / –	↓ / –	No

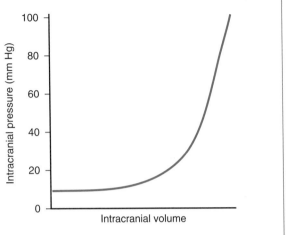

FIG. 10.2
Figure demonstrates capacity of cranial vault, under normal conditions, to tolerate large increases in volume with minimal effect on ICP. *(From Bendo AA, Kass IS, Hartung J, Cottrell JE: Anesthesia for neurosurgery. In Barash PG, Cullen BF, Stoelting RK: Clinical Anesthesia, Philadelphia: Lippincott Williams & Wilkins, 2006, pp 746–752.)*

3. Once this capacity is exceeded (e.g., rapidly expanding mass), small increases in volume produce large increases in ICP.

F. **INTRACRANIAL CONTENTS AND TREATMENT OPTIONS TO DECREASE VOLUME**
1. Surgical decompression of brain tissue, tumor, blood clot.
2. Diuretics and steroids to reduce cerebral fluid.
3. CSF drainage.
4. Decrease in arterial BP will decrease CBF.
5. Reduction in CVP will improve cerebral venous drainage.

G. **CBF CONTROL** (Table 10.2)

II. NEUROSURGICAL PROCEDURES
A. **CRANIOTOMY**
1. Indications.
a. Removal of benign or malignant tumor.
b. Evacuation of hemorrhage or abscess.
c. Seizures refractory to medical therapy.

TABLE 10.2

CBF CONTROL

Factor	Effect on CBF
$CMRO_2$	Changes in $CMRO_2$ are directly proportional to changes in CBF.
Hypothermia	$CMRO_2$ decreases by 6%–7% per degree Celsius of temperature reduction and thus decreases CBF.
$PaCO_2$	CBF changes linearly 1–2 mL/100 g/min for each 1 mm Hg change in $PaCO_2$.
PaO_2	CBF increases rapidly with PaO_2 < 60 mm Hg.
Rheologic	Polycythemia decreases CBF; anemia increases CBF.
Neurogenic	Intense increases in sympathetic output cause vasoconstriction and decreased CBF.
Autoregulation	The ability of cerebral circulation to rapidly adjust CVR to maintain constant CBF over a wide range of MAPs. • Autoregulation is blunted by high-dose volatile anesthetics and intracranial pathology; thus, CBF is dependent on adequate CPP. • Above and below autoregulatory plateau, cerebral vasculature is maximally vasoconstricted or vasodilated, respectively, and CBF becomes CPP dependent. • Cerebral regulation curve shifts to the right with chronic hypertension.

$CMRO_2$, Cerebral metabolic rate of O_2; CBF, cerebral blood flow; $PaCO_2$, partial pressure of CO_2 in arterial blood; PaO_2, partial pressure of O_2 in arterial blood; CVR, cerebrovascular resistance; MAP, mean arterial pressure; CPP, cerebral perfusion pressure.

d. Resection of arteriovenous malformation (AVM).
e. Clipping of intracranial aneurysm.
f. Treatment of movement disorders.

2. Preoperative assessment and plan.
a. Assess neurologic status prior to induction of anesthetic.
   i. Include upper- and lower-extremity strength.
b. Avoid anxiolytics such as midazolam if pt has altered mental status.

3. Anesthetic considerations for craniotomy.
a. Vascular access.
   i. Two large-bore peripheral IVs (18–16 G).
   ii. ±Central venous catheter, depending on pt status and IV access needs.
   iii. Arterial catheter for continuous BP measurement and ABGs.
b. IV fluid—NS.
   i. Slightly hyperosmolar (308 mOsm/L).
   ii. Decreases serum osmolarity and brain edema.
c. Induction.
   i. Maintain baseline MAP to avoid changes in CPP.
   ii. Intubate with complete muscle relaxation.
      • Coughing increases ICP.
      • Succinylcholine use can transiently increase ICP.

d. Maintenance.
   i.   Mechanical ventilation to maintain $PaCO_2$ at 25 to 30 mm Hg.
   ii.   Use of N_2O is controversial.
   iii.   Volatile anesthetic or IV anesthesia can be used.
   iv.   Short-acting opiates to allow fast emergence.
   v.   Barbiturates (thiopental) can be used to quickly lower ICP.
   vi.   Antiemetic to prevent postoperative N/V.
   vii.   Have vasopressors and beta blockers available.
   viii.   Mannitol and/or furosemide to reduce ICP.
   ix.   Seizure prophylaxis.
      • Fosphenytoin, phenytoin (Dilantin), or levetiracetam (Keppra) infusion.
      • Do not bolus phenytoin; can result in severe hypotension and bradycardia.
   x.   Maintain muscle relaxation.
   xi.   Caution using peripheral vasodilators.
      • Nitroprusside and nitroglycerin increase CBF and ICP.
   xii.   Fluid therapy.
      • Minimize fluids: 1 to 3 mL/kg/hr.
   xiii.   Lower-body warming blanket.
      • Maintain normothermia unless deliberate hypothermia is planned.

e. Emergence.
   i.   Give full reversal.
      • If pt's head is pinned, give reversal after pins are removed.
   ii.   Check neurologic exam prior to extubations.
      • Confirm exam with neurosurgery team prior to extubation.
      • Compare baseline neurologic function to postsurgical neurologic function.

f. Transport to ICU.
   i.   Bring reintubation equipment and emergency drugs for transport, including an induction agent that lowers ICP, a vasopressor, and a beta blocker.

4. Awake craniotomy.
a. Indications.
   i.   Facilitate intraoperative electrocorticography.
   ii.   Provide opportunity for mapping eloquent brain function (motor, speech).
   iii.   Minimize neurologic injury.
b. Anesthetic objectives.
   i.   Minimize pt discomfort.
   ii.   Ensure pt responsiveness and compliance.
   iii.   Produce minimal inhibition of spontaneous seizure activity.
c. Management.
   i.   Minimal sedation versus deep sedation versus asleep-awake-asleep technique ±LMA.
   ii.   Dexmedetomidine infusion.

10

NEUROANESTHESIA

- Provides sedation without respiratory depression.
- Very short $t_{1/2}$ allows quick emergence and neurologic exam.
  iii. Pain management.
  - Narcotics—bolus vs. infusion.
  - Scalp block.
    - Scalp supplied by branches of trigeminal nerve and the cervical plexus.
    - Draw circular line from glabella to occiput.
    - Divide into four parts at the intersection of sagittal and frontal plane.
    - Local anesthetics (bupivacaine and/or lidocaine) do not interfere with electrocorticography.
  iv. Complications.
  - Seizures.
    - Maintain airway protective measures.
    - Immediate administration of barbiturates, benzodiazepines, or propofol.
    - Administration of anticonvulsant medications.

5. Craniotomy for aneurysm or AVM.
a. Aneurysms.
  i. Hunt-Hess classification (Table 10.3).
  ii. Unruptured aneurysms (grade 0) are treated with elective clipping or coiling.
  iii. Ruptured aneurysms are treated emergently.
b. Risk factors for aneurysm.
  i. Hypertension.
  ii. Smoking.
  iii. Family history.
c. Pt considerations.

TABLE 10.3		
HUNT-HESS CLASSIFICATION FOR INTRACRANIAL ANEURYSMS		
Grade	Criteria	Perioperative Mortality
0	Unruptured aneurysm	0%–5%
I	Asymptomatic or mild headache Slight nuchal rigidity	0%–5%
II	Moderate-to-severe headache Nuchal rigidity Possible cranial nerve palsy	2%–10%
III	Moderate focal neurologic deficits Somnolence, confusion	10%–15%
IV	Stupor, vegetative disturbances Moderate-to-severe hemiparesis Possible early decerebrate rigidity	60%–70%
V	Deep coma, moribund appearance Decerebrate rigidity	70%–100%

i. Ruptured aneurysm presents as subarachnoid hemorrhage.
ii. Monitor MAP closely; hypertension can trigger rerupture.
iii. Myocardial effects.
- Transient ECG changes are common.
- Myocardial ischemia or troponin leak may be seen.
- With higher Hunt-Hess grade rupture:
    - Myocardial stunning with low ejection fraction.
    - Neurogenic pulmonary edema or acute respiratory distress syndrome.

4. Anesthetic considerations.
i. Closely monitor MAP intraoperatively to maintain CPP.
ii. Avoid hypertension; risk of rerupture.
iii. Seizure prophylaxis (see earlier under Craniotomy); postoperative seizures are possible.
iv. SSEP and EEG monitoring are commonly used (see later under Special Monitoring for Neurosurgical Procedures).
v. Burst suppression of EEG may be requested.
- If aneurysm reruptures.
- During temporary clipping of feeding vessels.
vi. Pay close attention to MAP during emergence.
- Perform neurologic exam when responsive.

5. **Craniotomy for seizure disorder.**
a. Pt considerations.
i. Seizures may be congenital; usually present in infancy or childhood.
ii. Seizures in infants and children can also be triggered by fever (febrile seizures).
iii. Adult-onset seizures are most commonly due to malignancy.
b. Anesthetic implications of seizure therapy.
i. Seizure medications may interact with anesthetic agents.
- Phenytoin (Dilantin).
- Levetiracetam (Keppra).
- Carbamazepine (Tegretol).
- Valproic acid.
c. Surgery for seizure disorders.
i. Offered to pts refractory to medical therapy.
ii. Hemispherectomy.
- Used to treat pts with severe epilepsy.
- Damaged cerebral hemisphere is removed.
iii. Corpus callosectomy.
- Used to treat children with severe epilepsy.
- Cuts fibers that connect the two cerebral hemispheres.
iv. Temporal lobectomy.
- Brain mapping is often performed prior to resection to identify area that triggers seizures.
- Requires separate surgical procedure to place mapping grid over cerebral cortex.

- Pt is monitored continuously for areas of brain activity during seizure.

7. Deep brain stimulation (DBS) for movement disorders.

a. Treatment for Parkinson disease or essential tremor.
   i.   Can reduce the magnitude of tremors.
b. Pt is placed in frame under MRI guidance ("stereotactic surgery").
c. Electrodes are placed into brain.
   i.   Usually thalamus, subthalamic nucleus, or globus pallidus.
   ii. Targeted area is stimulated to reduce tremor.
d. Neurostimulator device is implanted in chest wall (similar to pacemaker).
   i.   Battery in neurostimulator requires replacement periodically.
e. Thalamotomy or pallidotomy may be performed if pt is not a candidate for DBS.
   i.   Electrode is heated to ablate area associated with tremor, in lieu of stimulator placement.
f. Anesthesia for DBS.
   i.   Electrodes are placed into brain under LA.
   ii. Pt is awake to allow monitoring of tremor.
   iii. GA is induced for placement of neurostimulator into chest.
   iv. GA or IV sedation is used for battery changes.
g. Risks of DBS.
   i.   Agitation due to frame.
   ii. Artifact on ECG and pulse oximetry due to tremor.
   iii. Seizures.
   iv. Hemorrhage.
      - Can trigger seizure, altered mental status.
   v.   GA may be required for airway protection if seizure or hemorrhage occurs.

B.   ELECTROCONVULSIVE SHOCK THERAPY (ECT)

1. General.

a. Treatment for depression, bipolar disorder, and mania refractory to medical therapy.
b. Also used for the treatment of schizophrenia.
c. Electric current delivered to scalp in order to trigger a tonic-clonic seizure.
d. 30-sec seizure is therapeutic; treatment duration is 5 to 10 min.
e. Pts receive multiple treatments 2 to 3 times/wk.

2. Anesthesia for ECT.

a. General anesthesia via mask.
b. Short-acting induction agents used.
   i.   Methohexital: preferred; only barbiturate that lowers seizure threshold.
   ii. Propofol.
c. Succinylcholine is used as muscle relaxant.

     i.   Used to blunt magnitude of seizure.

     ii.   Half induction dose is given; do not want to block entire seizure.

d. Elderly pts and certain medications (lithium, anticonvulsants) may make seizure induction difficult.

e. Hyperventilation or caffeine administration can help to augment seizure response.

3. Potential contraindications to ECT.

a. Pt with space-occupying intracranial lesion.

     i.   ECT increases ICP.

b. Pts with cardiac disease should be cleared by cardiology prior to ECT.

     i.   Pacemakers are usually safe with ECT.

        • May need to be converted to fixed rate.

     ii.   Automatic internal cardiac defibrillators (ICD) may need to be deactivated prior to procedure.

        • If deactivated, will need continuous ECG monitoring and defibrillator pads attached until ICD reactivated.

c. Pregnancy.

     i.   Considered safe but may require fetal monitoring pre- and post-ECT.

4. Potential complications.

a. Prolonged seizure.

     i.   Benzodiazepines to halt seizure.

     ii.   Propofol will also halt seizure.

5. ECG changes.

a. Shock initially triggers parasympathetic response.

     i.   Can cause bradycardia or asystole.

     ii.   Usually short lived but may require atropine.

b. Secondary sympathetic response during and after seizure.

     i.   Tachycardia—may require beta blockers.

     ii.   Hypertension—may require therapy if persistent.

c. Sympathetic response can trigger myocardial ischemia in pts at risk.

6. Aspiration.

a. Airway not protected during seizure.

b. Increased secretions due to parasympathetic stimulation.

7. Muscle soreness.

a. Pts may experience muscle aches despite partial paralysis during ECT.

8. Nausea postprocedure.

a. Caused by stimulation of vagus nerve during ECT.

9. Soft-tissue injury.

a. Soft bite block used during procedure to protect pt from biting tongue or lips.

C. SPINAL SURGERY

1. Cervical spine surgery.

a. Performed for stenosis, disk herniation, and chronic pain.

b. May be performed via anterior, posterior, or combined approach.

10

NEUROANESTHESIA

    c. Consider staged extubation in ICU if combined approach (airway edema)
    d. Difficult airway common in these pts:
        i.   Unstable cervical spine.
        ii.   Rheumatoid arthritis, ankylosing spondylitis.
        iii. Neurologic deficits due to disease or trauma.
        iv. Presence of cervical collar or cervical traction.
    e. If arms are tucked during surgery, IV will be difficult to access.
    f. Anterior cervical fusion.
        i.   Consider in-line stabilization during intubation.
        ii.   Consider awake intubation if neck unstable or difficult airway.
        iii. Orogastric tube placement can help surgeons identify esophagus.
        iv. Cervical traction may be used by surgeons to improve exposure.
        v.   Neurologic monitoring, fluoroscopy may be used.
        vi. Potential complications.
            • Esophageal injury.
            • Recurrent laryngeal nerve injury.
            • Venous air embolism.
            • Airway edema due to retraction, external pressure on trachea.
            • Postoperative bleeding can cause airway compromise.
            • Reintubation may be challenging because of edema.
    g. Posterior cervical fusion.
        i.   Pt usually placed on chest rolls with head in pins.
        ii.   Ventilation may be difficult in obese pts.
        iii. Consider invasive BP monitoring because of positioning.
        iv. Swelling around airway more common than anterior approach.

2. Thoracolumbar spine surgery.

    a. Surgery performed for stenosis, scoliosis, nerve compression, chronic pain, tumors.
    b. Hardware may be placed to stabilize spine.
    c. Chronic pain with high narcotic requirements common.
    d. Blood loss can be significant.
        i.   Often multiple spinal levels involved.
        ii.   Scar tissue from previous fusions may be present.
        iii. Corpectomy (removal of vertebral body) can increase blood loss.
    e. Electromyelography or motor evoked-potential monitoring is often performed.
    f. Surgery performed in supine or prone position, or both.
        i.   High anterior thoracic procedures may require double-lumen tube to deflate lung for spinal exposure.
        ii.   Close attention to positioning is important for prone position to reduce risk of injury.
            • Arms may be tucked or at 90° on armboards.
            • Eyes and nose protected by open areas on special head pillows.
            • Vigilant checking during case to confirm no pressure on eyes.
            • Surgical beds (Jackson table, Wilson frame).
              - Designed to decrease pressure on abdomen.

. Spine tumors.
   i.   Most tumors to spine caused by metastatic disease.
- Intrinsic tumors: chordoma, meningioma, ependymoma.
   ii.   Anesthetic considerations.
- Assess preoperative neurologic deficit.
- Anticipate significant blood loss if metastatic tumor or AVM.
- Postprocedure neurologic exam required.
- Neurologic monitoring commonly used.
- If tumor in sacral region, special bed and positioning required.
- Andrews frame may be used to position pt with legs below sacrum for optimal exposure.
  - Venous pooling in legs can decrease cardiac output.

. Potential complications.
   i.   Coagulopathy due to significant blood loss.
   ii.   Venous air embolism (see below).
- Surgical field above heart.
- Vascular plexuses around spine can be difficult to control.
- Risk of injury to large blood vessels.
- Difficult to treat in prone pt.
   iii. Intraoperative hypotension or anemia.
- May decrease cord perfusion, resulting in postoperative neurologic deficits.
- May decrease perfusion to retina, resulting in postoperative blindness.
   iv. Prolonged prone position.
- Facial and airway edema may require postoperative intubation.
- Skin breakdown due to pressure points from positioning.

D. NEUROLOGIC TRAUMA SURGERY
1. Spinal trauma.
a. Spine can be injured by falls, MVA, or gunshot wounds.
b. Cervical spine is assumed to be injured after trauma until cleared.
c. Cervical spine precautions during intubation.
   i.   Do not remove cervical collar unless pt cleared by surgery.
   ii.   Use in-line cervical stabilization/traction during intubation.
   iii. Consider alternate methods of intubation that limit neck motion.
   iv. Avoid succinylcholine in spinal cord injury if >24 hr since injury.
- Risk of hyperkalemia.
  - Risk persists for several months after acute injury.
d. Close attention to MAP to maintain spinal cord perfusion.
e. Spinal shock may be present.
- Hypotension, vasodilation, flaccid paralysis below level of injury.
- Bradycardia, autonomic dysregulation if injury at T6 or higher.
- Hypoventilation, hypoxemia if cervical or high thoracic injury.
- Injury at C5 or higher may require urgent intubation.

f. Use of high-dose steroids controversial but common.
  i. 30 mg/kg bolus over 30 min.
  ii. 5.4 mg/kg/hr for 23 hr.
g. Autonomic hyperreflexia.
  i. Seen in chronic spinal cord injury at T6 or higher.
  ii. Can present within weeks to months of acute injury.
  iii. Spinal cord reflex due to stimulus below level of injury.
  iv. Triggers hypertension, bradycardia, vasodilation above level of injury, vasoconstriction below injury.
  v. Can be triggered by pain, bladder distention.
  vi. Treat hypertension, remove painful stimulus.
  vii. Important to provide adequate anesthesia during painful procedures.

2. Head trauma.
a. Hemorrhage.
  i. Epidural or subdural hemorrhage usually requires urgent surgery.
  ii. Arterial BP monitoring indicated for close MAP control.
  iii. Assume increased ICP: gentle intubation, hyperventilation.
  iv. Confirm that blood products are available.
  v. Assess for other injuries (C-spine, other fractures, abdominal injury).
  vi. Pts on anticoagulants at increased risk.
b. Closed head injury.
  i. Often treated expectantly in ICU.
  ii. May require decompressive craniectomy if ICP is elevated.
  iii. Hyperventilate to decrease CBF.
  iv. Mannitol and steroids to decrease cerebral edema.
  v. Severe cases may require barbiturate coma.

III. SPECIAL MONITORING FOR NEUROSURGICAL PROCEDURES

A. SOMATOSENSORY-EVOKED POTENTIALS (SSEP)
1. Monitors dorsal columns of the sensory spinal cord.
2. Peripheral sensory stimulus delivered through small needles.
3. Pt is used as own control; signals are compared every 10 min.
4. Time from stimulus to response (latency) and size of response (amplitude) are measured.
a. 50% change is considered significant.
b. Sensitive to high levels of inhalational anesthetics (>1 minimum alveolar concentration), >50% N_2O.
c. Commonly used in craniotomy and spine surgery.

B. MYOGENIC MOTOR-EVOKED POTENTIALS (MEP)
1. Measures the sensory component of the motor response (corticospinal tracts).
2. Used in high-risk spine surgery.
3. Stimulus is delivered over scalp; response is measured in periphery (arms and legs).

4. Pt is used as own control, signals run q 10 min.
5. Latency and amplitude are measured as with SSEP; 50% change is deemed significant.
6. Very sensitive to anesthetics; total IV anesthesia (TIVA) often preferred.
7. Requires incomplete or no paralysis (two to four muscle twitches).

C. EEG
1. Measures electric responses of cerebral cortex.
2. Indicator of global cerebral perfusion.
3. Commonly used in neurovascular surgery (aneurysm surgery).
4. Not significantly affected by anesthetics, provided that perfusion is maintained.
5. Burst suppression.
a. Suppression of EEG spikes is associated with decrease in global cerebral metabolic demand.
b. May be protective if vascular supply to brain is occluded.
c. May be requested during aneurysm surgery if temporary occlusion of cerebral artery is needed.
d. Propofol or etomidate may be used to achieve burst suppression.

D. ELECTROMYELOGRAPHY
1. Measures muscle responses.
a. Spontaneous firing of muscles that are innervated by nerves involved in surgery (e.g., spine surgery) is measured.
b. Also used to identify nerves (e.g., facial nerve during ear surgery) when surgeon is close to the nerve.
    i. Muscle response is detected when nerve is stimulated.
2. Requires incomplete or no paralysis (two to four muscle twitches via nerve stimulator).

E. BRAINSTEM AUDITORY-EVOKED RESPONSES
1. Monitor cranial nerve VIII (vestibuloacoustic nerve).
2. Used in acoustic neuroma resection surgery and brainstem surgery.
3. Auditory stimulus is delivered into ear; auditory waveforms are measured bilaterally q 10 min.
4. Not significantly affected by anesthetics.

F. VENOUS AIR EMBOLISM (VAE) MONITORING, PREVENTION, AND TREATMENT
1. Venous air embolism can occur when the pressure within an open vein is subatmospheric.
2. May exist in any position with any procedure when the wound is ≥5 cm above the right atria.
3. Low pressure in veins and large cerebral venous sinuses increase risk.

10

NEUROANESTHESIA

4. Consequences depend on volume, rate of air entry, and presence of a probe-patent foramen ovale.
5. Pathophysiology includes intense vasoconstriction of pulmonary circulation → ventilation/perfusion mismatch → interstitial pulmonary edema → reduced cardiac output.
6. Procedures with greatest risk of VAE are listed in Table 10.4.
7. Sources of critical VAE.
a. Major cerebral venous sinuses (transverse, sigmoid, posterior half of the sagittal sinus).
b. Emissary veins, near suboccipital musculature.
c. Diploic space of the skull (violated by both the craniotomy and pin fixation).
d. Cervical epidural veins.
8. Detection of VAE (Fig. 10.3).
9. Physiologic effects related to VAE volume and rate (Fig. 10.4).
10. Treatment of VAE.
a. Notify surgeon to flood or pack surgical field, or use bone wax to occlude air entry sites.
b. Lower the head of the pt.
c. Apply jugular compression.
   i. Bilateral jugular vein compression may ↑CVP, may slow air entrainment, and may cause back bleeding.
d. Discontinue N_2O if being used.
e. Administer 100% oxygen.
f. Infuse volume to increase CVP.
g. Aspirate via a right heart catheter if in place.
   i. Neurosurgical indications for right heart catheter.
      • All pts who undergo sitting posterior fossa.
      • Nonsitting positions, depending on procedure and the pt's physiologic reserve.
   ii. Catheter placement.
      • Place via jugular or brachial veins.
      • Position multi-orifice catheter tip 2 cm below the SVC-atrial junction.

TABLE 10.4	
PROCEDURES WITH GREATEST RISK OF VAE	
Procedure	Associated Risk
Posterior fossa procedures with pt in sitting position	40%
Posterior fossa procedures with pt in nonsitting positions	12%
Cervical laminectomy (dissection of suboccipital muscle may open emissary veins to the atmosphere)	<12%
Supratentorial procedures (parasagittal or falcine meningiomas near posterior half of the sagittal sinus; craniosynostosis procedures)	<12%
Pin sites and trapped gas under pressure	<1%

Most sensitive

☐ Transesophageal echocardiography
- Detects air bubbles as small as 0.25 mL.
- Has advantage of identifying right-to-left shunting of air.

☐ Precordial Doppler
- Placed over right atrium between the third and sixth ribs.
- Interruption of Doppler pulsation by sporadic roaring sounds indicates VAE.

☐ Pulmonary artery catheter
- Pressure increases proportionally to amount of air entrained.

☐ Expired CO_2 monitoring
- Decrease in E_TCO_2 proportional to increase in pulmonary dead space.

☐ Decrease in pulse oximetry

☐ Changes in BP and heart sounds (mill wheel murmur)

Least sensitive

FIG. 10.3

Detection of venous air embolism (VAE).

- Position single-orifice catheter with the tip 3 cm above the SVC-atrial junction.
  iii. Confirmation of catheter placement.
- Radiographic.
- Pull back from the RV while monitoring intravascular pressure.
- Intravascular ECG.
  - Increasing positivity as the developing P-wave vector approaches.
  - Increasing negativity as the wave of atrial depolarization passes and moves away from it.
h. Administer vasopressors and/or inotropes to improve cardiac output.
i. Use PEEP to increase CVP, but this may promote paradoxical embolism.
j. Persistent circulatory arrest necessitates the supine position and CPR.

11. Potential complications of VAE
a. Paradoxical air embolism.
  i. Usually only in the context of major air embolic events.

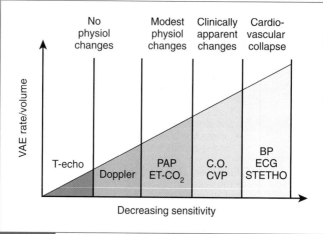

FIG. 10.4

Physiologic effects related to VAE volume and rate. CV, Cardiovascular; T-echo, transesophageal echocardiography; PAP, positive airway pressure; ETCO$_2$, end-tidal carbon dioxide; CO, cardiac output; CVP, central venous pressure; BP, blood pressure; ECG, electrocardiogram; STETHO, stethoscope. *(From Drummond JC, Patel PM: Neurosurgical anesthesia. In Miller RD: Miller's Anesthesia, 6th ed. Philadelphia: Churchill Livingstone, 2005. With permission.)*

    ii. May result in CVA or coronary artery occlusion.
    iii. Avoid PEEP, which may increase right atrial pressure greater than left.
    iv. Reduced by generous fluid administration.
  b. Transpulmonary passage of air.
    i. Usually with large volumes of air.
    ii. N$_2$O should be discontinued; air may reach the left-sided circulation through pulmonary vascular bed.

REFERENCES

Barash PG, Cullen BF, Stoelting RK: Clinical Anesthesia, Philadelphia: Lippincott Williams & Wilkins, 2006.

Miller RD: Miller's Anesthesia, Philadelphia: Churchill Livingstone, 2005.

Taylor S: Electroconvulsive therapy: A review of history, patient selection, technique, and medication management. South Med J 2007; 100(5):494–498.

Intraoperative Care for Specific Disorders and Procedures

Nadya Averback, MD, Jeffrey Bolka, MD, Rabi Panigrahi, MD, and Alok Sharma, MD
Edited by Jose M. Rodriguez-Paz, MD, and Kelly Grogan, MD

I. ANESTHETIC CONSIDERATIONS FOR PATIENTS WITH DRUG ADDICTION (Table 11.1)

A. WIDESPREAD PROBLEM THAT ESPECIALLY AFFECTS YOUNGER PATIENTS

11

B. DIFFICULT TO ASSESS—PTS MOST OF THE TIME HIDE THEIR ADDICTIONS OR UNDERESTIMATE THEIR INTAKE

C. ASSOCIATED WITH OTHER MEDICAL PROBLEMS
1. Hepatitis B and C.
2. HIV.
3. Malnutrition.
4. Difficult vein access.

D. IMPORTANT PREOPERATIVE QUESTIONS
1. What substance?
2. Route of administration?
3. Frequency?
4. Last use?

E. IF NOT EMERGENCIES, ALL CASES OF PTS WITH ACUTE INTOXICATION SHOULD BE POSTPONED

F. ALCOHOL
1. Alcoholism affects 15% of US population and 50% of these pts have problems related to alcohol consumption.
2. Acute alcohol use decreases minimum alveolar concentration (MAC) of GA.
a. Chronic use increases MAC.
3. Same trend is seen with other drugs used during GA: opioids, benzodiazepines, and barbiturates.
4. Chronic use affects liver function and all drugs metabolized by the liver (e.g., succinylcholine).
a. Liver dysfunction may affect the volume of distribution of any drug.
5. Other considerations in alcoholic pts.
a. Electrolyte abnormalities (hypokalemia, hyponatremia, hypoglycemia, etc.).
b. Macrocytic anemia.

TABLE 11.1

EFFECTS OF VARIOUS DRUGS ON MAC

	Acute Use	Chronic Use
Opioids	↓	↑
Cocaine	↓	↔
ETOH	↓	↑
Barbiturates	↑	↓
Benzodiazepines	↓	↓
Amphetamine	↑	↓
Cannabis	↓	unknown
Solvents	unknown	unknown

  c. Coagulopathy and thrombocytopenia.
  d. Dilated cardiomyopathy.
  e. Delirium tremens.

G. OPIOIDS
1. Prescribed opioids and heroin are commonly used drugs.
2. Chronic use requires higher doses of induction agents (especially barbiturates; less with propofol and volatile agents).
3. Risk for withdrawal when stopped abruptly (20% of daily requirements are needed to avoid withdrawal).

H. COCAINE
1. Cocaine can be used via multiple routes (not only the nose).
  a. Crack is derived from cocaine but is of greater purity.
2. Causes central and peripheral adrenergic stimulation.
  a. By inhibiting presynaptic reuptake of dopamine and noradrenaline and increasing levels of free catecholamines, all of which causes:
      i.   Myocardial ischemia.
      ii. Hypertensive crisis.
      iii. Dysrhythmias.
      iv. Alveolar hemorrhage.
      v.   Pulmonary edema.
      vi. Hepatic failure.
      vii. Disseminated intravascular coagulopathy (DIC).
3. Avoid using ephedrine (increases levels of norepinephrine) and selective β blockers because of their unopposed α effect (labetalol is recommended).
4. Halothane and isoflurane increase the risk of dysrhythmia.
5. Cocaine has an intrinsic muscular blockade property.

II. HEMATOLOGY
A. ANEMIA
1. The main function of RBCs is to transport oxygen from the lungs to the peripheral tissues, and that capacity is determined by the amount of Hb.

a. Once Hb reaches a critical threshold, any further decrease in Hb causes DO_2 to decrease and results in a decrease of VO_2 and hypoxia.

2. Definition anemia in adults.

a. Hb level <13.0 g/dL for men and <12.0 g/dL for women.

3. In the US, 4% of men and 8% of women are anemic.

4. Physiologic response to anemia.

a. Prior to changing cardiac output, the change in Hb produces decreases in the blood viscosity that cause increased blood flow.

b. Increase in cardiac output favors the coronary and cerebral circulations at the expense of the splanchnic vascular beds to maintain VO_2 (oxygen delivery).

c. Right shift in oxyhemoglobin dissociation curve and increased oxygen extraction ratio.

d. Increased diphosphoglycerate (2,3-DPG).

5. Anemia is more prevalent in older population (marked decrease in Hb after age 65), most likely secondary to decline in renal function.

6. 33% of pts have preoperative anemia (prevalence among surgical pts varies from 5% to 75%).

7. Etiology (the most common cause is blood loss due to injury or malignancy).

a. Hemorrhage.

b. Chronic disease.
   i. Renal disease.
   ii. Hepatic.
   iii. Chronic infections.
   iv. Malignancy (30%–90% of pts with cancer).
   v. Critical illness.

c. Infections.
   i. Hepatitis.
   ii. Mononucleosis.
   iii. CMV.
   iv. Malaria.
   v. Toxoplasmosis.
   vi. Clostridia.
   vii. Gram-negative sepsis.

d. Nutritional.
   i. Iron-deficiency anemia.
   ii. Vitamin B_{12} deficit.
   iii. Folate deficiency.
   iv. Malnutrition.

e. Genetic.
   i. Hemoglobinopathies.
   ii. Thalassemias.
   iii. Fanconi anemia.

f. Other causes of bleeding.
   i. Coagulopathy.
   ii. Recurrent phlebotomies while hospitalized.

    iii. Burns.

    iv. Prosthetic valves and surfaces.

    v. Drugs (aplastic anemia).

8. Anemia develops in the postoperative period (blunted erythropoietic response and perioperative blood losses) in a larger number of pts (>80%).

9. Linear association exists between decreased Hb levels and increased mortality and morbidity.

10. Preoperative and postoperative anemia and transfusion rates are associated with increased mortality, increased serious infection in the form of pneumonia, and increased lengths of stay.

11. A preoperative Hb level of <8 g/dL is associated with 16-fold increased mortality.

12. Postoperative infection increases up to 5.3% in direct proportion to the rate of transfusion, with most infections occurring in anemic pts, who receive five times more blood than nonanemic pts.

13. Transfusion of >4 units can increase the risk of infection ninefold and the risk of dying almost threefold.

14. Both postoperative anemia and the number of units of blood transfused correlate with length of stay, with a mean difference of 12 additional days for transfused versus nontransfused pts.

15. In cardiac pts, preoperative transfusion to correct anemia does not decrease perioperative mortality associated with anemia (anemia reflects an underlying process that must be addressed).

16. Diagnosis.

a. Origin of the anemia (losses, decreased production, or destruction of RBCs) may be confirmed by:

    i. Peripheral blood smear.

    ii. Reticulocyte count.

    iii. Folate level.

    iv. Serum iron and ferritin level.

    v. Serum haptoglobin level.

    vi. Bilirubin.

17. The main goal, based on available evidence, is to minimize the transfusion and maintain adequate intravascular volume perioperatively.

18. Alternatives to transfusion.

a. Recombinant human erythropoietin—a number of studies have documented that its use preoperatively significantly decreases the need for transfusion.

b. Iron/folate/vitamin B_{12}.

19. Pts with comorbidities, especially CV, are more susceptible to anemia, although it seems that it is not because of low Hb.

20. In pts with coronary artery disease (CAD), lower Hb level is an independent risk factor for death from associated compensatory changes.

a. Anemia increases myocardial oxygen consumption.
b. Owing to flow limitations, pts are unable to compensate.
21. Current practices follow more restrictive triggers for blood transfusion, unless pt has active CAD.
22. Indications for RBC transfusion.
a. Cardiac function must be a central consideration in decisions regarding transfusion in anemia.
b. In otherwise stable pts, if the Hb level is <7 g/dL.
c. In pts with CV disease, if the Hb level is <9 to 10 g/dL.
d. In bleeding pts, if anticipated blood loss will result in Hb level falling below the transfusion thresholds above.
e. In pts with symptomatic anemia.

B. COAGULATION FACTOR DEFICIENCIES
1. Coagulation defects during perioperative period are a considerable challenge for anesthesiologists.
2. Only traces of factor VII are needed to activate coagulation cascade.
3. Evaluation of the coagulation.
a. CBC.
b. ABO group.
c. PT and PTT.
d. Thrombin clotting time and fibrinogen.
e. von Willebrand disease screen (factor VIII, von Willebrand factor [vWF] antigen).
f. Platelet aggregation panel.
g. Renal, liver, and thyroid function tests.
4. For most coagulation factors, a minimum of 30% of their levels is required for normal function of the coagulation cascade.
5. Hemophilias A and B.
a. Factor VIII deficiency (hemophilia A) and factor IX deficiency (hemophilia B) are X-linked recessive diseases (hemophilia A, 1 : 5000 males; hemophilia B, 1 : 30,000).
b. Severe bleeding diatheses.
    i. Major risk during perioperative period.
c. Correction of deficiencies with the appropriate factor to obtain levels of 100% preoperatively has no impact on outcome.
d. Pts commonly develop neutralizing antibodies, making the replacement ineffective.
e. If bleeding does not respond to replacement, administer recombinant activated factor VII (raFVII).
6. Hemophilia C.
a. Factor XI deficiency.
b. Common among Ashkenazi Jewish population.
c. Autosomal pattern (1 : 1,000,000 births) both in males and females.

11

INTRAOPERATIVE CARE

   d. Normal level of activity ranges between 70% and 150%.
      i. Deficiency may be partial (activity 20%-70%) or severe (<15% activity).
   e. Normally, no spontaneous bleeding but increased risk of perioperative bleeding.
   f. Treatment.
      i. Plasma transfusion to achieve levels of activity of 30% to 45% (levels >70% may carry risk of perioperative thrombotic events).
   g. Inhibitors rarely occur.
   h. Consider also raFVII therapy.

7. von Willebrand disease.
   a. Most common inherited bleeding disorder (1% of the population).
   b. Autosomal-dominant inheritance.
   c. Type 1 (70%, quantitative defect).
   d. Type 2 (20%-25%).
      i. Type 2A.
         • Multimers are smaller than usual or break down easily.
      ii. Type 2B.
         • Factor sticks to platelets too well, leading to clumping of platelets, which can cause a low platelet number.
   e. Type 3 (rare, 1/500,000; but pts have no vWF levels).
      i. Because vWF transports factor VIII, pts also have very low levels of factor VIII.
         • Bleeding happens often and, if untreated, can be serious.
   f. Acquired von Willebrand disease.
      i. Fluoroquinolones.
      ii. Starches.
      iii. Hypothyroidism.
      iv. Uremia is associated with vWF defects.
      v. Aortic stenosis is associated with type 2A.
   g. Treatment.
      i. Type 1.
         • Desmopressin (DDAVP) 0.3 mcg/kg 90 min before surgery.
           - Risk for hyponatremia.
      ii. Types 2 and 3.
         • Factor VIII concentrates (contain vWF) or cryoprecipitate.

8. Factor V Leiden mutation.
   a. Most common inherited risk for thrombosis, although its relevance for perioperative thrombotic risk is unclear.
   b. Causes resistance to activated protein C.
   c. Mutation of arginine to glutamine in factor V.

9. Protein S deficiency.
   a. Important anticoagulant (cofactor of protein C).
   b. 1% to 7 % of the population.
   c. Deficiency causes thrombosis.
   d. Treatment—FFP.

10. Protein C deficiency.
a. Very important anticoagulant.
b. In 1:200 to 1:500 pts.
c. If homozygous, life-threatening thrombosis occurs.
d. Treatment—FFP.

C. DISSEMINATED INTRAVASCULAR COAGULATION

1. Activation of coagulation cascade, which leads to formation of thrombi and vessel occlusion (due to intravascular fibrin deposits), accompanied by consumption of platelets and coagulation factors, which leads to hemorrhage
2. Underlying conditions.
a. Trauma.
b. Sepsis.
c. Obstetric complications.
d. Malignancy.
e. Transfusion of incompatible blood products.
3. Physical examination.
a. Spontaneous bruising.
b. Extravasation from venipuncture sites.
c. Spontaneous hemorrhage (pulmonary, GI, intracranial).
4. Diagnosis—no single laboratory study; however, a conglomerate of several abnormal values points toward the diagnosis.
a. Prolonged clotting times.
b. Platelet count < 100,000.
c. Low fibrinogen.
d. Presence of fibrin-split products.
5. Clinical picture of vascular thromboses.
a. Developing gangrene.
b. Renal and hepatic failure.
c. Edema.
d. Hypotension.
6. Management.
a. Treat underlying disorder.
b. Supportive measures: ventilatory support, dialysis as necessary.
c. Platelets/FFP proven beneficial only in pts with low platelet counts and coagulation factors.
7. Carries high mortality rate and remains a treatment challenge.

D. SICKLE CELL ANEMIA

1. Genetic disorder characterized by the presence of Hemoglobin S (HbS).
2. Autosomal recessive disease (both parents with HbS or one parent with HbS and the other with other abnormal Hb).
3. Affects 1:375 blacks (0.5% are homozygous and 8% of blacks carry the trait) and 1:50,000 whites.

4. HbS differs from normal Hb (HbA) only in the substitution of valine for glutamic acid at the sixth position (β chain).
   a. Causes the affinity for oxygen to diminish ($P_{50} = 31$ mm Hg) and decreased solubility.
5. With deoxygenation, HbS polymerizes and precipitates in the red cell (crescent or sickle shape).
   a. The red cell eventually recovers but, with time, gets permanently damaged, and hemolysis occurs (anemia).
6. HbF (fetal) is protected from sickling.
7. Red cell survival is reduced to 10 to 15 days from the normal 120.
8. The sickling of the RBC causes:
   a. Obstruction of capillaries with tissue injury and microinfarctions (pain of soft tissues and bone, abdominal pain, acute chest pain, CV accident, priapism, renal dysfunction).
   b. Bacterial infection.
   c. Splenic sequestration.
   d. Aplastic crisis with profound anemia.
9. Diagnosis.
   a. Clinical suspicion and solubility test (exposure of pt blood to hypertonic solution).
10. Treatment.
   a. Normally detected in early stages of life.
   b. Avoid triggers: hypoxemia, acidosis, dehydration, hypothermia, and hyperthermia.
   c. Supportive treatment.
   d. Adequate analgesia.
11. Anesthesia management.
   a. Adequate oxygenation perioperatively.
   b. Euvolemia.
   c. Transfusion if needed (partial-exchange transfusion is an option), with goal hematocrit of 35% to 40% (50% of HbA).
   d. Avoid hypothermia, acidosis, hypotension, and/or hypovolemia.
   e. Avoid use of a tourniquet.

E. THROMBOCYTOPENIA
1. Definition: platelets < 150,000.
2. Most common cause of abnormal bleeding.
3. Normal cycle—1/3 of platelets are contained in the spleen, and platelets have a lifespan of 9 to 10 days.
   a. Every day, normally 15,000 to 45,000 platelets are produced per cubic milliliter of blood, or ~200 billion platelets per day, because of stimulation of bone marrow by thrombopoietin.
4. Etiology.
   a. Artifactual.
      i. Pseudothrombocytopenia (platelet clumping).
      ii. Giant platelets.

b. Production deficit.
   i. Megakaryocyte hypoplasia.
      • Leukemias.
      • Lymphomas.
      • Toxins (insecticides).
      • Medications (anticonvulsants, thiazides, chemotherapy, alcohol).
   ii. Ineffective thrombopoiesis.
      • Increase in megakaryocyte mass but low number of new platelets.
   iii. Hereditary thrombocytopenia.
      • May-Hegglin anomaly.
      • Wiskott-Aldrich syndrome.
c. Increased destruction.
   i. Acute idiopathic thrombocytopenic purpura (ITP).
      • Acute onset of thrombocytopenia, with platelet counts as low as 1000.
      • 80% of pts have history of recent viral infection.
      • 90% of cases resolve spontaneously.
   ii. Chronic ITP.
      • Platelet count ranges from 20,000 to 100,000.
      • Bone marrow biopsy may be useful to rule out other hematologic problems.
      • First-line treatment is steroids (clinical response starts within 48 hr).
      • Splenectomy should be considered in cases of ITP that are unresponsive to steroids with platelet counts < 10,000.
      • In life-threatening emergencies that require surgery, IV IgG can be administered followed by platelets.
      • ITP during pregnancy occurs in up to 10% of pregnancies.
        - Can cause bleeding in the fetus.
        - Can be treated with steroids of IgG.
d. Secondary to other factors and disease states.
   i. Infections (30% of septic pts).
   ii. Pregnancy.
   iii. Vascular disorders.
   iv. Drugs (heparin, gold salts, sulfa drugs, H_2 blockers, rifampin, carbamazepine, valproic acid) through an idiosyncratic reaction.
   v. Transfusion.
      • Post-transfusion purpura.
      • Massive transfusions.
   vi. Hypothermia.
   vii. Spleen disorders.
   viii. Microangiopathies.
   ix. DIC.
   x. TTP (treatment may require plasmapheresis, with 80% survival; alternative is to give FFP and avoid platelet transfusion).

11

INTRAOPERATIVE CARE

xi. Hemolytic uremic syndrome (common in children; linked to *E. coli* infection).

F. HEPARIN-INDUCED THROMBOCYTOPENIA (HIT)
1. Epidemiology.
a. 10% to 15% of pts receiving heparin (dose independent) and LMWH.
b. Up to 10% of pts will develop antibody associated with HIT without thrombocytopenia.

2. Etiology.
a. Two etiologic syndromes.
   i. HIT Type I.
      - 10% of pts.
      - Non-immune mediated.
      - Direct interaction of heparin with the platelet membrane, causing increased platelet aggregation.
      - Common after a few days of exposure.
      - Platelet count normally does not go below 100,000.
      - Resolves even in the presence of heparin.
   ii. HIT Type II.
      - 5% of pts.
      - Immune mediated.
      - More common with bovine lung heparin and unusual with LMWH (interacts less with PF4).
         - Heparin reacts with PF4 and forms complexes that bind antibodies (IgG), which bind platelet membrane receptors (FcγRIIA), causing platelet activation and a cascade of more platelet activation and thrombosis (white thrombosis syndrome).

3. Clinical presentation.
a. Type I HIT.
   i. Self-limited and no increased bleeding or thrombosis.
b. Type II HIT.
   i. Requires time to develop (4–20 days).
   ii. Commonly occurs between days 5 and 12 after exposure—or immediately if re-exposed.
   iii. Platelets <100,000 (rarely <20,000) or decreased by at least 30%.
   iv. Type II HIT is a thrombotic disorder; may result in:
      - Thrombosis (venous and arterial).
      - Embolism.
      - DIC.
      - Skin necrosis.
      - Myocardial infarction.
   v. Mortality in up to 30%.

4. Diagnosis.
a. Exclude other causes of thrombocytopenia.

b. No specific tests for Type I HIT.
  i. Demonstrate presence of heparin-dependent antibodies by platelet activation tests (antiheparin/PF4 antibodies are not specific for HIT).
  ii. Aggregation assay.
    • Uses donor platelets, pt serum, and heparin.
    • Sensitivity is low.
  iii. Serotonin release assay (SRA).
    • Uses donor platelets labeled with 14C-serotonin and heparin.
    • Sensitivity depends on control platelets used for assay (50%-80%).
    • Takes longer to obtain results.
  iv. ELISA assay for anti-PF4-heparin antibodies.
    • Sensitivity up to 90%.
    • A positive assay is not completely specific for HIT (up to 25% of pts during bypass have antibodies).
  v. It is recommended to run an aggregation assay and SRA or ELISA for definitive diagnosis.

5. Treatment.
a. Discontinuation of any type of heparin.
b. If anticoagulation is needed, other anticoagulants should be used.
  i. Argatroban.
  ii. Lepirudin.
  iii. Danaparoid.
c. LMWH should not be used because of cross-reactivity with the HIT antibody in 90% of cases.
d. If pt has history of HIT and requires CPB:
  i. Danaparoid and hirudin may be used.
  ii. If antibody is no longer detected, standard heparin can be used for the case.

III. ENDOCRINE SYSTEM

A. ADRENAL

1. Physiology.
a. The adrenal cortex produces glucocorticoids (cortisol), mineralocorticoids (aldosterone), and androgens (dehydroepiandrosterone and androstenedione).
b. Glucocorticoids both promote and inhibit gene transcription in many cells and organ systems.
  i. Cause anti-inflammatory actions and increased hepatic gluconeogenesis.
c. Mineralocorticoids regulate electrolyte transport across epithelial surfaces, particularly renal conservation of Na^+ in exchange for K^+.
d. Adrenal androgens' chief physiologic activity occurs after conversion to testosterone and dihydrotestosterone.
e. Adrenal medulla synthesizes and secretes catecholamines (epinephrine) and peptides (hormones).

11

INTRAOPERATIVE CARE

TABLE 11.2

RELATIVE POTENCY AND EQUIVALENT DOSES FOR COMMONLY
USED GLUCOCORTICOIDS

Steroids	Relative Glucocorticoid Potency	Equivalent Glucocorticoid Dose (mg)
SHORT-ACTING		
Cortisol (hydrocortisone)	1.0	20.0
Cortisone	0.8	25.0
Prednisone	4.0	5.0
Prednisolone	4.0	5.0
Methylprednisolone	5.0	4.0
INTERMEDIATE-ACTING		
Triamcinolone	5.0	4.0
LONG-ACTING		
Betamethasone	25.0	0.60
Dexamethasone	30.0	0.75

  f. Most deficiency syndromes affect output of all adrenocortical
      hormones.
      i.   Hypofunction may be primary (Addison disease) or secondary.
  g. Hyperfunction.
      i.   Glucocorticoids (Cushing syndrome) and aldosterone,
           (hyperaldosteronism) with overlapping features.
      ii. Excess quantities of epinephrine and norepinephrine are produced
           in pheochromocytomas.
  h. Relative potency and equivalent doses for commonly used
      glucocorticoids are listed in Table 11.2.

2. Addison disease.
  a. Hypofunctioning of the adrenal cortex.
  b. Symptoms are hypotension and hyperpigmentation.
  c. Can lead to adrenal crisis with CV collapse.
  d. Diagnosis is made by elevated plasma ACTH with low plasma cortisol.
  e. 70% of cases in the US are idiopathic (autoimmune processes).
  f. Hypoadrenocorticism may be induced by etomidate.
  g. Mineralocorticoids and glucocorticoids are deficient.
  h. Severe dehydration, plasma hypertonicity, acidosis, decreased
      circulatory volume, hypotension, and eventually, circulatory collapse.
  i. Hyperpigmentation is characterized by diffuse tanning of exposed skin.
  j. Glucocorticoid deficiency contributes to hypotension and produces
      severe insulin sensitivity and disturbances in carbohydrate, fat, and
      protein metabolism.
  k. Resistance to infection, trauma, and other stress is diminished.
  l. Adrenal crisis is characterized by profound asthenia; severe pain in the
      abdomen, lower back, or legs; peripheral vascular collapse; and finally,
      renal shutdown with azotemia.

m. Partial loss of adrenal function (limited adrenocortical reserve).
   i. Pts appear well but experience adrenal crisis when under physiologic stress (e.g., surgery, infection, burns, critical illness).
n. Elevated ACTH (≥50 pg/mL) with low cortisol (<5 mcg/dL [<138 nmol/L]) is diagnostic, particularly in pts who are severely stressed or in shock.
o. ACTH-stimulation testing in adults is performed by injecting cosyntropin (synthetic ACTH) 250 mcg IV or IM.
   i. Normal preinjection plasma cortisol ranges from 5 to 25 mcg/dL (138 to 690 nmol/L) and doubles in 30 to 90 min, reaching at least 20 mcg/dL (552 nmol/L).
p. For adults, 10 mg hydrocortisone PO is usually given in the morning, with half as much at lunchtime and again in the early evening.
   i. The total daily dose is usually 15 to 30 mg.
   ii. Additionally, fludrocortisones, 0.1 to 0.2 mg PO q d, is recommended to replace aldosterone.
q. Normal hydration and absence of orthostatic hypotension are evidence of adequate replacement therapy.
r. Adrenal crisis.
   i. Treatment.
      • Fluids.
      • Steroid replacement (100–150 mg hydrocortisone IV; then, 30–50 mg q 8 hr).
      • Inotropes as necessary.
      • Electrolyte correction.
s. Anesthetic considerations.
   i. Essential to ensure adequate steroid replacement therapy during the perioperative period.
   ii. If unstressed, glucocorticoid-deficient pts usually have no perioperative problems; they have acute adrenal crisis with minor stress.
   iii. Treatment of hypovolemia, hyperkalemia, and hyponatremia is important.
t. Guidelines for adrenal supplementation in adults are listed in Table 11.3.

3. Cushing syndrome.
a. Symptoms.
   i. Truncal obesity and skinny extremities.
   ii. Thin skin.
   iii. Easy bruising.
   iv. Striae.
   v. Muscle wasting.
   vi. Proximal muscle weakness.
   vii. Osteopenia.
   viii. Fluid retention and HTN.
   ix. Possibly also hyperglycemia.

11

INTRAOPERATIVE CARE

TABLE 11.3	
GUIDELINES FOR ADRENAL SUPPLEMENTATION THERAPY	
Medical or surgical stress	**Corticosteroid dosage**
MINOR	
Inguinal hernia repair	25 mg of hydrocortisone or 5 mg of
Colonoscopy	methylprednisolone IV on day of procedure
Mild febrile illness	only
Mild-to-moderate N/V	
Gastroenteritis	
MODERATE	
Open cholecystectomy	50–75 mg of hydrocortisone or 10–15 mg of
Hemicolectomy	methylprednisolone IV on day of procedure
Significant febrile illness	Rapid taper over 1–2 days to usual dose
Pneumonia	
Severe gastroenteritis	
SEVERE	
Major cardiothoracic surgery	100–150 mg of hydrocortisone or 25–30 mg
Whipple procedure	of methylprednisolone IV on day of procedure
Liver resection	Rapid taper to usual dose over next 1–2 days
Pancreatitis	

- b. Most common cause.
    - i. Administration of glucocorticoids.
- c. Anesthetic consideration.
    - i. Pts tend to be volume overloaded and have hypokalemic metabolic alkalosis.
    - ii. Spironolactone will stop the potassium loss and help to mobilize excess fluid.
    - iii. Preoperative weakness may indicate increased sensitivity to NMB agents.
    - iv. Bilateral adrenalectomy in pts with Cushing syndrome is associated with a high incidence of postoperative complications (mortality rate of 5%–10%).

4. Mineralocorticoid excess.

- a. Intrinsic causes.
    - i. Unilateral adenoma.
    - ii. Bilateral hyperplasia
    - iii. Carcinoma of adrenal gland.
    - iv. Primary hyperaldosteronism (Conn syndrome).
    - v. 0.5% to 1% of idiopathic hypertensive pts.
- b. Clinical presentation.
    - i. Potassium depletion.
    - ii. Sodium retention.
    - iii. Muscle weakness.
    - iv. HTN.
    - v. Tetany.

     vi. Polyuria.

     vii. Inability to concentrate urine.

     viii. Hypokalemic alkalosis.

c. Treatment.

     i. Spironolactone causes intravascular fluid volume, electrolyte concentrations, and renal function to be restored to normal limits.

5. Pheochromocytoma.

a. <0.1% of all cases of HTN.

b. 25% to 50% of hospital deaths in pts with pheochromocytoma occur during induction of anesthesia or during operative procedures.

c. These tumors may be found anywhere.

     i. 10% to 15% are malignant.

     ii. 10% to 15% are bilateral.

     iii. 10% are extra-adrenal.

d. Localization of tumors can be achieved by (in decreasing order of combined sensitivity and specificity) MRI or CT scans, metaiodobenzylguanidine (MIBG) nuclear scanning, ultrasonography, or IV pyelography studies.

e. Paroxysmal headache, sweating, and HTN are the most sensitive and specific indicators of the disease.

f. Preoperative evaluation and preparation.

     i. Adrenergic block and volume replacement.

- α-Adrenergic receptor blockers (prazosin or phenoxybenzamine).
  - Reduce complications of hypertensive crisis and myocardial dysfunction.
- α-Adrenergic receptor blockade restores plasma volume, often followed by a decrease in hematocrit.
  - Phenoxybenzamine for adults is usually started in doses of 20 to 30 mg/70 kg orally once or twice per day (60–250 mg/day).
- Administer β-adrenergic receptor blockade (propranolol) if persistent dysrhythmias or tachycardia.
  - DO NOT use β-adrenergic receptor blockade without concomitant α-adrenergic receptor blockade.
- Clinical end points of therapy.
  - BP < 165/90 mm Hg (48 hr before surgery).
  - Orthostatic hypotension (not <80/45 mm Hg).
  - No ST-T changes or significant dysrhythmias on ECG.

g. Anesthesia considerations.

     i. Avoid hypotension or increased sympathetic outflow (may lead to adrenergic crisis).

- Painful or stressful events such as intubation may result in an exaggerated stress response.

     ii. Desflurane may precipitate non-neurogenic catecholamine release.

     iii. Vasoactive agents are used to treat hypotension and hypertension.

     iv. Use labetalol for severe tachycardia.

11

INTRAOPERATIVE CARE

v.   Blood glucose should be monitored frequently.
vi. Usually after the venous supply is secured and pt is euvolemic, BP returns to normal values.
  • In some cases, hypotension may occur, requiring infusions of catecholamines.
vii. Postoperatively, 50% of pts remain hypertensive for 1 to 3 days.
viii. ICU care is usually required in the postoperative period.

B. DIABETES MELLITUS
1. Pathophysiology.
a. Relative or absolute lack of insulin.
b. Multitude of hormone-induced metabolic abnormalities, resulting in diffuse microvascular lesions and long-term end-organ complications.
2. Diagnosis.
a. Diagnosed by a fasting blood glucose level >125 mg/dL (7.0 mmol/L).
b. Impaired glucose tolerance is diagnosed if the fasting level is <125 mg/dL (7.0 mmol/L) but >110 (6.1 mmol/L).
c. Plasma insulin levels are normal or elevated in type 2 diabetics but are relatively low for the level of blood glucose.
d. Types (both share similar end-organ abnormalities).
  i.   Type 1 is associated with autoimmune diseases.
    • Pt is insulin deficient and susceptible to ketoacidosis if insulin is withheld.
  ii. Type 2 (accounts for >90% of the over 18 million diabetics in the US).
    • Peripheral insulin resistance.
    • Susceptibility to the development of a hyperglycemic-hyperosmolar nonketotic state.
  iii. Gestational diabetes develops in >2% of all pregnancies and increases the risk for type 2 diabetes to 17% to 63% within 15 years.
e. Acute presentations.
  i.   Diabetic ketoacidosis.
    • Insulin therapy is initiated with insulin 0.3 Units/kg IV bolus, followed by continuous insulin infusion.
    • During the first 1 to 2 hr of fluid resuscitation, glucose level may fall precipitously.
    • When serum glucose reaches 250 mg/dL, IV fluid should include 5% dextrose.
    • Volume of fluid required for therapy in adults varies with overall deficit, ranging from 3 to 5 L, and may be as high as 10 L.
    • Monitor sodium levels.
      - Plasma sodium concentration decreases by ~1.6 mEq/L for every 100 mg/dL increase in plasma glucose above normal.
      - ~1/3 of the estimated fluid deficit is corrected during the first 6 to 8 hr, and the remaining 2/3 is corrected over the next 24 hr.

- The degree of acidosis is determined by measurement of ABGs and detection of an increased anion gap.
- Persistent ketosis with a serum bicarbonate <20 mEq/L in the presence of a normal glucose concentration is an indication of the continued need for intracellular glucose and insulin for reversal of lipolysis.
- Depletion of potassium may occur in diabetic ketoacidosis, with deficits ranging from 3 to 10 mEq/kg body weight.

ii. Hyperosmolar, non-ketotic hyperglycemia.
- Glucose >500 mg/dL with osmotic diuresis and hypovolemia and altered sensorium.
- Unlike ketoacidosis, insulin is sufficient to avoid ketosis.
- Treatment.
  - Volume resuscitation with NS.
  - Insulin infusion and electrolyte replacement.

3. Treatment.
a. Exercise and diet.
  i. For type 2 diabetes.
     - Associated with normalization of fasting blood glucose levels and delay of glucose intolerance in >50% of subjects.
b. Oral hypoglycemic medications.
  i. Stimulate the release of insulin by pancreatic β cells and improve tissue responsiveness to insulin.
     - Tolazamide (Tolinase) and tolbutamide (Orinase).
     - Sulfonylureas.
       - Glyburide (Micronase), glipizide (Glucotrol), and glimepiride.
     - Metformin.
       - Decreases hepatic glucose output and may increase peripheral responsiveness to glucose.
       - Associated with lactic acidosis if pt becomes dehydrated.
     - Acarbose.
       - Decreases glucose absorption.
     - Thiazolidinediones (rosiglitazone and pioglitazone).
       - Increase peripheral responsiveness to insulin.
c. Insulin (Table 11.4).
  i. Increasingly more pts are arriving to the OR with implantable insulin pumps; thus, it is imperative to know their settings and normal blood sugar levels.

4. Anesthesia considerations.
a. Surgical mortality rates in the diabetic population are on average higher than rates in the nondiabetic population.
  i. Blood sugars >250 mg/dL are more likely to be associated with adverse outcomes.
b. The major risk factors for diabetics undergoing surgery are related to the end-organ diseases associated with diabetes.
  i. CV dysfunction.

11

INTRAOPERATIVE CARE

TABLE 11.4			
INSULIN PHARMACOKINETICS			
Agent	Onset (hr)	Peak Effect (hr)	Duration (hr)
SHORT-ACTING			
Lispro (Humalog)	≤0.25	1–2	4–6
Aspart (NovoLog)	≤0.25	1–2	4–6
Regular	0.25	2–4	6–10
Glulisine (Apidra)	≤0.25	1–2	4–6
INTERMEDIATE-ACTING			
NPH	0.5–3	6–12	12–18
Lente	2–4	6–15	22–28
LONG-ACTING			
Ultralente	1–6	10–30	≥36
Glargine (Lantus)	2–8	No peak	20–24
Detemir (Levemir)	2–4	No peak	20–22

   ii. Renal insufficiency.
   iii. Periperal neuropathies.
   iv. Joint abnormalities ("stiff joint syndrome").
- Limitation in neck extension and decreased atlantoaxial mobility may increase risk of difficult airway.
- Pt inability to approximate palms and fingers together (called the "prayer sign") may indicate potential difficult intubation.
   v. Gastroparesis increases risk of aspiration.
   vi. Autonomic dysfunction.
- 20% to 40% of diabetics.
- Orthostatic changes in BP, loss of normal respiratory variations of HR, and resting tachycardia.
- Typical clinical findings of myocardial ischemia/infarction absent.
- Intraoperative BP lability, hypothermia, and increased risk of sudden cardiorespiratory arrest.

  c. Preoperative insulin/hypoglycemic agent management.
   i. Basal insulin requirements should be continued (1/2–2/3 of usual insulin dose as intermediate insulin the evening before surgery and in the morning of surgery).
   ii. Oral agents should be held the day of surgery.
- Metformin should be stopped 48 hr prior to surgery, especially if pt has altered renal function.

5. Intraoperative blood glucose management.
  a. Goal: To safely achieve a serum glucose level <180 mg/dL with either SQ insulin aspart or IV regular insulin.
   i. Tight postoperative glycemic control that maintains blood glucose in the range of 80 to 120 mg/dL is being studied to determine association with decreased mortality when compared with traditional, less aggressive glucose management.

b. Pts require frequent blood glucose monitoring and treatment of hyperglycemia.
c. Pts who would benefit from IV insulin management (vs. SQ administration) have **EITHER**:
   i. ONE of the following clinical scenarios:
      - Pt is significantly edematous, resulting in poor/unreliable SQ absorption.
      - Pt is on high-dose inotropes, resulting in poor/unreliable SQ absorption.
      - Pt has failed SQ management (two glucose values greater than 4 hr apart, with glucose >220 mg/dL).
   ii. **OR** TWO or more of the following clinical scenarios:
      - Is an insulin-dependent diabetic.
      - Is undergoing partial or complete pancreatectomy.
      - Is undergoing surgical procedure in which large volume shifts are anticipated.
      - Initial glucose is >250 mg/dL.
      - Has an SCII pump that will be turned off during procedure.
      - Will be admitted to the ICU postoperatively.
d. IV Insulin infusion guidelines (Table 11.5).
   i. Insulin adjustments should be based on observed changes in glucose levels rather than on absolute glucose level.
   ii. When deciding how much to adjust infusion rate, it is important to consider the rate of glucose change, the absolute level of glucose, and the infusion rate.
      - For example, a pt with an insulin infusion rate of 10 U/hr whose glucose has decreased from 200 mg/dL to 130 mg/dL will have a different treatment than a pt who is also on 10 U/hr but whose glucose has dropped from 140 mg/dL to 130 mg/dL.
      - The absolute level of glucose is not the sole determinant; trends and clinical judgment must be used.
   iii. Bolus dosing of insulin is at physician discretion, with recommended dosages provided in the insulin titration algorithms (Table 11.5).
   iv. Insulin drips, in general, should not be increased by more than 5 U in any given hour.
   v. All insulin infusions must be administered via an infusion pump, using low absorbing tubing.
   vi. Suggested insulin concentration is 1 U/mL.
   vii. Because it can absorb insulin, the IV tubing should be primed with 20 mL of the insulin infusion, clamped for 10 min, and flushed through and discarded before starting the infusion.
   viii. The IV rate and dosage should be verified by a second anesthesia provider upon initiation of the infusion and with any rate changes or boluses.

11

INTRAOPERATIVE CARE

TABLE 11.5

INTRAVENOUS INSULIN MANAGEMENT GUIDELINES FOR ADULTS

Insulin Loading Doses and Initial Infusion Rate

Glucose (mg/dL)	Recommended Action	
	Loading Dose (units)	Infusion Rate (units/hr)
>300	8	5–6
271–300	6	4–5
241–270	4	3–4
211–240	2	2–3
181–210	0	1–2
150–180	0	0.5–1

Insulin Doses for Infusion Titration Based on Hourly Glucose Monitoring (i.e., after patient is already on drip)

Glucose (mg/dL)	Rising Glucose (units)		Falling Glucose	
	Re-bolus	Increase Rate	Hold Infusion (min)	Decrease Rate (%)
>350	6	3–4	—	0
301–350	4	2–3	—	0
251–300	3	2–3	—	0
201–250	2	1–2	—	0–10
161–200	0	1–2	—	0–25
121–160	0	No change	0–30	0–50
81–120	0	No change	0–60	50–75
61–80	0	No change	60	75–100
<60	• Stop Infusion • Administer ½ amp D50 • Recheck glucose in 20 min			
If glucose remains <60	• Administer 1/2 amp D50 • Start glucose infusion of D10 at 10 mL/hr • Recheck glucose every 20 min until glucose >60 mg/dL • Once >60, recheck q 1 hr × 3			

NOTE: This algorithm is provided as a **guideline only**. Physicians should use their experience and clinical judgment in titrating the insulin drip to achieve the glucose goal.

ix. Serum glucose levels must be checked at least every hour while pt is on infusion.

x. Insulin dose should not be increased more frequently than every hour.

xi. Serum glucose levels should not be drawn from any line containing a dextrose-containing solution.

xii. Consider rechecking serum glucose if a significant increase from previous glucose value is observed when no significant management change (i.e., steroid administration or initiation of inotropes) has occurred prior to treatment.

xiii. DO NOT DELAY TREATMENT OF HYPOGLYCEMIA OR SUSPECTED HYPOGLYCEMIA FOR CONFIRMATION BY SERUM GLUCOSE LABORATORY VALUE.

TABLE 11.6

SUBCUTANEOUS INSULIN MANAGEMENT IN ADULTS

Glucose Value (mg/dL)	Aspart Insulin Dosage (units)
61–150	None
151–190	2
191–230	4
231–270	6
271–310	8; consider using insulin drip
311–350	10; consider using insulin drip
>350	12; consider using insulin drip

e. SQ insulin infusion guideline (Table 11.6).
   i. Blood serum glucose levels can be obtained from intravascular catheter, venipuncture, or finger stick.
   ii. If blood is drawn from an indwelling vascular catheter, ensure that it does not have a glucose-containing solution.
   iii. Check glucose levels at least every 4 hr.
   iv. SQ insulin administration should not occur any more frequently than every 4 hr, to avoid insulin stacking.
f. Management of hypoglycemia in ALL pts.
   i. Do not delay treatment of hypoglycemia or suspected hypoglycemia while waiting for laboratory value confirmation.
   ii. If glucose falls below 60 mg/dL:
      • Discontinue any insulin management.
      • Administer 1/2 amp D50.
      • Recheck glucose in 20 min.
   iii. If glucose remains <60 mg/dL:
      • Administer 1/2 amp D50 (25 g).
      • Start glucose infusion of D10 at 10 mL/hr.
      • Ensure that no other source of insulin is being administered.
      • Recheck glucose every 20 min until glucose is >60 mg/dL.
      • Once glucose is >60 mg/dL, recheck q 1 hr for 3 hr.

C. THYROID DISEASES
1. Physiology.
a. Thyrotropin-releasing hormone (TRH) is secreted from the hypothalamus and passes via the portal system to the anterior pituitary, where thyroid-stimulating hormone (TSH) synthesis and release are stimulated.
b. The glycoprotein TSH then stimulates receptors on the thyroid gland.
c. The active form of thyroid hormone is triiodothyronine (T_3), which is mainly produced in peripheral tissues from the hormone thyroxine (T_4) (via specific nuclear receptors).
d. T_3 and T_4 are bound to proteins and stored within the thyroid.

11

INTRAOPERATIVE CARE

e. Several drugs inhibit thyroid peroxidase, notably propylthiouracil (PTU), methimazole, and carbimazole.

    i. PTU also has peripheral actions (inhibits 5'-deiodinase), which methimazole and carbimazole do not have.

f. Thyroid function tests.

    i. The best test is to check TSH levels, which are often high or low long before clinical correlates of hypothyroidism or hyperthyroidism are noted.

    ii. In most laboratories, a normal TSH is in the range of ~0.3–5 mIU/L.

2. Hyperthyroidism (thyrotoxicosis).

a. Hypermetabolism and elevated serum levels of free thyroid hormones.

b. Etiology.

    i. Graves disease (toxic diffuse goiter).

    ii. Toxic multinodular goiter.

    iii. Thyroiditis.

    iv. Inappropriate TSH secretion.

    v. Molar pregnancy.

    vi. Choriocarcinoma.

    vii. Hyperemesis gravidarum.

c. Clinical presentation.

    i. Tachycardia.

    ii. Fatigue.

    iii. Weight loss.

    iv. Tremor.

    v. Many common symptoms and signs of hyperthyroidism are similar to those of adrenergic excess.

d. Infiltrative ophthalmopathy is specific to Graves disease and can occur years before or after hyperthyroidism.

e. Diagnosis is clinical and with thyroid function tests.

f. Thyroid storm.

    i. Acute form of hyperthyroidism precipitated by infection, trauma, surgery, embolism, diabetic ketoacidosis, or toxemia of pregnancy.

    ii. Abrupt florid symptoms of hyperthyroidism with one or more of the following.

        • Fever.

        • Marked weakness and muscle wasting.

        • Extreme restlessness with wide emotional swings.

        • Confusion.

        • Psychosis.

        • Coma.

        • N/V.

        • Diarrhea.

        • Hepatomegaly with mild jaundice.

    iii. The pt may present with CV collapse and shock.

    iv. Thyroid storm is a life-threatening emergency that requires prompt treatment.

g. Treatment.
   i. Treatment depends on cause.
   ii. Iodine.
      - Iodine in pharmacologic doses inhibits the release of T_3 and T_4 within hours and inhibits the organification of iodine (a few days to a week).
      - For emergency management of thyroid storm, for hyperthyroid pts undergoing emergency nonthyroid surgery, and (because it decreases the vascularity of the thyroid) for preoperative preparation of hyperthyroid pts undergoing subtotal thyroidectomy.
      - Usual adult dosage is two to three drops (100–150 mg) of a saturated potassium iodide solution PO tid or qid or 0.5 to 1 g sodium iodide in 1 L 0.9% saline solution given IV slowly q 12 hr.
   iii. Propylthiouracil and methimazole block thyroid peroxidase, decreasing the organification of iodide and impairing the coupling reaction.
      - Usual starting adult dose of propylthiouracil is 100 to 150 mg PO q 8 hr.
      - Usual starting adult dose of methimazole is 5 to 20 mg tid.
      - Higher doses are used for thyroid storm.
   iv. β blockers.
      - Propranolol improves tachycardia, tremor, mental symptoms, heat intolerance, and sweating.
      - Do not affect thyroid gland function but do decrease the peripheral conversion of T_4 to T_3.
h. Treatment of thyroid storm (adults).
   i. Iodine.
      - Five drops saturated solution of potassium iodide PO tid or 10 drops Lugol solution PO tid.
      - **OR** 1 g sodium iodide slowly by IV drip over 24 hr.
      - **OR** iopanoic acid 0.5 g bid.
   ii. Propylthiouracil (adult dose).
      - 600 mg PO given before iodine, then 400 mg q 6 hr.
   iii. Propranolol (adult doses).
      - 40 to 80 mg PO qid.
      - Rapid treatment—1 mg/min IV, max 10 mg, under close monitoring; may repeat in 4 to 6 hr.
   iv. Supportive treatment for all other symptoms and treatment of underlying disease, such as infection.
   v. Corticosteroids (adult dose).
      - 100 mg hydrocortisone IV q 8 hr or dexamethasone 8 mg IV once/day.
   vi. Definitive therapy after control of the crisis consists of ablation of the thyroid with ^{131}I or surgical treatment.
i. Anesthetic considerations.

11

INTRAOPERATIVE CARE

i. Preoperative.
  - All elective surgical procedures, including subtotal thyroidectomy, should be postponed until pt is rendered euthyroid with medical treatment.
  - Assessment should include H&P, and thyroid function test.
  - Antithyroid medications and β-adrenergic antagonists are continued through the morning of surgery.

ii. Intraoperative.
  - No anesthetic drug has advantage over any other for surgical pts who are hyperthyroid.
  - CV function and body temperature should be closely monitored.
  - Eyes of pts with exophthalmos should be well protected.
  - Pt with large goiter can be handled in the same way as any other pt with difficult airway management.
  - Thiopental may be the induction agent of choice, as it possesses antithyroid activity.
  - Avoid sympathetic stimulants (ketamine, pancuronium).
  - Hyperthyroid pts sometimes can be chronically hypovolemic, vasodilated, and prone to exaggerated hypotension with induction.
  - Hyperthyroidism does not increase anesthetic requirements.
  - Thyrotoxicosis is sometimes associated with an increased incidence of myopathies and myasthenia gravis.
    - Muscle relaxants should be used cautiously.
  - Regional anesthesia may be beneficial in thyrotoxic pts.
    - **AVOID** epinephrine.

iii. Postoperative.
  - Postoperative complications.
    - Thyroid storm.
    - Bilateral recurrent nerve trauma.
    - Hypocalcemic tetany.
    - Bleeding.
    - Nerve injuries.
    - Metabolic abnormalities.
  - Recurrent laryngeal nerve palsy will result in hoarseness (unilateral) or stridor (bilateral) and laryngeal obstruction as a result of unopposed adduction of the vocal cord and closure of the glottic aperture.
    - Unilateral recurrent nerve injury often goes unnoticed because of compensatory over-adduction of the normal cord.
  - Hypoparathyroidism may result from unintended removal of the parathyroid glands.
    - Symptoms of acute hypocalcemia usually manifest within 24 to 72 hr.
  - Hematoma formation may cause airway compromise.
    - Immediate treatment includes opening the neck wound and evacuating the clot.
    - Early intubation is usually warranted.

3. Hypothyroidism.

a. Thyroid hormone deficiency.
   i. Occurs in ~10% of women and ~6% of men >65.
   ii. Difficult to diagnose in elderly pts.
b. Primary hypothyroidism.
   i. TSH is increased.
   ii. The most common cause is probably autoimmune, from Hashimoto thyroiditis.
   iii. Also common after radioactive iodine therapy or surgery for hyperthyroidism or goiter.
   iv. Iodine deficiency decreases thyroid hormonogenesis.
      • TSH is released and goiter results.
   v. Endemic cretinism is the most common cause of congenital hypothyroidism in severely iodine-deficient regions.
c. Secondary hypothyroidism.
   i. Hypothalamus produces insufficient TRH, or the pituitary produces insufficient TSH.
d. Clinical presentation.
   i. Often subtle and insidious.
   ii. Cold intolerance.
   iii. Constipation.
   iv. Forgetfulness.
   v. Personality changes.
   vi. Modest weight gain (secondary to fluid retention and decreased metabolism).
   vii. Paresthesias of the hands and feet are common by deposition of proteinaceous ground substance in the ligaments around the wrist and ankle.
   viii. Menorrhagia or secondary amenorrhea in women.
   ix. Facial expression is dull, voice is hoarse, and speech is slow; facial puffiness and periorbital swelling, hair is sparse, coarse, and dry; skin is coarse, dry, scaly, and thick.
   x. Relaxation phase of deep tendon reflexes is slowed.
   xi. Hypothermia is common.
   xii. Dementia or psychosis (myxedema madness) may occur.
   xiii. Deposition of proteinaceous ground substance in the tongue may produce macroglossia.
   xiv. Bradycardia due to decrease in both thyroid hormone and adrenergic stimulation.
   xv. Pericardial, pleural, or abdominal effusions may be found.
   xvi. Myxedema coma.
      • Life-threatening complication of hypothyroidism.
      • Usually occurs in pts with a long history of hypothyroidism.
      • Coma with extreme hypothermia (temperature 24°–32.2°C), areflexia, seizures, and respiratory depression with CO_2 retention.
      • Rapid diagnosis based on clinical judgment.

11

INTRAOPERATIVE CARE

- H&P is imperative because death is likely without rapid treatment.
- Precipitating factors include illness, infection, trauma, drugs that suppress the CNS, and exposure to cold.
e. Diagnosis.
  i. Serum TSH is the most sensitive test.
  ii. In primary hypothyroidism, serum TSH is always elevated, and serum free T_4 is low.
  iii. In secondary hypothyroidism, free T_4 and serum TSH are low (sometimes, TSH is normal but with decreased bioactivity).
  iv. Circulating levels of T_3, are near normal; therefore serum T_3 is not sensitive for hypothyroidism.
  v. Anemia is often present.
  vi. Serum cholesterol is usually high in primary hypothyroidism but less so in secondary hypothyroidism.
f. Treatment.
  i. Thyroid hormone replacement.
    - Synthetic preparations of T_4 (L-thyroxine) and T_3 (liothyronine combinations of the two synthetic hormones and desiccated animal thyroid extract).
  ii. L-thyroxine is preferred.
    - Average maintenance dose is 75 to 125 mcg PO once/day.
    - Therapy is begun with low doses, especially in the elderly—usually 25 mcg once/day.
    - Dose is adjusted q 6 wk until maintenance dose is achieved.
    - Maintenance dose may need to be decreased in elderly pts and increased in pregnant women.
  iii. Secondary hypothyroidism.
    - L-Thyroxine should not be given until evidence is seen of adequate cortisol secretion (or cortisol therapy is given) because L-thyroxine could precipitate adrenal crisis.
  iv. Myxedema coma.
    - Large initial dose of T_4 (300–500 mcg IV) or T_3 (25–50 mcg IV).
    - Maintenance dose of T_4 is 75 to 100 mcg IV once/day.
    - Maintenance dose of T_3 is 10 to 20 mcg IV bid until T_4 can be given orally.
    - Corticosteroids are also given because the possibility of central hypothyroidism usually cannot be initially ruled out.
    - Pt should not be rewarmed rapidly, as this may precipitate hypotension or dysrhythmias.
    - Because hypoxemia is common, PaO_2 should be monitored.
    - The precipitating factor should be rapidly and appropriately corrected.
    - All drugs should be given cautiously because they are metabolized more slowly than in healthy people.
g. Anesthetic considerations.

i. Preoperative.
  - Euthyroid state is ideal for elective procedures, though mild-to-moderate hypothyroidism does not appear to be an absolute contraindication.
  - Pts with severe hypothyroidism or myxedema coma should not undergo elective surgery.
  - Administer normal dose of levothyroxine on the morning of surgery.
  - Do not use high doses of sedation.
  - Delayed gastric emptying remains an issue; due consideration should be given.

ii. Intraoperative.
  - Pt may present a difficult airway because of a large tongue.
  - Drug metabolism is anecdotally reported to be slow.
  - Increased susceptibility to hypotensive effect of anesthetic agents (blunted baroreceptor reflex) is possible.
  - Addison disease is more common in hypothyroidism.
    - These pts are treated with stress dose of corticosteroids perioperatively.
  - Decreased cardiac output may slow induction with IV agents.
  - Because body heat mechanisms are inadequate in these pts, temperature should be monitored and maintained.

iii. Postoperative.
  - Recovery from GA may be delayed in these pts; they often require prolonged mechanical ventilation.
  - Nonopioid analgesics are advocated in view of risk of respiratory depression.

IV. LIVER

A. ACUTE HEPATOCELLULAR INJURY
1. Can be due to viral infection (hepatitis A-E, Epstein-Barr virus, cytomegalovirus, herpes simplex virus), drugs (alcohol, phenytoin, acetaminophen), and inborn errors of metabolism (Wilson disease and α_1-antitrypsin deficiency).

B. CHRONIC PARENCHYMAL DISEASE
1. Can lead to cirrhosis, which may be due to chronic active hepatitis, alcoholism, hemochromatosis, primary biliary cirrhosis, or some congenital disorders.

C. HYPERBILIRUBINEMIA IS AN IMPORTANT MARKER FOR HEPATOBILIARY DISEASE
1. Unconjugated hyperbilirubinemia is due to excess bilirubin production (massive transfusion or hemolysis) or impaired uptake of unconjugated bilirubin by the hepatocyte (Gilbert syndrome).

2. Conjugated hyperbilirubinemia generally occurs with hepatocellular disease (alcoholic or viral hepatitis, cirrhosis), disease of the small bile ducts (primary biliary cirrhosis, Dubin-Johnson syndrome), or obstruction of the extrahepatic bile ducts (gallstones, pancreatic carcinoma, cholangiocarcinoma).

D. CHOLESTASIS IS USUALLY DUE TO CHOLELITHIASIS
1. Other less frequent causes are primary biliary cirrhosis and primary sclerosing cholangitis.

E. END-STAGE HEPATIC DISEASE
1. End-stage hepatic disease eventually leads to portal HTN and esophageal varices.
2. Complications of portal HTN and decreased hepatic function include ascites, coagulopathy, GI bleeding, and encephalopathy.
3. Surgical procedures to reduce manifestations of portal HTN are:
a. Orthotopic liver transplantation.
b. Splenorenal shunt.
c. Transjugular intrahepatic portocaval shunt.
d. LeVeen shunt.
4. Advanced hepatic dysfunction can produce the following body system disturbances:
a. Encephalopathy/coma.
b. Asterixis.
c. Cerebral edema/elevated ICP.
d. Extreme hyponatremia.
e. Central pontine myelinolysis.
f. Hyperdynamic circulatory state/decreased SVR/elevated cardiac output.
g. Tachycardia.
h. Arteriovenous shunts AND spider angiomata in the skin can be present in almost all vascular beds.
i. Decreased effective intravascular volume due to vasodilation and portosystemic shunting.
j. Increased total body fluid volume.
k. Ascites, edema/anasarca.
5. Anesthetic implications of advanced hepatic dysfunction.
a. Increased risk of excessive sedation because of alterations in mental status and reduced metabolism of medications.
b. Increased risk for aspiration due to altered mental status or ascites.
c. Chronic hypoxemia from many causes (e.g., ascites, pleural effusions, atelectasis) may be present at baseline, and desaturation on induction may be rapid.
6. Diminished hypoxic pulmonary vasoconstriction results in ventilation-perfusion mismatch and intrapulmonary shunting.
a. Variceal bleeding may occur.

b. Prerenal azotemia, metabolic alkalosis, hypokalemia, and hyponatremia.
c. Hepatorenal syndrome—renal failure in the presence of hepatic failure.
d. Coagulopathy may be caused by several factors.
   i.   Synthesis of clotting factors and anticoagulants (proteins C and S) is impaired in liver failure and vitamin K deficiency; thrombocytopenia may also be present.
   ii. Preoperative correction of clotting abnormalities with administration of FFP or vitamin K.
e. Hypoglycemia and nutritional deficiencies may be present.

V. OTOLARYNGOLOGY/HEAD AND NECK SURGERY

11

INTRAOPERATIVE CARE

A. LASER SURGERY

1. General considerations.
a. Laser may be used for a variety of ENT procedures such as supraglottoplasty or excision of laryngeal lesions.
b. Fire hazard is minimal in absence of combustible material (i.e., plastic).
c. May use FiO_2 of 1.0 if not using plastic ETT.
d. Use lowest possible FiO_2 when plastic ETT is in place (air or O_2/air mixture).
e. For certain laser procedures around glottis, a metal-wrapped ETT may be used.

2. Hazards of lasers.
a. Atmospheric contamination.
   i.   Dispersion of diseased particulate matter.
b. Fire.
   i.   0.5% to 1.5% reported risk of ETT fires with laser surgery.
c. Embolism.
   i.   Venous gas embolism (rare) associated with Nd:YAG lasers.
d. Ocular damage.
   i. CO_2 lasers cause corneal opacification.
   ii. Nd:YAG lasers cause damage to retina.
e. Perforation.
   i.   Viscus or blood vessel.
   ii. May occur days later when edema and tissue necrosis are increased.

3. Management of airway fire.
a. Stop ventilation.
b. Disconnect oxygen.
c. Remove ETT.
d. Flood surgical field with saline.
e. Mask-ventilate pt with 100% oxygen; then reintubate.
f. Use rigid laryngoscopy/bronchoscopy with jet ventilation to assess damage and remove debris.

g. Administer short-term steroids.
h. Provide ventilatory support and antibiotics if needed.

B. RADICAL NECK DISSECTION
1. Consists of complete cervical lymphadenectomy, resection of supraclavicular muscle, internal jugular vein, and cranial nerve XI.
2. If bilateral neck dissection, consider tracheostomy to avoid problems secondary to airway edema.
3. Watch for bradycardia w/dissection around carotid bulb.
a. Provide therapy with LA or IV atropine.
4. Complications.
a. Bleeding (rarely, can see sudden large blood loss from internal jugular vein at skull base).
b. Infection.
c. Cranial nerve injury.
d. Pneumothorax.
e. Diaphragmatic paralysis.
5. Control BP to decrease complications from bleeding.
6. Use of muscle relaxation is often determined by the surgeon.
7. Smooth emergence necessary.
8. May consider extubating over tube exchanger if worried about airway edema or recurrent laryngeal nerve damage.

C. SUSPENSION MICROLARYNGOSCOPY
1. Provides means of assessing supraglottic structures and glottic opening.
2. Aids in removal of laryngeal lesions (i.e., papillomas, nodules, polyps).
3. Involves suspension of laryngoscope from Mayo stand or OR table.
4. Goals.
a. Provide surgeon with clear view and immobile field.
5. Avoid routine premedication.
6. May administer antisialagogue to dry oral secretions.
7. Airway management.
a. Endotracheal intubation.
   i. Use small, long ETT with high-pressure, low-volume cuff to improve surgeon's view.
   ii. Advantages.
      • $ETCO_2$ monitoring, positive-pressure ventilation, airway protection.
b. Jet ventilation.
   i. Ventilation without ETT provides surgeon unobstructed view of larynx.
   ii. Keep jet tip within laryngoscope to avoid barotraumas.
   iii. Vocal cords must be completely relaxed.
   iv. Contraindicated in children and pts with morbid obesity, bullous emphysema, and large tumors of the airway.
c. Intermittent apnea.

    i.   Intermittent removal of ETT during endoscopy.

    ii. Useful in children.

d. For relaxation, may use succinylcholine infusion or nondepolarizing NMB if procedure is to last at least 30 min.

e. If laser is used, low FIO_2 is necessary to minimize the risk of airway fire.

D. TRACHEOSTOMY

1. Performed as part of procedure (i.e., laryngectomy) or emergently.
2. Indications.
   a. Laryngeal fractures.
   b. Severe sleep apnea.
   c. Inability to intubate.
   d. Prolonged ventilatory assistance.
3. Tracheostomy under LA preferred in pts with upper airway obstruction.
4. In elective situations, performed under GA.
   a. Airway devices used in tracheostomy include ETT, rigid bronchoscope, facemask, LMA, glottic aperture seal airway.
      i.   Intubate with fiberoptic scope or intubating LMA.
      ii. No muscle relaxants.
5. Early complications.
   a. Tube malposition.
   b. Pneumothorax.
   c. Pneumomediastinum.
   d. Hemorrhage.
   e. Tube misplacement.
   f. Occlusion of tracheostomy tube (secretions, mucous plug, blood, or tube malposition).
   g. Airway fire.
6. Late complications.
   a. Tracheal stenosis.
      i.   Use of high-pressure, low-volume cuffs minimizes this risk.
      ii. Cuffless tracheostomy tubes may be used but offer no protection from aspiration.
7. Postoperative care.
   a. Humidify oxygen.
   b. Suction secretions.
   c. Maintain cuff pressures at 15 to 20 mm Hg.
   d. Stoma tract is not fully established for 5 to 7 days.
      i.   It is recommended to wait for at least 7 days before changing the tracheostomy tube.

VI. ORTHOPEDIC SURGERY

A. PREOPERATIVE ASSESSMENT

1. Crucial to formulation and execution of anesthetic plan.

11

INTRAOPERATIVE CARE

2. Evaluation of preexisting medical problems, potential airway difficulties, and previous anesthetic and complications.
3. CAD is common in elderly population.
a. Difficult to assess exercise tolerance because of limitations in mobility.
b. Pharmacologic functional CV testing may be warranted.
4. Overall, orthopedic surgery is considered intermediate risk for perioperative cardiac complications.

B. PT POSITIONING

1. Improper positioning may result in intraoperative or postoperative problems.
a. Air embolism can occur when the operative field is above the level of the heart (e.g., surgery of c-spine, shoulder in sitting position, lumbar spinal surgery in prone position).
b. Stretch or malposition of joints may occur during anesthesia.
c. Direct pressure over bony prominences can cause:
   i. Tissue ischemia or necrosis, especially after prolonged surgery when hypotensive anesthesia is used.
   ii. Postoperative neurapraxia.
   iii. Prolonged venous obstruction may lead to compartment syndrome with edema, neurapraxia, elevation of creatine phosphokinase level, and myoglobinuria.
d. Special problems of prone positioning include:
   i. ETT kinking or dislodgement.
   ii. Edema of upper airway in prolonged cases, causing postoperative respiratory obstruction.
   iii. Increased abdominal pressure, which can cause elevation of epidural venous pressure, contributing to intraoperative bleeding during spine surgery.
   iv. Retinal injury (due to compression) and blindness.

C. ANESTHETIC TECHNIQUE

1. Choice of regional or GA in orthopedics depends on:
a. Pt's preference.
b. State of health of the pt.
c. Expertise of the anesthesiologist.
d. Duration of procedure.
e. Surgeon's preference.
2. Most extremity procedures can be performed using regional anesthesia alone with light sedation (concern over inability to detect compartment syndrome postoperatively).
3. More complicated operations such as allograft replacements, major tumor surgery, reconstructive procedures, and repair of major trauma may be performed using GA alone.
4. Combining techniques that use continuous regional anesthesia supplemented with GA via an LMA may be particularly useful.

D. **SPECIAL CONSIDERATIONS**

1. Tourniquet problems.

a. Tourniquets are applied around upper or lower extremities to decrease intraoperative bleeding.

b. Physiologic changes include:

   i. Application >60 min—tourniquet pain and HTN.

   ii. Application >2 hr—muscle dysfunction and potential postoperative neurapraxis.

c. Metabolic acidosis after releasing the tourniquet, with transient increase in E_TCO_2.

2. Bone cement.

a. Made of polymethylmethacrylate.

b. Regularly used for arthroplasties (most frequently with femoral prosthesis).

c. The process of cement hardening causes intramedullary HTN that may cause fat embolization, cement embolization.

d. May cause systemic vasodilation, platelet aggregation, and microthrombus that lead to hemodynamic instability, hypoxia, dysrhythmias, and pulmonary HTN.

e. Prevention.

   i. Increase FiO_2 and maintain euvolemia or slight hypervolemia during cementing.

   ii. The surgeons may use cementless prosthesis (especially in younger pts).

f. Treatment.

   i. Supportive.

3. Fat embolism.

a. Rare but very serious complication (mortality up to 20%).

b. Within 72 hr after long bone or pelvic fracture.

c. Classic presentation.

   i. Dyspnea, petechiae, and confusion.

d. Increased fatty acids in plasma cause release of vasoactive substances.

   i. ARDS-like syndrome.

   ii. Capillary damage to cerebral circulation.

e. During GA.

   i. Decline in E_TCO_2 and PaO_2.

f. Treatment.

   i. Supportive.

E. **ARTHROSCOPY**

1. Important to evaluate medical comorbidities and adjust anesthetic technique.

2. Many of these procedures are done as outpatient surgery, and the anesthesia technique must be tailored to permit the quick recovery of the pt.

11

INTRAOPERATIVE CARE

3. In many cases, these procedures can be performed with a regional technique and sedation.
4. In major arthroplasties (knee and shoulder), pts may require good postoperative analgesia.
a. If a regional technique is used, pts will benefit from continuous analgesia (catheters).
5. Intraarticular injection of LAs and opioids may offer advantages over systemic injection of opioids.
6. Minimal blood loss.

F. BONE TUMORS

1. Mostly affects younger pts.
2. Resection of these tumors may require extensive surgeries and possible reconstruction.
3. Most of these tumors have extensive vascularization.
a. Resection may be accompanied by large blood loss, aggressive fluid resuscitation, and transfusion of blood products (especially pelvic tumors).
4. Some of these pts will undergo embolization of vascular access to tumor prior to surgery (minimize blood loss).
5. Multiple large-bore IVs are needed for these procedures.
6. Multiple anesthesia techniques may be used, but adequate postoperative analgesia is critical for quick recovery.
7. Air and fat embolisms are possible.
8. Pts may have received chemotherapy and/or radiotherapy prior to surgery.
a. It is essential to obtain information regarding these techniques and their influence over the anesthetic plan.

G. SCOLIOSIS AND SPINAL SURGERY

1. Scoliosis can be congenital, idiopathic, or traumatic.
2. Preoperative assessment requires pulmonary function tests (to assess restrictive patterns), especially in those pts with major deformities.
3. If pulmonary function is restricted, over time most pts will develop hypoxia and pulmonary HTN.
4. In children, pts with scoliosis due to muscular dystrophy are prone to malignant hyperthermia.
5. Some of these pts may have altered spine mobility that affects the cervical spine.
a. It is important to assess airway to establish a plan to secure it.
6. Special neurophysiology monitoring is normally used in extensive procedures (somatosensory- and motor-evoked potentials).
a. Alternatively, an intraoperative wake-up test can be performed to assess lower extremity function.
7. Generally done with pt in prone position.

8. Extensive surgeries are generally associated with large volume shifts and blood loss.
9. Good IV access is mandatory in these cases.
a. Invasive monitoring (arterial line) and central line are often required for managing these pts.
10. Prolonged surgeries will require that pts be kept intubated postoperatively.

H. TOTAL HIP REPLACEMENT

1. Anesthetic management of total hip replacement varies according to the complexity of the surgery and the medical status of the pt.
2. Anesthetic management.
a. Invasive hemodynamic monitoring is used perioperatively in the elderly, medically compromised pt or in revision surgery.
b. Most pts are elderly; difficult to assess CV status.
c. Fluid administration must be carefully managed.
d. Regional technique is associated with better outcomes, most likely secondary to reduction in thromboembolic disease.
   i. Epidural anesthesia offers the advantage of good postoperative pain control and less delirium.
e. Use of hypotensive or regional (epidural or spinal) anesthesia reduces the blood loss by 30% to 50%.
f. Blood loss during total hip replacement is significantly greater during revision surgery.
g. Lateral decubitus position.
   i. Potential ventilation-perfusion mismatch, with resultant hypoxemia.
h. Intraoperative hypotension.
   i. Profound hypotension immediately after insertion of cemented femoral prostheses has resulted in cardiac arrest and death.
   ii. Aggressive and effective treatment of hypotension is necessary.
i. Postoperative pain management may be accomplished by multiple modalities.

VII. PLASTIC SURGERY
A. FLAPS

1. Pt population.
a. Cancer pts after major cancer resection.
b. Those who sustained deforming injuries as a result of trauma/burns.
c. Pts with congenital defects.
2. Preoperative assessment.
a. Possible prior radiation and/or chemotherapy may have effects on respiratory and CV systems.
b. Anemia is possible as a result of illness and treatment.
c. Anticoagulation is sometimes used prior to a case or during the procedure (Dextran).
3. Intraoperative challenges.

11

INTRAOPERATIVE CARE

a. Often long case duration, with multiple surgical teams involved.
b. Positioning is the key.
   i. Place lines and leads to avoid surgical field.
   ii. Plan ahead for ETT placement and possible tracheostomy in head and neck cases.
   iii. Pad pressure points thoroughly.
c. Expect and prepare to counteract possible hypothermia due to long case duration and large body surface area (BSA).
d. Muscle relaxation is usually necessary after a standard induction.
e. Arterial lines are often necessary for blood draws and close monitoring.
4. Postoperative monitoring is often carried out in the ICU setting.
a. These pts are often subject to return trips to the OR because of flap compromise.

B. BREAST RECONSTRUCTION
1. Defects are mostly due to breast cancer.
a. Rarely, pts with Poland syndrome are encountered.
2. Reconstructive options.
a. Tissue expanders.
b. Soft tissue reconstruction using latissimus dorsi flap, TRAM flap, free TRAM flap, or DIEP flap.
   i. With free TRAM flap and DIEP flap, microscopes are utilized for creation of vascular anastomoses.
3. Special considerations.
a. Refer to "Flaps" (section A, above) for pulmonary and CV considerations.
b. Reconstruction often immediately follows mastectomy.
   i. Consider muscle relaxation once mastectomy and node dissection are complete.
c. Maintain appropriate hydration and normothermia for adequate graft perfusion.
d. Position pt in accordance with surgeon's request and secure arms.
   i. The results of reconstruction are often primarily reviewed intraoperatively by sitting the pt up.

C. BURNS
1. Classified based on:
a. Total BSA involved (rule of nines—surface area of one palm is equal to 1%).
b. Depth (1st degree limited to epithelium, 2nd degree extends into dermis, 3rd degree destroys the full thickness of epidermis, 4th extends into muscle and fascia).
2. Initial airway assessment.
a. Assess extent and mechanism of injury and overall health status.
   i. Consider cervical spine injury.

b. Evaluate for presence of inhalational injury immediately (stridor, hoarseness, facial burns, soot, carbon monoxide levels) and at 12- to 24-hr mark (increasing shunting, increased A-a gradient).

c. Immediate intubation for hemodynamic instability, respiratory compromise, altered mental status, massive burn, head/neck burns.

d. Succinylcholine is appropriate for pts with acute burns at <48 hr.
   i. Select induction agent based on CV factors/stability.

e. Expect ventilation and oxygenation issues 24 to 48 hr after the insult due to:
   i. Pulmonary edema.
   ii. Decreased chest wall compliance due to circumferential injury.
   iii. Tracheobronchitis.
   iv. Atelectasis.

3. CV considerations.
a. Significant fluid shifts from intravascular to interstitial space.
b. Massive vasodilation.
c. Large evaporative heat loss.
d. Depressed myocardial function → "burn shock" followed by hypermetabolic phase 72 hr later.
e. Treatment.
   i. Initial fluid resuscitation with crystalloid according to Parkland formula (LR at 4 mL/kg/% total BSA in the first 24 hr.
   ii. Monitor urine output with Foley catheter.

4. Hematologic considerations.
a. Assess estimated blood loss as closely as possible.
b. Discuss the expected area of excision/grafting with surgeons to plan fluid resuscitation.
c. Consider possibility of coagulopathy.
   i. Decreased survival of platelets, fibrinogen, factors V and IX.

5. Renal.
a. Acute renal failure (ARF) is possible owing to early hypovolemia and multi-organ system failure and/or sepsis.
b. Electrolyte derangements include hyperkalemia in the initial stages.
c. Consider hypokalemia at later stage; possibly myoglobinuria if electric injury was present.

6. CNS.
a. Plan for management of hypermetabolic state that ensues with increased levels of "stress response," leading to hyperthermia, HTN, tachycardia, hyperglycemia.

7. Intraoperative considerations for burn pts.
a. Induction.
   i. Propofol/thiopental if volume is resuscitated; otherwise, use etomidate or ketamine.
   ii. Up to 1.5× the usual intubating dose of muscle relaxants may be necessary.

b. Maintenance.
   i. Usually higher PEEP and higher minute ventilation are required.
c. Monitoring.
   i. Obtain central venous access for CVP monitoring.
      • Anticipate extensive blood loss.
   ii. Establish arterial access for close monitoring and blood draws.
   iii. Maintain urine output at 0.5 to 1 mL/kg/hr.
   iv. ECG monitoring may require needle electrodes.
   v. Monitor core temperature and warm the room and fluids; use warming blankets if possible.
d. Prior to extubation, assess possible airway edema.

VIII. RENAL SYSTEM
A. END-STAGE RENAL DISEASE (ESRD)
1. ARF (Table 11.7).
a. Decrease in renal function over 24 to 72 hr.
   i. Creatinine increase by 0.5 mg/dL, creatinine increase by 50% or creatinine >2 mg/dL, and possible oliguria (<20 mL/hr)
b. Prerenal azotemia due to renal hypoperfusion (may progress to ARF).
   i. Hypovolemia.
   ii. Hypotension.
   iii. Low cardiac output.
   iv. Increased renal vascular resistance (e.g., embolus).
c. Postrenal azotemia due to obstruction or compression of urinary tract (may progress to ARF).
d. Intrinsic renal failure due to direct renal injury, ischemia (acute tubular necrosis), prolonged obstruction to urinary flow, drugs/contrast, toxic exposures, or nephritis/nephrosis.
e. Diagnosis.
   i. Clinical features include hypervolemia, peripheral edema, electrolyte disturbances, impaired excretion of drugs and toxins, progression to chronic renal failure.
f. Treatment.
   i. Correction of the cause.

TABLE 11.7

URINARY AND SERUM INDICES IN THE DIAGNOSIS OF ACUTE RENAL FAILURE

	Prerenal	Renal	Postrenal
Specific gravity	>1.018	<0.012	
Osmolality (mmol/kg)	>500	<350	<350
Urine/plasma urea nitrogen ratio	>8	<3	<3
Urine/plasma creatinine ratio	>40	<20	<20
Urine/sodium (mEq/L)	<10	>40	>20
Fractional excretion of sodium (%)	<1	>3%	>2%
Renal failure index	<1	>1	

ii. Diuresis.
  • Maintaining urine flow with diuretics remains controversial.
iii. Correction of electrolyte abnormalities.
iv. Fluid restriction.
v. Possible dialysis (intermittent hemodialysis vs. continuous renal replacement therapy).
g. Indications for dialysis.
  i. Fluid overload.
  ii. Severe acidosis.
  iii. Hyperkalemia.
  iv. Metabolic encephalopathy.
  v. Pericarditis (uremia).
  vi. Drug toxicity.

2. Chronic renal failure.
a. Progressive, irreversible decline in renal function of >3 to 6 mo.
b. Causes.
  i. HTN.
  ii. Chronic glomerulonephritis.
  iii. Polycystic kidney disease.
  iv. Renovascular disease.
c. Characterized by:
  i. Uremia, usually evident by the time GFR drops below 25 mL/min.
  ii. Metabolic abnormalities.
    • Hyperkalemia.
    • Hypophosphatemia.
    • Hypermagnesemia.
    • Hyponatremia.
    • Hypocalcemia.
    • Hypoalbuminemia.
  iii. Metabolic acidosis.
  iv. Uremic pericarditis/pericardial effusion/tamponade.
  v. Hypervolemia, HTN, leading to possible LV hypertrophy, CHF, or pulmonary edema.
  vi. Anemia due to undersecretion of erythropoietin.
  vii. Dysfunctional platelets due to uremia.
  viii. Immunosuppression.
  ix. Metabolic bone disease due to secondary hyperparathyroidism with hypercalcemia.
  x. CNS depression ranging from altered mentation to severe encephalopathy.
  xi. Peripheral neuropathy.
d. Treatment involves dialysis (intermittent hemodialysis or peritoneal dialysis) and transplantation.

3. Approach to the pt with ESRD.
a. Confirm etiology of renal disease.

11

INTRAOPERATIVE CARE

b. Order serum chemistries to evaluate electrolyte status, specifically Na^+/K^+ owing to risk of cardiac dysrhythmias.

c. Order ABG to help evaluate acid-base status.

d. Evaluate for signs and symptoms of uremia; treat reversible causes; delay elective cases until diagnosis is made and treatment, if possible, is initiated.

e. Pt should have dialysis on the day of or the day prior to surgery.

f. Evaluate vascular access (central access, AV fistula) for patency.

   i. Monitoring and procedures should be done on opposite side of AV fistula.

g. Calculate creatinine clearance to determine GFR and renal reserve.

   i. May have to adjust drug doses in relation to creatinine clearance (CrCl).

$$CrCl = [(140 - age) \times weight\ (kg)] / [72 \times serum\ creatinine\ (mg/dL)]$$

h. Order hematologic studies to evaluate Hb, platelet count, qualitative platelet function, and coagulation.

   i. Type and crossmatch for blood if major blood loss is anticipated.

i. Obtain ECG to evaluate cardiac effects of electrolyte derangement or ischemia.

j. Echocardiogram may help to assess cardiac status and the presence of pericardial effusion.

   i. Obtain CXR to evaluate for fluid overload/pulmonary edema, cardiomegaly, pericardial effusion.

k. Establish invasive monitoring to monitor BP in those with poorly controlled HTN, or central venous/pulmonary artery catheter monitoring if large fluid shifts are anticipated.

l. Succinylcholine is acceptable if serum K^+ is <4 mEq/L.

m. Prolongation of narcotic and muscle relaxant medications is likely.

n. Avoid hypoventilation and hypercarbia that may worsen preexisting acidosis.

B. RETROPUBIC RADICAL PROSTATECTOMY

1. **Prostatectomy through abdominal incision, usually performed with pelvic lymph node dissection.**

a. Prostate is removed en bloc with ejaculatory ducts, seminal vesicles, and part of bladder neck.

   i. Remaining bladder is anastomosed to urethra over Foley catheter.

b. Indigo carmine is injected to visualize urethra.

   i. May cause hypotension/hypertension and pulse oximetry aberrations.

c. May be done with regional, general, or combined techniques.

   i. Spinal or epidural may be used.

      • T6-level block is necessary.

   ii. Sedation is usually necessary because of positioning.

1. Prepare for significant blood loss (>500 mL).
2. Central venous monitoring and/or arterial BP monitoring should be in place in pt with significant CV comorbidities.
3. Typed and crossmatched blood or autologous blood should be available.
4. Increased risk of DVT due to dissection around pelvic veins.

C. CYSTOSCOPY
1. May be diagnostic or therapeutic.
2. Indications include hematuria, urinary obstruction, resection of tumor, and ureteral stent placement.
3. Can be done under topical, regional, or general anesthesia.
4. Must be careful with positioning.
   a. Lithotomy position is associated with decreased functional residual capacity, atelectasis, and hypoxia.
   b. These can be accentuated by Trendelenburg position.
5. Trendelenburg and flattening of the OR table may be associated with hypertension/hypotension secondary to increased/decreased venous return, which, in turn, may worsen preexistent CHF.
6. Compression of peroneal nerves by stirrups can cause foot drops.
7. Prolonged lithotomy position can cause rhabdomyolysis and compartment syndrome of lower extremities.
8. Hands may get caught in OR table with position changes.
9. Compression of saphenous nerve may cause medial thigh numbness; thigh flexion may cause sciatic nerve stretch.

D. LITHOTRIPSY
1. Focuses shock waves at kidney stones.
   a. May be electrohydraulic, piezoelectric, or electromagnetic energy.
2. Stones in upper 2/3 of ureters or kidneys are treated with extracorporeal shock-wave lithotripsy (ESWL).
3. Changes in acoustic impedance at tissue/stone or tissue/air interfaces cause shearing and tearing forces.
   a. Contraindications include inability to place lung or intestine outside the shock-wave focus, bleeding, infection, pregnancy, and urinary obstruction below the stone.
   b. Presence of aortic aneurysm or orthopedic prosthesis near the stone is a relative contraindication.
4. Pts with implanted cardiac devices or history of cardiac dysrhythmia are at increased risk of having cardiac dysrhythmias or dislodgement of intracardiac devices during lithotripsy.
5. Immersion into water bath (rarely used currently) can cause vasodilation, possibly leading to hypotension.
   a. Redistribution of blood causes increased venous blood return and decreased functional residual capacity.
   b. These can exacerbate CHF and/or cause hypoxemia.

11

INTRAOPERATIVE CARE

6. Can be performed under regional anesthesia with epidural or spinal technique.

7. Adequate fluid loading with 1 to 1.5 L crystalloid can help with postural hypotension associated with being seated in water bath.

8. Light sedation may be helpful.

9. Avoid using large amounts of air for loss of resistance in epidural, as air/tissue interface can promote nerve damage.

a. Difficult-to-control regional techniques are associated with movement of the stone due to diaphragmatic excursion.

10. GA with muscle relaxation can control diaphragmatic excursion during ESWL.

11. Muscle relaxation can also help with preventing movement with positioning.

12. Fluid loading with 1 L of crystalloid can help to prevent postural hypotension.

13. MAC with opioid supplementation for pain control may be used for ESWL.

14. Close ECG and pulse oximetry monitoring for dysrhythmia and hypoxemia is indicated.

15. Large amounts of IV fluid are indicated to promote good urinary flow.

E. **TRANSURETHRAL PROSTATECTOMY (TURP)/TRANSURETHRAL RESECTION OF BLADDER TUMOR (TURBT)**

1. Performed through a transurethral resectoscope and wire-loop cautery.

2. May be performed with GA or regional anesthesia with a T6-T10-level block.

3. Regional anesthesia may be preferable owing to less incidence of DVT and decreased likelihood of masking the diagnosis of TURP syndrome or bladder perforation.

4. Prostatic venous sinuses opened during surgery promote absorption of irrigant and release of urokinase from prostate.

5. Quantity of fluid absorbed is determined by irrigant hydrostatic pressure, duration of surgery, irrigation flow rate, venous sinuses opened, and peripheral venous pressure.

6. Electrolyte solutions are well tolerated but not used because of dispersion of electrical current.

7. Water provides best visibility, but excess absorption may lead to water intoxication.

8. Slightly hypotonic solutions such as 1.5% glycine or 2.7% sorbitol and 0.54% mannitol can be used.

a. Significant water intoxication risk exists.

b. Solute absorption toxicity may occur.

c. Glycine toxicity may result in N/V, visual disturbances, or transient blindness.

8. Hepatic metabolization may cause elevated serum ammonia levels, leading to CNS toxicity.

9. Marked hypo-osmolality and hyponatremia may occur, leading to CNS toxicity and possible hemolysis.

10. Urokinase release from prostate may lead to DIC.

a. Treat with ε-aminocaproic acid.

11. Dilutional thrombocytopenia may occur.

12. TURP syndrome is a group of symptoms caused by excess absorption of irrigant.

a. Hypervolemia and subsequent hyponatremia and hypo-osmolality may occur.

b. Intraoperatively or several hours later, awake pts may develop CNS symptoms such as headache, dizziness, convulsions.

c. May progress to coma and CV collapse.

d. Under GA, pts may develop refractory bradycardia, hypoxemia, hemodynamic instability, ST elevations, QRS widening, or V-tach/V-fib.

e. Careful monitoring of pulse oximetry and ECG is indicated.

13. Treatment depends on symptom severity.

a. Correct hypoxia and hypoperfusion.

b. Loop diuretics and fluid restriction.

c. Hypertonic saline.

d. Control seizure activity with benzodiazepines or phenytoin for sustained anti-seizure activity.

14. Bladder perforation may manifest as sudden hypotension/hypertension, generalized abdominal pain (in awake pts), and nausea.

15. Hypothermia may occur as the result of heat loss from prolonged bladder irrigation.

a. Monitor temperature closely.

16. Monitor for septicemia from bacteremia following prostatic manipulation.

17. Prostatic bleeding may be difficult to control through the resectoscope.

a. Crossmatched blood should be available for pts with large prostate glands or those with anemia or increased risk for bleeding.

IX. TRANSPLANTATION

A. MANAGEMENT OF THE ORGAN DONOR

1. Main goal—optimization of organ retrieval and viability of the organ/s.

a. Maintain oxygen delivery to tissues with lowest FiO_2 possible and aggressively treat any metabolic disarrangements (avoiding high doses of vasopressors and inotropes).

   i. Drugs of choice—dopamine and vasopressin.

b. Maintain body temperature, urine output, hematocrit >25%, while minimizing blood transfusions.

11

INTRAOPERATIVE CARE

   c. Use volatile anesthetics to maintain BP.
   d. Use NMB agents to control any motor activity.
2. Cadaveric donation.
   a. Brain death must be established following well-defined criteria.
   b. Brain death causes multiple physiologic derangements.
      i. Autonomic dysfunction.
      ii. Dysrhythmias.
      iii. Hemodynamic instability.
      iv. Problems with body temperature regulation.
   c. Surgical procedure.
      i. Starts with organ dissection.
      ii. Once completed, donor receives full heparinization, and aorta is crossclamped.
   d. Generally, kidneys are first, followed by liver and heart (simultaneously).
      i. Ventilation must be maintained until lungs are flushed with preservative solution and trachea is clamped.

B. LIVER TRANSPLANT
1. Preoperative considerations.
   a. End-stage liver disease presents with a constellation of systemic diseases.
      i. CNS—encephalopathy.
      ii. CV—decreased SVR, hyperdynamic circulation, blunted response to pressors/inotropes.
      iii. Pulmonary—hypoxia, hepatopulmonary syndrome (portopulmonary HTN).
      iv. GI—bleeding, ascites, delayed gastric emptying.
      v. Decreased synthesis of clotting factors.
      vi. Renal failure (hepatorenal syndrome).
2. Preoperative assessment.
   a. MELD score—prognostic scoring system that predicts 90-day mortality using creatinine, bilirubin, and INR.
   b. Pharmacologic stress test, echocardiography, and catheterization are used to evaluate CAD.
      i. Severe CAD that requires a CABG is usually a contraindication to liver transplantation.
   c. Echocardiography may also evaluate the extent of pulmonary HTN.
      i. Mean pulmonary artery pressures >50 mm Hg and/or PVR >250 dynes•s•cm^{-5}.
       • Epoprostenol and sildenafil can be used to treat pulmonary HTN.
   d. Extent of renal involvement should be evaluated.
      i. Hepatorenal syndrome.
       • Type I—acute, creatinine > 2.5 mg/dL, rapidly fatal.
       • Type II—chronic, creatinine > 1.5, GFR < 40.
3. Intraoperative management.

a. Very complex management.
   i. Significant physiologic changes require understanding of pharmacology during end-stage liver disease.
b. It is very important to establish good IV access.
   i. At least three- to four-bore IVs; at least 2 IVs should be 8.5F sheath introducers.
   ii. Strict aseptic technique.
c. Standard ASA monitors plus pulmonary artery catheter and possibly TEE.
d. Thromboelastogram should be used for coagulation management.
e. Blood bank should be notified of potential large volume of transfusions.
f. Rapid-sequence induction indicated owing to gastroparesis and increased intra-abdominal pressure from ascites.
g. In most cases, vasopressors and inotropes are needed.

4. Phases of transplant.
a. Pre-anhepatic.
   i. Includes hepatectomy, gallbladder resection, and resection of hepatic veins and IVC.
   ii. Main concerns.
       • Portal HTN.
       • Hemodynamic instability.
       • Oliguria.
       • Thrombocytopenia/coagulopathy.
       • Bleeding.
b. Anhepatic.
   i. Starts with crossclamp of portal vein/IVC and ends with the release of the clamps.
   ii. Surgeons flush the preservation fluid out of the new graft.
   iii. Different surgical technique that may require venovenous bypass.
   iv. Clamping of the IVC determines most of the physiologic derangements that require careful correction.
       • Metabolic acidosis.
       • Hypocalcemia.
       • Coagulopathy.
       • Hypothermia.
       • Renal dysfunction.
c. Postanhepatic.
   i. Includes reperfusion of the graft after release of clamps.
   ii. Reperfusion of the graft causes major physiologic instability.
       • Hyperkalemia.
       • Metabolic acidosis.
       • Reperfusion syndrome.
       • Bleeding.
       • Fibrinolysis.
       • Hemodynamic instability.
       • Hypothermia.

11

INTRAOPERATIVE CARE

- Oliguria.
- Hypocalcemia.

iii. Early, aggressive correction of these derangements is mandatory to avoid severe hemodynamic collapse.

5. Good early signs of adequate graft function.

a. Reduced need for calcium with transfusion (citrate metabolism).

b. Metabolic alkalosis.

c. Bile production.

d. Improved coagulation.

6. Liver transplant is performed under GA.

a. Drugs used during the anesthetic may have altered pharmacokinetics because of liver failure.

b. Drugs metabolized independent of liver function include:

   i. Remifentanil.

   ii. Cisatracurium.

   iii. Esmolol.

   iv. Succinylcholine.

c. Because conjugation is relatively preserved in liver failure, opioids and propofol may be better tolerated.

d. Any volatile agent can be used.

7. Goals are to correct INR to 1.5, keep platelets >50,000/mm^3, and keep fibrinogen >100 mg/dL.

C. KIDNEY TRANSPLANT

1. Preoperative management.

a. Renal transplant pts usually have significant CV morbidity.

b. ECG and echocardiogram to evaluate cardiac function.

c. PFT indicated in lung disease.

d. Establish good glucose control in diabetic pts.

e. Perform dialysis prior to surgery.

f. Obtain hematologic studies to assess degree of anemia and coagulation.

2. Intraoperative management.

a. GA.

   i. Rapid-sequence induction is indicated, especially if pt has diabetes (gastroparesis).

   ii. Delayed gastric emptying is common in ESRD.

b. Use of combined spinal-epidural anesthetic has been reported

c. Arterial catheter is needed for close hemodynamic monitoring ± central catheter for CVP monitoring.

d. It is important to maintain hemodynamic stability and adequate renal blood flow.

   i. Use isotonic fluids, pressors, and anesthetics to maintain BP goals.

e. Cisatracurium for paralysis.

    i. Vecuronium or rocuronium may be safely used; duration may be
        prolonged after repeated doses.
  . Diuretics are used per surgeon preference.
    i. Mannitol and furosemide.
  3. Manage electrolyte disturbances.
    i. Maintain blood glucose in normal range (80–110).
  1. Have blood available to manage anemia/blood loss.
    i. Administer immunosuppression in the OR.
3. Postoperative management.
  a. Maintain adequate pain control with IV PCA or epidural PCA.

D. PANCREATIC TRANSPLANT
1. Normally performed in conjunction with renal transplant.
2. Native pancreas is left in place.
3. Major anesthetic concern is related to glucose management.
  a. Frequent measurements are required.
  b. Special attention is necessary after reperfusion of new pancreas.
4. New pancreas is anastomosed to the bladder.

**E. ANESTHESIA MANAGEMENT FOR PTS WITH A TRANSPLANTED
   ORGAN**
1. Requires good understanding of the altered physiology of the
   transplanted graft, associated risks of these pts (mainly infections),
   and pharmacology of immunosuppressants.
2. It is important to know what immunosupressants the pt is taking.
  a. Most drugs can be stopped during perioperative period, but
     cyclosporine and tacrolimus must be restarted as soon as possible.
3. Assess function of the graft and any physiologic derangements (renal,
   hepatic, cardiac, etc.) through physical, laboratory tests, and other
   studies (e.g., ultrasound, echocardiography).
4. The level of physiologic alterations and the organs affected will
   determine the type of anesthetic technique.
5. Maximize sterility of any procedure.
6. In case of pregnant transplanted pt, any of the techniques used in OB
   anesthesia can be safely used.

11

INTRAOPERATIVE CARE

REFERENCES
Angelini Giuditta A, Ketzler JT, Coursin DB: Perioperative care of the
   diabetic patient. ASA Refresher Courses Anesthesiol 2001;29(1):1–9.
Bartholomew JR: The incidence and clinical features of heparin-induced
   thrombocytopenia. Sem Hematol 2005;42(Suppl 3):S3–S8.
Blanding R, Stiff J: Perioperative anesthetic management of patients with
   burns. Anesthesiol Clin North America 1999;17(1):237–250.
Borgeat A, Ekatodramis G: Orthopaedic surgery in the elderly. Best Pract
   Res Clin Anaesthesiol 2003;17:235–244.

Braunfeld M: Anesthesia for liver transplantation. ASA Refresher Courses Anesthesiol 2001;29(1):83–96.

Brown CJ, Buie WD: Perioperative stress dose steroids: Do they make a difference? J Am Coll Surg 2001;193(6):678–686.

Buckenmaier CC: Anaesthesia for outpatient knee surgery. Best Pract Res Clin Anaesthesiol 2002;16(2):255–270.

Cavaliere F, Iacobone E, Gorgoglione M, et al: Anesthesiologic preoperative evaluation of drug addicted patient. Minerva Anestesiol 2005;71(6):367–371.

Chelly JE, Ben-David B, Williams BA, Kentor ML: Anesthesia and postoperative analgesia: Outcomes following orthopedic surgery. Orthopedics 2003;26(8 Suppl):s865-s871.

Cheng DC: The drug addicted patient. Can J Anaesth 1997;44:R101-R111.

Cobas M: Preoperative assessment of coagulation disorders. Int Anesthesiol Clin 2001;39(1):1–15.

Comunale ME, Van Cott EM: Heparin-induced thrombocytopenia. Int Anesthesiol Clin 2004;42(3):27–43.

Connery LE, Coursin DB: Assessment and therapy of selected endocrine disorders. Anesthesiol Clin North Am 2004;22(1):93–123.

Connoly D: Orthopaedic anaethesia. Anaesthesia 2003;58:1189–1193.

Dempfle CE: Disseminated intravascular coagulation and coagulation disorders. Curr Opin Anaesthesiol 2004;17(2):125–129.

Dierdorf SF: Anesthesia for patients with diabetes mellitus. Curr Opin Anaesthesiol 2002;15(3):351–357.

Ehrenwerth J, Seifert HA: Fire safety in the operating room. ASA Refresher Courses Anesthesiol 2003;31(1):25–33.

Graham GW, Unger BP, Coursin DB: Perioperative management of selected endocrine disorders. Int Anesthesiol Clin 2000;38(4):31–67.

Gulur P, Nishimori M, Ballantyne JC: Regional anaesthesia versus general anaesthesia, morbidity and mortality. Best Pract Res Clin Anaesthesiol 2006;20:249–263.

Hahn RG: Transurethral resection syndrome after transurethral resection of bladder tumours. Can J Anaesth 1995;42(1):69–72.

Hernandez M, Birnbach DJ, Van Zundert AAJ: Anesthetic management of the illicit-substance-using patient. Curr Opin Anaesthesiol 2005;18(3):315–324.

Hébert P, Van der Linden G, Biro L, et al: Physiologic aspects of anemia. Crit Care Clin 2004;20:187–212.

Hilton PJ, Hepp M: The immediate care of the burned patient. CEPD Reviews. 2001;4:113–116.

Hoogwerf BJ: Perioperative management of diabetes mellitus: How should we act on the limited evidence? Cleve Clin J Med 2006;73(Suppl 1):S95-S99.

Inzucchi SE: Glycemic management of diabetes in the perioperative setting. Int Anesthesiol Clin 2002;40(2):77–93.

acober SJ, Sowers JR: An update on perioperative management of diabetes. Arch Intern Med 1999;159(20):2405–2411.

Koehntop DE, Beebe DS, Belani KG: Perioperative anesthetic management of the kidney-pancreas transplant recipient. Curr Opin Anaesthesiol 2000;13(3):341–347.

Krohner RG: Anesthetic considerations and techniques for oral and maxillofacial surgery. Int Anesthesiol Clin 2003;41(3):67–89.

Lameire N, Vanholder R: New perspectives for prevention/treatment of acute renal failure. Curr Opin Anaesthesiol 2000;13(2):105–112.

Lange RA, Hillis LD: Cardiovascular complications of cocaine use. N Engl J Med 2001;345:351–358.

Leung LL: Perioperative evaluation of bleeding diathesis. Hematology Am Soc Hematol Educ Program 2006;457–461.

Levi M, ten Cate H: Disseminated intravascular coagulation. N Engl J Med 1999;341:586–592.

Lineaweaver WC, Hui K, Jaffe RA, et al: Functional restoration—microsurgery. In Jaffe RA, Samuels SI (eds): Anesthesiologist's Manual of Surgical Procedures, 2nd ed, Philadelphia: Lippincott Williams & Wilkins, 1999, pp 839–847.

Lineaweaver WC, Hui KCW, Jaffe RA, Samuels SI: Functional restoration-microsurgery. In Jaffe RA (ed): Anesthesiologist's Manual of Surgical Procedures, 2nd ed. Philadelphia: Lippincott Williams and Wilkins, 1999, pp 841–844.

Madjdpour C, Spahn DR, Weiskopf RB: Anemia and perioperative red blood cell transfusion: A matter of tolerance. Crit Care Med 2006;34(5 Suppl):S102-S108.

Mahon P, Shorten G: Perioperative acute renal failure. Curr Opin Anaesthesiol 2006;19(3):332–338.

Mayhew JF: Airway management for oral and maxillofacial surgery. Int Anesthesiol Clin 2003;41(3):57–65.

Mentzelopoulos SD, Tzoufi MJ: Anesthesia for tracheal and endobronchial interventions. Curr Opin Anaesthesiol 2002;15(1):85–94.

Merritt WT: Perioperative concerns in acute liver failure. Int Anesthesiol Clin 2006;44(4):37–57.

Morgan GE, Mikhail MS, Murray MJ: Anesthesia for the trauma patient. In Morgan GE, Mikhail MS, Murray MJ (eds): Clinical Anesthesiology, 4th ed. New York: McGraw-Hill, 2006, pp 861–873.

Morozowich ST, Donahue BS, Welsby IJ: Genetics of coagulation: Considerations for cardiac surgery. Semin Cardiothorac Vasc Anesth 2006;10:297–313.

Napolitano LM: Perioperative anemia. Surg Clin North Am 2005;85(6):1215–1227.

Neligan PMA: Renal replacement therapy in perioperative medicine. ASA Refresher Courses Anesthesiol 2006;34(1):105–114.

Nielsen KC, Steele SM: Management of outpatient orthopedic surgery. Curr Opin Anaesthesiol 2001;14(6):611–616.

11

INTRAOPERATIVE CARE

Nielsen KC, Tucker MS, Steele SM: Outcomes after regional anesthesia. In Anesthesiol Clin Regional 2005;43(3):91–110.

Park KW: Sickle cell disease and other hemoglobinopathies. Int Anesthesio Clin 2004;42(3):77–93.

Planinsic RM, Lebowitz JJ: Renal failure in end-stage liver disease and liver transplantation. Int Anesthesiol Clin 2006;44(3):35–49.

Puyo C: Thrombocytopenia. Int Anesthesiol Clin 2001;39(1):17–34.

Rampil IJ: Anesthetic considerations for laser surgery. Anaesth Analg 1992;74:424–435.

Sadovnikoff N: Perioperative acute renal failure. Int Anesthesiol Clin 2001;39(1):95–109.

Schiff RL, Welsh GA: Perioperative evaluation and management of the patient with endocrine dysfunction. Med Clin North Am 2003;87(1):175–192.

Schlendel SA, Samuels SI, Jaffe RA: Functional restoration. In Jaffe RA (ed): Anesthesiologist's Manual of Surgical Procedures, 2nd ed, Philadelphia: Lippincott Williams and Wilkins, 1999, pp 832–835.

Sinatra RS, Torres J, Bustos AM: Pain management after major orthopaedic surgery: Current strategies and new concepts. J Am Acad Orthop Surg 2002;10(2):117–129.

Spijkstra JJ, Thijs LG: Adrenal dysfunction in critical illness: A clinical entity that requires treatment? Curr Opin Anaesthesiol 2000;13(2):99–103.

Sprung J, Kapural L, Bourke DL, et al: Anesthesia for kidney transplant surgery. Anesthesiol Clin North Am 2000;18(4):919–951.

Steadman RH: Anesthesia for liver transplant surgery. Anesthesiol Clin North Am 2004;22(4):687–711.

Steinberg MH: Management of sickle cell disease. N Engl J Med 1999;340(13):1021–1030.

Stolzenburg JU, Aedtner B, Olthoff D, et al: Anaesthetic considerations for endoscopic extraperitoneal and laparoscopic transperitoneal radical prostatectomy. BJU Int 2006;98(3):508–513.

Strumper-Groves D: Perioperative blood transfusion and outcome. Curr Opin Anaesthesiol 2006;19(2):198–206.

Tasch MD: Corticosteroids and anesthesia. Curr Opin Anaesthesiol 2002;15(3):377–381.

Toivonen HJ: Anaesthesia for patients with a transplanted organ. Acta Anaesthesiol Scand 2000;44(7):812–833.

Triplett DA: Coagulation and bleeding disorders: Review and update. Clin Chem 2000;46(8 Pt 2):1260–1269.

Whalley DG, Berrigan MJ: Anesthesia for radical prostatectomy, cystectomy, nephrectomy, pheochromocytoma and laparoscopic procedures. Anesthesiol Clin North Am 2000;18:899–917.

Obstetric Anesthesia

David Kim, MD, Jamie Murphy, MD, and Michael Phelps, MD
Edited by Andrew Harris, MD

I. PREGNANCY
A. PHYSIOLOGY (Table 12.1)

B. ABNORMALITIES
1. Preeclampsia.
a. Multisystem disorder.
b. New-onset elevated BP (>140/90) after 20 wk, with proteinuria and edema.

c. Affects 2% to 8% of pregnancies.
d. Risk factors.
   i. First pregnancy, maternal age >40, personal or family history of preeclampsia, obesity, multiple pregnancies.
e. Potential complications.
   i. Intracerebral hemorrhage.
   ii. Seizures.
   iii. Blindness.
   iv. HELLP (*h*emolysis, *e*levated *l*iver enzymes, *l*ow *p*latelets) syndrome.
   v. Hepatic rupture.
   vi. Laryngeal edema.
   vii. Renal injury.
   viii. Placental abruption.
   ix. Pulmonary edema.
   x. Fetal demise.
   xi. Intrauterine growth restriction.
f. Prophylaxis.
   i. Low-dose aspirin.
g. Treatment.
   i. Ultimate treatment is delivery of placenta.
   ii. Antihypertensives (labetalol, methyldopa, calcium-channel blockers).
   iii. Magnesium sulfate around time of delivery to use as prophylaxis against seizures (eclampsia).

2. Eclampsia.
a. Preeclampsia with associated seizures.
b. Risk significantly (>50%) reduced by magnesium sulfate.

3. Pregnancy-induced hypertension.
a. New-onset hypertension (>140/90) after 20 wk of gestation WITHOUT proteinuria.
b. Resolves within 3 mo after delivery.

3. Gestational diabetes.
a. Incidence in Europe 2% to 6% of pregnancies.

TABLE 12.1

SUMMARY OF PHYSIOLOGIC CHANGES ASSOCIATED WITH PREGNANCY

Organ System	Property	Direction of Change	Magnitude of Change (%)
Respiratory	FRC	Decrease	20
	Oxygen consumption	Increase	20
	Minute ventilation	Increase	30–40
	Tidal volume	Increase	30–40
	RR	Increase	
	PaCO$_2$	Decrease	
CV	Cardiac output	Increase	30–50
	Stroke volume	Increase	30
	Heart rate	Increase	15–20
	Plasma volume	Increase	40–50
	SVR	Decrease	20–30
GI	Lower esophageal sphincter	Decrease	
	Gastric volume	Increase	
	Gastric pH	Decrease	
	Gastric emptying	Decrease	
Hematologic	RBC production	Increase	
	Hct	Net decrease	
	Clotting factors	Increase	
CNS	MAC	Decrease	30–40
Renal	GFR	Increase	50
Musculoskeletal	Joint relaxation	Increase	
	Sensitivity to nondepolarizing muscle relaxants	Increase	

FRC, Functional residual capacity; *RR*, respiratory rate; *CV*, cardiovascular; *GI*, gastrointestinal; *CNS*, central nervous system; *MAC*, minimal alveolar concentration; *GFR*, glomerular filtration rate.

b. 70% risk of developing diabetes within 10 yr.

4. Placenta previa.

a. Placenta overlies internal os of cervix.

b. Four types.
    i. Complete (completely overlies os).
    ii. Partial (partially overlies os).
    iii. Marginal (just reaches internal os).
    iv. Low-lying (extends to lower uterine segment but does not reach os).

c. Risk factors.
    i. Prior C-section or uterine surgery.
    ii. Smoking.
    iii. Increasing age.
    iv. Multiparity.
    v. Cocaine.

d. Prevalence—0.3% to 0.5% of pregnancies.

e. High risk of bleeding (relative risk 9.81).

. Management.
   i.   C-section.
   ii. Ensure good IV access.
   iii. Type and cross in blood bank.

5. Placenta accreta.
a. Abnormally adherent placenta to the uterus (invaded myometrium).
b. Risk factors.
   i.   Placenta previa.
   ii. Prior C-section.
   iii. History of dilatation and curettage procedures.
c. Can lead to massive obstetric hemorrhage.
   i.   Average blood loss at delivery is 3000 to 5000 mL.
d. Management.
   i.   Typically, total abdominal hysterectomy with C-section.
   ii. Anticipate heavy blood loss.
   iii. Good IV access; blood products available.

C. LABOR
1. Stages.
a. First.
   i.   Onset of true labor to complete cervical dilation.
   ii. Latent phase (to ~4 cm dilation).
        • T11-T12 nerve roots convey most of the pain in this phase.
        • Considered prolonged if >20 hr (nulliparous) or >14 hr (multiparous).
   iii. Active phase (~4 cm dilation to 10 cm).
        • Visceral fibers via T10-L1 nerve roots.
        • Increased rate of cervical dilation.
b. Second.
   i.   Full cervical dilation to delivery of fetus.
   ii. Sensory innervation extends to sacral (S2-S4) roots.
c. Third.
   i.   Delivery of baby to delivery of placenta.
2. Fetal heart monitoring.
a. Normal fetal HR is 120 to 160.
b. Acceleration.
   i.   Reassuring if in response to fetal stimulus.
c. Persistent tachycardia.
   i.   Chronic fetal distress.
   ii. Maternal fever.
   iii. Chorioamnionitis.
   iv. Medication.
d. Bradycardia.
   i.   Congenital heart block.
   ii. Fetal hypoxia/acidosis.
e. Decelerations.

12

OBSTETRIC ANESTHESIA

   i. Early.
       • Deceleration >20 bpm with onset of uterine contraction; returns
         to baseline at end of contraction.
       • Caused by fetal head compression; usually benign.
   ii. Late.
       • Deceleration 20 to 30 sec after onset of uterine contraction;
         resolves after the contraction.
       • Caused by uteroplacental insufficiency.
  iii. Variable.
       • Variable in shape and onset; fetal HR <100 bpm and >15 bpm
         below baseline.
       • Caused by umbilical cord compression and, if prolonged, can
         result in fetal asphyxia.

3. Analgesia.
a. Systemic.
   i. Nitrous oxide.
   ii. Opioids.
       • Risk of maternal and fetal respiratory depression.
       • 10 to 25 mg meperidine IV q 1 to 2 hr.
       • 25 to 100 mcg fentanyl IV q 1 hr.
       • 2 to 5 mg morphine IV, 5 to 10 mg IM q 4 hr.
       • Remifentanil.
         - Consider PCA bolus, 0.5 mcg/kg, lockout 2 min.
         - Use when there is concern of sedating effects on the fetus, as
           duration of action is very short.
       • 1 to 2 mg butorphanol (Stadol) IV or IM q 4 hr.
         - Mixed agonist/antagonist; lasts 3 to 4 hr.
       • 10 mg nalbuphine (Nubain) IV or IM q 3 hr.
         - Mixed agonist/antagonist; lasts 3 to 6 hr.
       • Ketamine.
         - Low doses, 5 to 20 mg IV.
b. Epidural.
   i.   Can be utilized at almost any point in labor.
   ii. Advantages.
        • Can provide effective analgesia with minimal sedating effects for
          mother and baby.
        • Usable for Cesarean delivery.
        • Can reduce the risk of GA for urgent C-section.
   iii. Disadvantages.
        • Potential for hypotension.
        • Headache in 1% to 3% of pts.
        • Increases need for forceps or vacuum-assisted deliveries.
        • Increased maternal intrapartum fever.
        • Possibly prolonged second stage of labor.
   iv. Anticoagulation guidelines.

- SQ unfractionated heparin (prophylaxis dose) and NSAIDs (including aspirin) are safe with neuraxial anesthesia.
- LMWH.
  - Hold for 10 to 12 hr if on DVT prophylaxis doses after catheter removal.
  - Hold for 24 hr if on DVT treatment doses after catheter removal.
  - Hold first dose of LMWH for at least 2 hr after catheter removal.
- Antiplatelet agents (except NSAIDS).
  - Hold ticlopidine for 14 days prior to catheter placement.
  - Hold clopidogrel for 7 days prior to catheter placement.
  - Hold abciximab for 24 to 48 hr prior to catheter placement.
  - Hold eptifibatide or tirofiban for 4 to 8 hr prior to catheter placement.
v. Typically L3-L4 or L4-L5.
- Confirmation of correct placement.
  - Aspiration prior to injection to observe for blood or CSF.
- Test dose.
  - Typically 3 mL of lidocaine, 1.5% or 2% + 1:200,000 epinephrine.
  - Observe for HR increase >10 bpm and/or systolic BP increase >15 mm Hg, symptoms of LA intoxication (tinnitus, metallic taste), or signs/symptoms of intrathecal administration (dense motor block).
vi. PCEA.
- Frequently, 0.0625% to 0.125% bupivacaine or 0.0625% to 0.1% bupivacaine + opioid.
- Typical settings.
  - Continuous, 0 to 12 mL/hr.
  - Bolus, 4 to 12 mL.
  - Lockout, 6 to 24 min.
- Some studies suggest increased maternal satisfaction with higher bolus/longer lockouts.
vii. Continuous infusion
- 8 to 20 mL/hr of 0.0625% to 0.125% bupivacaine or 0.0625% to 0.1% bupivacaine + opioid.
viii. Bolus for analgesia (Table 12.2).
- 5 to 12 mL lidocaine 0.5% to 1%.
- 5 to 12 mL bupivacaine 0.0625% to 0.25%.
- 5 to 12 mL chloroprocaine 2%.
- 10 to 30 mcg sufentanil.
- 50 to 100 mcg fentanyl.
ix. Combined spinal/epidural.
- Advantages (versus epidural alone).

12

OBSTETRIC ANESTHESIA

TABLE 12.2
LOCAL ANESTHETICS COMMONLY USED IN OBSTETRIC ANESTHESIA

Local Anesthetic	Class	Onset	Duration Epidural (Spinal) (hr)	Max Dose (mg/kg) with epi	Nerve Block Concentration (%)	Epidural Concentration (Dose) (%)	Spinal Concentration (Dose) (%)
Lidocaine	Amide	Moderate	Moderate 0.5–1 (1–1.5)	7	1–1.5	1–2 (150–400 mg)	1.5–5 (50–70 mg)
Mepivacaine	Amide	Moderate	Moderate 0.75–1	7	15–1.5	1–2	1–4
Bupivacaine	Amide	Slow	Long 1.5–3 (2–4)	3	0.25–0.5	0.125–0.5 (25–150 mg)	0.5–0.75 (7.5–10.5 mg)
Ropivacaine	Amide	Slow	Long 2–5	3	0.25–0.5	0.25–0.5 (75–150 mg)	0.5–1
Chloroprocaine	Ester	Rapid	Short 0.25–0.5	12		2–3 (300–900 mg)	
Tetracaine	Ester	Slowest	Long (3–5)	3			0.25–1 (10–14 mg)

epi, Epinephrine.

    - Faster onset for analgesia.
    - No difference in risks of headache or hypotension compared
      with epidural alone.
    - Higher reliability of epidural functioning.
  • Disadvantages.
    - Potential for fetal bradycardia.
    - Uterine hypertonicity. Treat with 50 to 100 mcg nitroglycerin
      IV or sublingual nitroglycerin spray.
  x. Blocks.
    • Paracervical.
      - Adequate analgesia in 75% of cases.
      - Performed in the first stage of labor.
      - Risks include direct fetal injection, intravascular injection, and
        fetal bradycardia (15%).
    • Pudendal.
      - Performed during second stage of labor.
      - Adequate analgesia in 50% of cases.

D. C-SECTION
1. General
a. Can be elective, urgent, or emergent.
b. Higher risk of maternal mortality with GA.
2. Steps common to all anesthetic techniques.
a. Predelivery.
  i.   Minimize opioids and benzodiazepines.
  ii. Ketamine (10 to 20 mg IV up to 0.5 mg/kg) for patchy regional
       block.
b. After cord clamp.
  i.   Antibiotics, if indicated.
  ii. Begin oxytocin infusion.
    • 10 to 20 units added to 500 to 1000 mL IV bag.
  i.   Uterine constriction.
    • Use after delivery of baby.
    • Uterotonic agents (Table 12.3).
3. Regional techniques—need to block to T_4 level.
a. Spinal.
  i.   Bupivacaine 0.75% hyperbaric; inject a total of 12 mg.
  ii. Hypotension.
    • Both phenylephrine and ephedrine are acceptable pressors
      (phenylephrine may be pressor of choice).
    • Prophylaxis may be achieved by high-dose (100 mcg/min)
      phenylephrine infusion and/or fluid hydration.
  iii. Antiemetics.
    • 10 mg metoclopramide IV is effective with spinal anesthesia.
b. Epidural.
  i.   Can utilize preexisting epidural catheter.

TABLE 12.3

UTEROTONIC AGENTS

Uterotonic Drug	Dose	Comments
Oxytocin (Pitocin)	10–40 U/L IV infusion at 10 mL/min; 10–40 U IM	Never IV push; possible ADH effect, leading to volume overload/pulmonary edema if large doses are given.
15S-methyl prostaglandin F2α (Hemabate)	0.25 mg IM q 15–90 min, max of 8 doses	Not to be given to asthmatics or to pts with significant renal, hepatic, or cardiac disease.
Methylergonovine maleate (Methergine)	0.2 mg IM q 2–4 hr	Not to be given to pts with PEC/HTN/Raynaud phenomenon.
Prostaglandin E1 analog (Cytotec)	800–1000 mcg PR	Caution in renal, cardiac disease.

ADH, Antidiuretic hormone; *PEC*, preeclampsia; *HTN*, hypertension; *PR*, per rectum.

    ii. ~20 mL of lidocaine 2%, chloroprocaine 3%, or bupivacaine 0.5% required for T4 level.
    iii. Alkalinized LA.
       • 10% by volume of sodium bicarbonate added to LA (usually lidocaine 2%).
       • Decreased time to surgical anesthesia.
       • Stable for only 6 hr and may precipitate LA.
    iv. Usually less dense block than spinal.
    v. Can use for postoperative pain via PCEA.
       • Use lower dose settings than for labor PCEA and lower concentration of LA.
  c. Combined spinal/epidural.
    i. Combines denser spinal block with ability to augment block intraoperatively if necessary.
    ii. Can utilize epidural for postoperative analgesia.
4. GA.
  a. Higher risk of maternal mortality.
  b. Use if truly emergent or if there is contraindication to regional anesthesia.
  c. Predelivery.
    i. Prep and drape while preoxygenating.
    ii. Rapid-sequence induction with propofol, thiopental, or ketamine plus succinylcholine.
    iii. Volatile anesthetic ~0.7 MAC + O_2 until delivery.
    iv. OG tube/aspirate stomach.
  d. Postdelivery.
    i. Decrease volatile anesthetic to facilitate uterine tone.
    ii. Start nitrous oxide unless contraindicated.
    iii. Consider midazolam, analgesics.

    iv. May give small amount of medium-acting, nondepolarizing muscle relaxant (vecuronium, rocuronium, cisatracurium) or intermittent succinylcholine.

5. LA.

a. Mix 60 mL of 2% chloroprocaine with 60 mL NS.

b. Inject 10 mL in skin, 15 mL in fascia, and pour remainder into peritoneal cavity.

c. May need to use ketamine to supplement analgesia.

6. Postoperative pain management.

a. Epidural PCEA.

    i. Typically, utilizes lower concentration of LA compared with that used with labor (e.g., bupivacaine 0.0625%) and lower bolus doses (e.g., 4 to 6 mL).

b. Opioids.

    i. Intrathecal or epidural.

- 0.2 mg morphine intrathecally or 3 to 5 mg epidurally can provide up to 24 hr of analgesia.
- Increased risk of N/V and pruritus.
- IV and/or oral.
- Consider IVPCA if on IV opioids.
- NSAIDS (e.g., ketorolac 30 mg IV q 6 hr for up to 3–5 days).

7. Postpartum.

a. Common procedures include bilateral tubal ligation and dilatation and curettage.

b. Physiology.

    i. Return to non-pregnant physiology may take 6 to 8 wk.

    ii. Airway engorgement still present for several days postpartum.

c. Epidural

    i. Increased segmental epidural dose requirement 8 to 24 hr postpartum relative to antepartum.

    ii. Epidural significantly less likely to function adequately after >4 hr of nonuse.

II. OBSTETRIC EMERGENCIES

A. UTERINE RUPTURE

1. Establish large-bore IV access.

a. May need to transfuse large quantities of blood.

2. Consider invasive monitoring.

3. Consider aortic crossclamp.

B. FETAL DISTRESS

1. May need urgent or emergent C-section.

2. May require repositioning of parturient.

C. UTERINE PROLAPSE

1. Incidence 1/2000 deliveries.

2. Consider 50 mcg nitroglycerin IV or volatile anesthetics to facilitate uterine relaxation.

D. VAGINAL TWIN DELIVERY
1. May require 50 mcg nitroglycerin IV or volatile anesthetics to facilitate uterine relaxation.

E. AMNIOTIC FLUID EMBOLISM
1. Incidence between 1/8000 and 1/83,000 live births, with mortality of 61% to 86%.
2. Rapid CV collapse, hypotension, shock, hypoxia, DIC, altered mental status, and pulmonary edema are often seen.
3. May be related to intense inflammatory response.
4. Aggressive and supportive treatment is required, though maternal mortality remains high.

F. SEVERE POSTPARTUM HEMORRHAGE
1. Often due to uterine atony.
2. Risk factors.
a. Abnormal placental position.
b. Prior C-section.
c. Obesity.
d. Advanced maternal age.
e. Preeclampsia.
f. Augmentation of labor.
g. Instrumented vaginal delivery.
h. Multiple pregnancies.
3. Management.
a. Establish large-bore IV access.
b. Aggressive blood transfusions as needed.
c. Consider recombinant factor VII.
d. Consider invasive monitoring.

G. ECTOPIC PREGNANCY.
1. Indications for surgical treatment.
a. Ruptured ectopic pregnancy.
b. Contraindications to, or failed medical therapy with, methotrexate.
c. Previous tubal sterilization.
d. Coexisting intrauterine pregnancy.
2. Be prepared for large blood loss.
a. Establish large-bore IV access.

H. LA TOXICITY
1. Seizures.
a. Consider 2 to 5 mg midazolam, 50 to 100 mg propofol, or 100 to 250 mg thiopental.

2. CV collapse.

a. Seen more commonly with bupivacaine, etidocaine, and ropivacaine.

b. Consider 20% lipid emulsion (intralipid) 1 mL/kg bolus, then 0.5 mL/kg/min.

c. Consider 40 units vasopressin and 1 mg epinephrine.

d. Consider CPB.

REFERENCES

Altabef KM, Spencer JT, Zinberg S: Intravenous nitroglycerin for uterine relaxation of an inverted uterus. Am J Obstet Gynecol 1992;166(4):1237–1238.

American Society of Regional Anesthesia (ASRA) Consensus Statement on Anticoagulation in Neuraxial Blocks. http://www.asra.com/consensus-statements/2.html.

Bernard JM, Le Roux D, Vizquel L, et al: Patient-controlled epidural analgesia during labor: The effects of the increase in bolus and lockout interval. Anesth Analg 2000;90:328–332.

Birnbach DJ, Gatt SP, Datta S: Textbook of Obstetric Anesthesia. Philadelphia: Churchill Livingstone, 2000, pp 86, 285.

Dufour P, Vinatier D, Puech F: The use of intravenous nitroglycerin for cervico-uterine relaxation: A review of the literature. Arch Gynecol Obstet 1997;261:1–7.

Franchini M, Lippi G, Franchi M: The use of recombinant activated factor VII in obstetric and gynaecological haemorrhage. BJOG 2007;114:8–15.

Hudon L, Belfort MA, Broome DR: Diagnosis and management of placenta percreta: A review. Obstet Gynecol Surv 1998;53:509–517.

Kaaja RJ, Greer IA: Manifestations of chronic disease during pregnancy. JAMA 2005;294(21):2751–2757.

Kee WDN, Khaw KS: Vasopressors in obstetrics: What should we be using? Curr Opin Anaesthesiol 2006;19:238–243.

Kee WDN, Khaw KS, Ng FF: Prevention of hypotension during spinal anesthesia for Cesarean delivery. Anesthesiology 2005;103:744–750.

Kee WDN, Khaw KS, Ng FF, Lee BB: Prophylactic phenylephrine infusion for preventing hypotension during spinal anesthesia for Cesarean delivery. Anesth Analg 2004;98:815–821.

Lam DT, Ngan Kee WD, Khaw KS: Extension of epidural blockade in labour for emergency Caesarean section using 2% lidocaine with epinephrine and fentanyl, with or without alkalinisation. Anaesthesia 2001;56(8):790–794.

Lieberman E, O'Donoghue C: Unintended effects of epidural analgesia during labor: A systematic review. Am J Obstet Gynecol 2002;186:S31-S68.

Moore J, Baldisseri MR: Amniotic fluid embolism. Crit Care Med 2005;33(10):S279-S285.

Moschini V, Marra G, Dabrowska D: Complications of epidural and combined spinal-epidural analgesia in labour. Minerva Anesthesiol 2006;72:47–58.

Norris MC: Are combined spinal-epidural catheters reliable? Int J Obstetric Anesthesia 2000;9:3–6.

Oyelese Y, Smulian JC: Placenta previa, placenta accreta, and vasa previa. Obstet Gynecol 2006;107(4):927–941.

Rosen MA: Nitrous oxide for relief of labor pain: A systematic review. Am J Obstet Gynecol 2002;186(5 Suppl Nature):S110-S126.

Rosenblatt MA, Abel M, Fischer GW, et al: Successful use of a 20% lipid emulsion to resuscitate patient after a presumed bupivacaine-related cardiac arrest. Anesthesiology 2006;105(1):217–218.

Volikas I, Male D: A comparison of pethidine and remifentanil patient-controlled analgesia in labour. Int J Obst Anesth 2001;10(2):86–90.

Pediatric Anesthesia

Joshua Dishon, MD, Jennifer Lee, MD, Justin Lockman, MD,
Michael Nemergut, MD, and Julie Williamson, DO
Edited by Marco Corridore, MD, Eugenie Heitmiller, MD, and
Deborah Schwengel, MD

I. AIRWAY

A. INFANT'S AIRWAY IS SIGNIFICANTLY ANATOMICALLY DIFFERENT FROM AN ADULT'S AIRWAY (Table 13.1)
1. The larynx is more cephalad—C2 (infants) versus C5 (adults).
2. As the laryngeal apparatus in infants is more cartilaginous, the arytenoid cartilages are very prominent.

B. SIZE IS AN OBVIOUS DIFFERENCE, REQUIRING THE ANESTHESIOLOGIST TO CHOOSE AIRWAY EQUIPMENT APPROPRIATELY
1. ETT sizes (Table 13.2).
2. Laryngoscope sizes (Table 13.3).
3. LMA sizes (Table 13.4).

C. ETT POSITION (RULES ARE SHOWN IN Box 13.1)
1. The ETT can quickly become displaced if the head is not in neutral position.
2. Remember—"The tube goes where the nose goes."
a. Neck flexion moves ETT deeper; extension moves ETT higher.

II. FLUID MANAGEMENT

A. WEIGHT
1. Except in adult-sized teens, fluid management and pharmacologic management are weight based (Table 13.5).

B. FLUID REQUIREMENTS
1. Hourly maintenance fluid requirements (Holliday-Segar Method) (Table 13.6).
2. By this method, a 28-kg child should receive:

$$10\,kg \times 4\,mL/kg/hr = 40\,mL/hr + 10\,kg \times 2\,mL/kg/hr$$
$$= 20\,mL/hr + 8\,kg \times 1\,mL/kg/hr = 8\,mL/hr = 68\,mL/hr$$
$$(\textit{Shortcut}: \text{if wt} >20\,kg, \text{then} = 40\,mL + wt)$$

3. During surgery, fluid requirements include maintenance (above) + deficits, insensible losses, and blood losses.
a. Deficits are number of hours of NPO × maintenance rate + stool, urinary, or evaporative losses prior to surgery.
b. Insensible losses are estimated based on size of incision, bowel exposure, presence of fever and respiratory rate. Insensible losses can reach 10 to 15 mL/kg/hr.

13

TABLE 13.1

ANATOMIC AIRWAY DIFFERENCES BETWEEN ADULT AND PEDIATRIC PATIENTS

Parameter	Difference	Anesthetic Implication(s)
Head size	Significantly larger overall in relation to rest of body; large occiput.	Careful consideration of head and neck alignment (may need shoulder roll).
Tongue size	Larger size relative to mouth.	Airway appears more anterior; oral airway may help with mask ventilation by displacing tongue from back of pharynx.
Airway shape	Narrow, longer, folded epiglottis; narrowest diameter at cricoid for children <8 yr.	Straight blade preferable in infants to lift epiglottis. Consider risks/benefits of uncuffed ETT. Check for a leak around the ETT; a leak <25 cm but >10 cm H_2O is preferable.

Adapted from Barash PG, et al. Clinical Anesthesia, 5th ed. Philadelphia: Lippincott Williams and Wilkins, 2006.

TABLE 13.2

USUAL ETT SIZES (INTERNAL DIAMETER)

Age	ETT Size (mm)
Preemie <2.5 kg	2.5
Term newborn	3.0
1–6 mo	3.5
6–18 mo	4.0
18–24 mo	4.5
3 yr	5.0
Equation for age >2 yr	(age in yr/4) + 4

If using cuffed tubes, size is reduced by 0.5 mm ID.

TABLE 13.3

LARYNGOSCOPES

Age	Type
Preemie or NB	Miller 0
0–6 mo	Miller 1
6–12 mo	Miller 1 or Wis-Hipple (WH) 1½
>12 mo	Mac 2, Miller 1, or WH 1½

Straight blades are best for infants <1 yr old.

TABLE 13.4

LARYNGEAL MASK AIRWAYS

LMA Size	1	1½	2	2½	3	4	5
Wt (kg)	<5	5–10	10–20	20–30	30–50	50–70	70–100
Max size ETT (ID) that will fit through LMA	3.5	4.0	4.5	5.0	6.0	6.0	7.0

BOX 13.1
TUBE POSITION FROM LIPS TO MID-TRACHEA
NEWBORN 1-2-3/7-8-9 RULE
1 kg → 7 cm
2 kg → 8 cm
3 kg → 9 cm
FORMULA FOR DETERMINING ORAL ETT DEPTH
ETT ID × 3
NASAL ETT DEPTH
Oral depth + 20%

13

PEDIATRIC ANESTHESIA

TABLE 13.5	
NORMAL AVERAGE WEIGHTS BY AGE	
Age	**Weight (kg)**
Newborn	3.5
3 mo	6
6 mo	7–8
9 mo	9
12 mo	10
2–9 yr	(age × 2) + 9

TABLE 13.6	
HOURLY MAINTENANCE FLUID REQUIREMENTS (HOLLIDAY-SEGAR METHOD)	
Body Weight	**mL/kg/hr**
First 10 kg	4
Second 10 kg	2
Each additional kg	1

c. Blood losses are replaced with crystalloid 3 × the blood loss.

4. For children who have been NPO for surgery:

a. It is generally advisable to administer a 10 mL/kg bolus of isotonic solution (NS or LR), followed by repletion of the remainder of the fluid deficit over 1 to 2 hr.

b. The decision to administer dextrose to prevent hypoglycemia in the NPO child depends on age and nutritional status (see below for guideline).

   i. The risk of hypoglycemia under anesthesia generally outweighs the risk of hyperglycemia in children.

   ii. Consider D2.5 in LR or NS (5 mL D50 + 95 mL LR/NS) as maintenance for children <20 kg or those who have fasted >12 hr.

   iii. Use LR or NS for bolus fluids and insensible losses.

   iv. Use a buretrol set for children <20 kg.

     • Fill volume chamber with no more than 10 mL/kg.

TABLE 13.7	
ESTIMATED BLOOD VOLUME	
Age	Blood Volume (mL/kg)
Preemie	100
Term neonate	90
3–12 mo	80
1 yr old	75
Teenager	65–70

    v.   If pt is receiving parenteral nutrition, continue infusion intraoperatively and check glucose.

    vi. De-air all IV tubing so that it is free of bubbles.

    vii. Use small-bore tubing (1.3–1.8 mL dead space) for infants.

5. Crystalloid/colloid administration.

a. Fluid bolus for hypovolemia.

    i.   10 to 20 mL/kg NS or LR.

b. Albumin.

    i.   5% → 10 mL/kg; 25% → 2–3 mL/kg.

c. Hetastarch.

    i.   10 mL/kg; no more than 35 mL/kg/day.

d. 2% and 3% buffered saline.

    i.   1/2 to 1 1/2 maintenance or 1 to 3 mL/kg bolus over 20 min.

    ii. Monitor serum sodium every hour.

    iii. 2% saline may be infused via peripheral IV.

    iv. 3% saline must be infused via CVC *only*.

C. BLOOD PRODUCT ADMINISTRATION (Tables 13.6, 13.7)

1. Maximum allowable blood loss (MABV).

$$MABV = \frac{estimated\ blood\ volume\,(EBV)\times (starting\ hematocrit - target\ hematocrit)}{(starting\ hematocrit + target\ hematocrit)/2}$$

2. RBCs.

a. 10 to 15 mL/kg will raise Hb by 1 to 2 g/dL.

3. Platelets.

a. 1 U/10 kg.

III. INVASIVE MONITORING CATHETER SIZES

A. ARTERIAL CATHETER (Table 13.8)

1. Sterile prep/drape.

a. Consider using a polyethylene 2.5 F, 2.5 cm catheter.

b. May use radial, dorsalis pedis, posterior tibial, femoral, axillary, or umbilical artery in neonates.

TABLE 13.8

ARTERIAL CATHETER SIZES

Age	Arterial Catheter Size (g)	Comments
Infant	24	Femoral okay if >5 kg
10–40 kg	22	Use 3 F; 5 cm
>40 kg	20	

TABLE 13.9

CVC SIZES

Weight (kg)	Catheter	Comments
<2–3	3 F; 5 cm	Single lumen only
3–4	4 F; 5 or 8 cm	Single lumen for volume or double-lumen 4 F.
5–10	4 F; 8, 9, or 12 cm	
10–12	5 F; 8 cm	*Length calculation (cm)*
12–40	5 F; 12 or 15 cm	Height <100 cm → (Height/10) – 1
>40	7 F; 15 cm	Height >100 cm → (Height/10) – 2

13

PEDIATRIC ANESTHESIA

B. CVC (Table 13.9)
1. Call critical care technician for assistance.
2. Use sterile prep and full-barrier precautions per vascular access device policy.
3. Ultrasound guidance is recommended.
4. Post-insertion CXR is required after placement.
5. Use polyurethane catheters for venous insertion.
6. Always pick appropriate catheter size and length for size of child, prior to insertion.

IV. ANESTHETIC MANAGEMENT

A. **PREOPERATIVE SEDATION**
1. Midazolam.
a. Most common sedation given to children.
b. Oral.
   i.   0.5 to 1 mg/kg; max 20 mg.
   ii. A premixed oral syrup can be used, or the IV formulation (5 mg/mL) can be mixed with 10 to 15 mg/kg acetaminophen to make it more palatable. It can also be mixed with apple juice or ginger ale, based on individual preference.
c. Rectal.
   i.   0.5 to 1 mg/kg is useful in young children. The IV formulation (5 mg/mL) is mixed with 5 mL of NS in a 10 mL syringe and is administered into the rectum via a 3- to 4-in segment of a lubricated 14 F suction catheter.

     ii.   Add enough air to push the solution through the catheter.

     iii. May need to hold buttocks together for a few minutes so that pt does not expel the solution.

     iv. This technique is usually reserved for children still in diapers.

d. Intranasal.

     i.   0.2 to 0.3 mg/kg.

     ii. The undiluted IV midazolam formulation (5 mg/mL) is dropped into the nostrils during inhalation.

     iii. Children often dislike the taste and sensation of the intranasal administration.

e. IV.

     i.   0.05 to 0.1 mg/kg increments.

f. IM.

     i.   0.1 to 0.2 mg/kg.

     ii. Stings on injection.

2. Ketamine.

a. Should be administered with an antisialagogue (0.02 mg/kg atropine) to prevent excessive secretions.

b. Ketamine produces dissociative anesthesia; eyes may remain open, but pt does not respond to stimulation.

c. Dosing.

     i.   IV.

         • 1 to 2 mg/kg.

     ii. IM.

         • Sedation—2 to 3 mg/kg.

         • GA—5 to 8 mg/kg.

         • Rapid sequence—10 mg/kg (with a rapid-acting IM NMB in pts who require emergent intubation and have no IV access.

            - Midazolam may be added at 0.1 to 0.15 mg/kg (stings with IM injection).

3. Oral sedation: "Ketazolam."

a. 6 mg/kg ketamine, 0.6 mg/kg midazolam, and 0.02 mg/kg atropine mixed with acetaminophen (10–15 mg/kg) or ibuprofen (10 mg/kg).

B. INDUCTION OF ANESTHESIA

1. General differences between children and adults.

a. When given the choice, most young children prefer an inhalational induction rather than having an IV placed.

b. If parents are allowed in the room for induction, they should be told preoperatively about the possibility of changes in respiration, coughing, and excitation during induction; parents may find it upsetting to watch.

c. The inside of the anesthesia mask may be scented with flavored lip balm, or prescented masks may be purchased,

2. Inhalational induction.

a. Rapid inhalational technique uses a high concentration of volatile agent, typically 8% sevoflurane and oxygen ± 70% N_2O.

    i. Prior to placement of the mask, the circuit is filled with the volatile anesthetic.

    ii. For an uncooperative child, the mask may be placed tightly on the face; within a few breaths or cries, the child typically loses consciousness.

    iii. A cooperative, older child may be able to take a deep breath, hold it, and then exhale as if to blow out birthday candles.

    iv. Loss of consciousness typically occurs within 30 sec.

b. A slower inhalational technique can be used if the child will tolerate a mask on his/her face.

    i. An initial 100% O_2 or 70/30 N_2O/O_2 mixture is used, and incrementally sevoflurane is increased by 0.5% to 1% until child loses consciousness.

c. During inhalational induction, a period of excitement may occur prior to complete loss of consciousness.

    i. To keep the anesthesia mask on the face, place hands on each side of the mask and allow the mask to move with the pt.

    ii. Another technique by which to control head movement is to hold the mask and mandible with the left hand and place the right hand behind the occiput to keep the head still.

d. With deepening anesthesia, the tongue and airway muscles will relax, tending toward upper-airway obstruction.

    i. Jaw thrusting and CPAP are very effective in promoting airway patency.

    ii. Oral airways may reduce obstruction from tongue and soft tissue.

    iii. N_2O should be discontinued and 100% O_2 used if airway obstruction occurs.

e. A peripheral IV is placed following inhalational induction for administration of fluids and medications.

f. If laryngospasm occurs prior to placement of the IV, 100% O_2 with positive pressure should be the first action to break laryngospasm.

    i. IM succinylcholine (4 mg/kg) and atropine (0.02 mg/kg) should be administered if laryngospasm is not immediately resolved.

3. IV induction.

a. Older children or those who do not like mask induction may have an IV placed after topical or SQ LA is applied to the insertion area, with or without IM sedation prior to placement.

b. After establishment of an IV, induction may proceed as in adults.

4. IM induction.

a. If IV access is very difficult, IM ketamine can be used with an IM NMB agent (succinylcholine, rocuronium).

5. Endotracheal intubation with/without muscle relaxant (see Table 13.1 for ETT sizes).

a. Whenever the head is turned and repositioned after intubation, bilateral breath sounds and E_TCO_2 should be confirmed, particularly in infants, in whom small movement of the ETT can result in a significant change

13

PEDIATRIC ANESTHESIA

in its position (too deep if chin is down; too high if chin is up; remember—"The tube goes where the nose goes"; the fulcrum is the C-spine—not the trachea).

C. REGIONAL ANESTHESIA
1. Important pediatric landmarks.
a. Iliac crest line is at L3-L4 in adults, L4-L5 in children, and L5-S1 in infants.
b. The spinal cord ends at ~L1 in adults versus L3 in infants <1 yr.
c. The dural sac ends at S2 in adults and S4 in infants.
d. Thoracic landmarks.
   i. Scapular spine is T3; inferior edge of scapula is T7.
2. Spinal anesthesia.
a. Specific pediatric indications include children with chronic tracheal or lung disease or cooperative children at risk for malignant hyperthermia.
b. Typically performed with a 22 G to 25 G spinal needle with pt in lateral decubitus position.
c. To achieve a T4-T6 level, 0.3 mg/kg of hyperbaric bupivacaine (0.75% concentration with 8.25% dextrose) is given.
d. In pediatric pts, the spinal dermatome levels recede more quickly than in adults.
3. Epidural or caudal anesthesia.
a. Used for intraoperative and postoperative pain management during GA; often placed after GA induction in pediatric pts.
b. A single caudal injection is typically given for short procedures below the umbilicus; for example, hernia repair and circumcision.
   i. 0.25% bupivacaine or 0.2% ropivacaine with 1:200,000 epinephrine is typically used.
   ii. Dose—0.5 to 1 mL/kg.
   iii. Always aspirate, inject a test dose, and wait 1 min, watching for signs of intravascular injection, before injecting the entire dose.
       • Test dose—0.1 mL/kg; max, 3 mL of LA with epinephrine 1:200,000.
   iv. Signs of V injection.
       • Increase or decrease in HR by 10 to 15 beats or more in first minute.
       • Increase in systolic BP by 15 mm Hg or more in first 2 min.
       • Change in T-wave amplitude of 25% (increase or decrease).
b. An epidural or caudal catheter is placed for longer procedures or planned postoperative pain management.
   i. A tunneled caudal or lumbar epidural catheter can be placed for pain management lasting 3 to 4 wk (e.g., bladder exstrophy repair with osteotomies)
   ii. Bolus dosing begins in the OR in the same manner as single caudal injections and is then redosed in 90 min with 1/2 to 2/3

TABLE 13.10

LAs FOR EXTREMITY BLOCKS		
Anesthetic	Plain (mg/kg)	With Epinephrine (mg/kg)
Lidocaine	5	7
Bupivacaine	2	3
Mepivacaine	5	6
Ropivacaine	3.5	3.5

Adjuncts, 1 to 2 mcg/kg clonidine, 1 to 2 mcg/kg fentanyl, or 30 mcg/kg morphine.

the original volume; a continuous infusion is started in the PACU or PICU after surgery (ordered by pediatric pain service).
iii. Infusion of 0.2 to 0.4 mg/kg/hr (bupivacaine); 0.8 to 1.6 mg/kg/hr (ropivacaine).

c. Penile block (Fig. 13.1).
   i. Used for circumcision or hypospadias repair.
   ii. A 22 G or 25 G needle is placed at base of penis, midline below the symphysis pubis.
   iii. 1% to 2% lidocaine or 0.25% bupivacaine is used. NO epinephrine.
   iv. Inject 2 to 3 mL at 2 and 10 o'clock.

d. Extremity blocks (Table 13.10).
   i. Bupivacaine dose is usually 0.5 to 1 mL/kg.
   ii. Care should be taken not to give a toxic dose, *especially* when doing multiple blocks.
   iii. Use a nerve stimulator (target 0.4–0.5 mA) and/or ultrasound.

V. COMMON SURGICAL PROCEDURES

A. STRABISMUS REPAIR

1. Most common pediatric eye surgery performed.
2. Goal is to correct ocular misalignment by weakening the muscles, strengthening the muscles, or transposing the muscles.
3. Surgical time is 60 min.
4. Outpatient procedure.
5. Complications

a. Oculocardiac reflex.
   i. Immediately treated by release of retraction of the eye muscle.
   ii. May be prevented by treatment with atropine.
   iii. Reflex may fatigue over time with repeated retraction of eye muscle.

b. Increased risk of PONV.
   i. Prophylaxis for PONV is recommended.

c. Eye pain.
   i. Usually treated with ketorolac and small doses of narcotics.

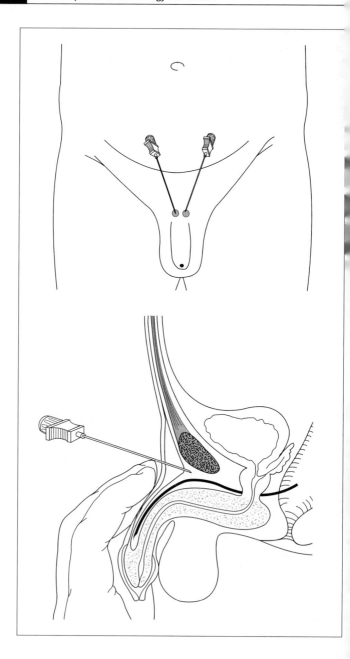

FIG. 13.1
A 22 G or 25 G needle is inserted almost perpendicular to the skin and caudally until it pierces Scarpa's fascia with a characteristic give at a distance of 10 to 25 mm. Because the subpubic space is frequently divided into two separate compartments by a medial division (the suspensory ligament of the penis), an injection is made on each side at approximately the 10 and 2 o'clock positions. The volume of 0.5% bupivacaine without epinephrine to be injected is 0.1 mL/kg per side up to a maximum of 5 mL per side. An alternative technique consists of performing a subcutaneous ring of local anesthetic at the base of the penis. *(From Dalens BJ: Regional anesthesia in children. In Miller RD: Miller's Anesthesia, 6th ed. Philadelphia: Churchill Livingstone, 2005. With permission.)*

13

PEDIATRIC ANESTHESIA

B. **MYRINGOTOMY WITH POSSIBLE TYMPANOSTOMY TUBE PLACEMENT**
1. Procedure typically performed for recurrent acute or chronic serous otitis media.
2. These children tend to have chronic, nonpurulent rhinorrhea.
3. Surgical time is <15 min.
4. Outpatient procedure.
5. Anesthetic technique.
a. GA with face mask is usually sufficient.
b. Nitrous oxide may be used.
c. Children with trisomy 21 may have small ear canals.
   i.   The procedure may be technically more difficult, and these children are at higher risk of obstructive sleep apnea (OSA) and airway obstruction.

C. **ADENOIDECTOMY**
1. Indications.
a. Recurrent otitis media not effectively treated by myringotomy and tubes.
b. Adenoidal hypertrophy.
2. Surgical technique.
a. Palate is elevated; nasopharynx is viewed with mirror through the mouth.
3. Surgical time is 20 min.
4. Anesthetic technique requires GA with use of oral RAE tube (see later for anesthetic technique for tonsillectomy).

D. **TONSILLECTOMY**
1. Indications.
a. Tonsillar hypertrophy.
b. OSA.
c. Chronic tonsillitis.

2. Surgical technique.
a. Mouth is opened with oral retractor.
b. Tonsils are removed through the mouth after cold knife excision or hot cautery excision.
3. Surgical time is ~20 min.
4. Outpatient procedure if OSA not severe and pt is ≥3 yr.
5. Anesthetic technique.
a. GA with inhalational induction for most; consider IV induction for pts with severe OSA.
b. Oral airway may be required to relieve soft tissue obstruction.
c. After peripheral IV line is placed, an oral RAE ETT is inserted.
d. Cuffed tube or uncuffed tube with minimal leak is used to avoid airway fire and blood entering the trachea.
   i. Reduce oxygen concentration to <30%, using air mixture to reduce risk of fire.
   ii. Nitrous oxide also supports combustion.
e. Opioid analgesia is usually given if LA is not injected by the surgeon.
   i. Some practitioners prefer to administer opioids after emergence.
f. Prior to emergence, an orogastric tube is used to suction bloody secretions from the stomach.
6. **Complications include airway obstruction and intraoperative or postoperative blood loss.**
7. **Pediatric OSA.**
a. Presentation—snoring, disrupted sleep, abnormal sleep positions, weight loss, hyperactivity, obesity in older children, associated with airway abnormalities and some syndromes.
b. Apnea-hypopnea Index scores of ≥10 constitute severe OSA.
c. Admit and monitor overnight following T&A because of higher risk of postoperative respiratory morbidity.
   i. Known or suspected severe OSA.
   ii. Significant comorbidities.
   iii. History of prematurity.
   iv. Age < 3 yr.
   v. Craniofacial abnormalities.

E. CLEFT LIP AND PALATE REPAIR
1. **Cleft lip is a craniofacial abnormality that can be unilateral or bilateral and can be associated with palatal clefts.**
a. Although most are not syndromic, facial abnormality may be part of a syndrome that includes airway anomalies (e.g., Pierre Robin, Treacher Collins) or congenital heart defects.
2. **Operative time can be 1 to 2 hr, depending on complexity.**
a. Surgeries are staged—first, lip adhesions; later, palate repairs.
3. **Typically, pt is admitted for overnight observation after palate repair.**
4. **Anesthetic technique.**
a. GA with ETT, typically an oral RAE.

b. Standard inhalational induction, maintaining spontaneous respiration.
c. Intubation is usually successful with laryngoscopy; may be difficult to visualize vocal cords in pts with micrognathia or small mouth opening.
d. Oropharyngeal packing is used to minimize bloody secretions from entering stomach and trachea.
5. Position pt for surgeon with neck extension, face exposed, and bed rotated 90° to surgeon.
6. At the end of the procedure, pt's arms should be secured with soft splints so that the child does not reach up to the face during or after emergence.

F. INGUINAL/UMBILICAL HERNIA REPAIR

1. Most inguinal hernias are indirect, occurring with a patent processus vaginalis.
a. Hernia occurs when neck of processus is large enough for passage of bowel.
b. Hydrocele occurs when only intraperitoneal fluid can accumulate.
2. ~80% of hydroceles may close spontaneously by 2 yr, and 95% of inguinal hernias by 5 yr of age.
a. They are repaired if persistent or large.
3. May be performed laparoscopically (see below).
4. Surgical time <60 min.
5. Anesthetic technique.
a. GA, typically with LMA for older infants and children for open inguinal hernia repair.
b. ETT for laparoscopic or umbilical hernia repair.
6. Regional blocks for pain management include caudal block (as described above) or ilioinguinal and iliohypogastric nerve blocks (Fig. 13.2).
7. Complications are higher in premature infants, particularly those with lung disease or cardiac disease.
a. Hb < 10 g/dL may be an independent risk factor for postoperative apnea in premature or young infants.

G. CIRCUMCISION/ HYPOSPADIAS REPAIR

1. Typically, circumcision procedures performed in the OR are performed free hand.
a. Clamps are used when circumcisions are performed in the newborn nursery.
2. Larger or proximal hypospadias repairs may require intraoperative placement of a urinary catheter.
3. Pts are typically otherwise healthy unless penile abnormality is part of a syndrome.
4. Surgical time for circumcision is ~30 min.
a. Amount of time necessary for hypospadias repair will depend on extent of correction needed.

13

PEDIATRIC ANESTHESIA

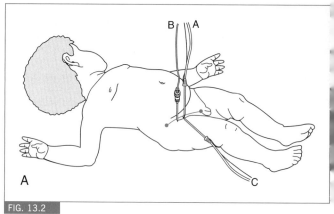

FIG. 13.2

(A) Sites for nerve blocks: specific femoral nerve block (A), fascia iliaca compartment block (B), and "3-in-1" block (C).

5. Circumcision is an outpatient procedure, whereas hypospadias repair may require hospital admission, depending on extent of correction and potential need for urethral catheterization.
6. Anesthetic technique.
a. GA with ETT, LMA, or mask.
b. GA is often combined with caudal block for postoperative pain management.

H. LAPAROSCOPIC PROCEDURES
1. Used for many general abdominal surgeries and urologic procedures in the pediatric population.
2. CO_2 is used to insufflate the peritoneum for laparoscopy.
3. Anesthetic technique.
a. GA to allow for positive-pressure ventilation and to protect airway from potential reflux and aspiration.
4. Peritoneal insufflation often impairs ventilation.
a. Increased abdominal pressure from insufflation and Trendelenburg positioning leads to atelectasis, decreased functional residual capacity (FRC), decreased tidal volumes, increased peak pulmonary inflation pressures, increased arterial partial pressure of CO_2, and decreased O_2.
   i. After insufflation, peak inspiratory pressure and respiratory rate should be increased to maintain O_2 saturation and CO_2.
b. Laparoscopy can decrease venous return by increasing intraperitoneal pressures.
5. Complications include difficult oxygenation and ventilation, hypotension, injury to abdominal organs, CO_2 embolus, and SQ emphysema.

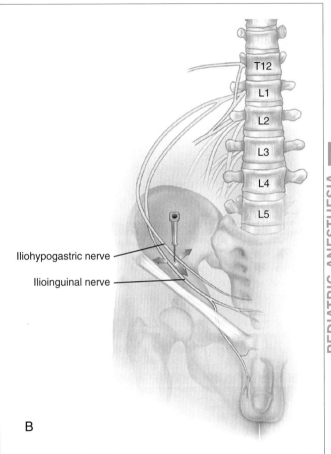

FIG. 13.2—cont'd

(B) Anatomy for ilioinguinal and iliohypogastric blocks. *(Modified from Dalens BJ: Regional anesthesia in children. In Miller RD: Miller's Anesthesia, 6th ed. Philadelphia: Churchill Livingstone, 2005; and Ross AK: Pediatric regional anesthesia. In: Motoyama EK, Davis PJ: Smith's Anesthesia for Infants and Children, 7th ed. Philadelphia: Mosby, 2006.)*

I. PYLOROMYOTOMY
1. Pyloric stenosis consists of circular thickening of the muscles of the pylorus, which causes gastric outlet obstruction.
2. Presentation: projectile, nonbilious vomiting; weight loss; hypochloremic, hypokalemic, metabolic alkalosis; young infants between 2 wk and 6 mo of age.

a. Hydrogen and chloride are lost from the vomitus.
b. Potassium is lost in the distal tubules owing to the increased bicarbonate load presented to the kidneys.
3. Anesthetic implications.
a. Fluid and metabolic management must take place prior to surgical correction.
   i.   Replete chloride with NS and give potassium if necessary.
b. Stomach should be decompressed with an oral or nasal gastric tube to reduce risk of aspiration.
c. Induction is usually IV with cricoid pressure, either a rapid sequence or modified rapid sequence.
   i.   Desaturation is likely unless infant is fully preoxygenated.
d. Opioids are usually avoided because of the short duration of the case (20–30 min, open; 45 min, laparoscopy).
e. LA is injected into the surgical wound(s).

VI. PAIN MANAGEMENT
A. KEY POINTS OF PEDIATRIC PAIN MANAGEMENT
1. Children as young as premature infants experience pain.
2. Extreme pain in the neonate may cause reorganization of the developing CNS, leading to lifelong enhanced reaction to painful stimuli.
3. In older children, a Visual Analog Scale (VAS) should be used for self-reporting of pain.
a. In young children, the Wong-Baker FACES pain rating scale may be used for self-reporting of pain.
b. Younger children require behavioral assessments because self-reporting is not possible.
4. Parent-controlled analgesia (PCA pump operated by a parent/ guardian) is controversial and may lead to overdose in an inappropriate setting.
a. Nurse-controlled analgesia (PCA pump operated by nurse) has been shown to be effective in children <6 yr of age.
5. Acetaminophen is a useful analgesic in children, and intraoperative rectal administration of 30 mg/kg (first dose only) has been shown to decrease narcotic requirements in the postoperative period.

VII. NEONATAL PHYSIOLOGY
The neonatal period is defined as the first 30 days of life; prematurity as <37 wk gestational age. Neonates are physiologically different from adults in many ways that can affect anesthetic management. These differences are summarized below.

A. CV
1. Neonatal O_2 consumption = 7 to 9 mL O_2/kg/min versus 3 mL/kg/min in adults.

2. Neonatal resting cardiac output (CO) is closer to maximum CO than in adults.
a. The neonatal heart possesses less contractile mass per gram of cardiac tissue than does the adult heart.

3. Anesthetic implications.
a. Neonatal CO is considered rate dependent because neonates have less compliant (stiffer) ventricles than do adults and limited ability to increase their stroke volume.
b. Neonates have limited cardiac reserve because of their elevated baseline CO.

B. PULMONARY

1. Tidal volumes, normalized to weight, are similar in neonates and adults (7 mL/kg/breath).
a. Therefore neonates require higher respiratory frequency (30–60 respirations/min vs.12–16 in adults), with resultant high minute ventilation to compensate for higher O_2 consumption.
b. FRC is similar in adults and children >1 yr of age.
  i. FRC is lower in infants, and when anesthetized, children lose more FRC than do young adults.
    • Anesthesia results in greater FRC in children versus adults because maintenance of FRC in infants is dynamic (auto-PEEP) and thoraces are more compliant in children and infants.
  ii. Neonates.
    • Minute ventilation/FRC is higher in neonates.
    • Neonates possess closing volumes that are within normal tidal-volume breaths.
    • Neonates possess a pliable ribcage, which is mechanically disadvantageous when increased respiratory effort is required.
    • The diaphragm of neonates has a relative paucity of type I, slow-twitch muscle fibers.

2. Anesthetic implications.
a. Higher O_2 consumption, lower FRC, and higher closing capacity render neonates susceptible to rapid desaturation.
b. Higher minute volume/FRC results in rapid induction of, and awakening from, inhalational anesthetics.
c. Loss of FRC can be combated with PEEP, longer inspiratory time, faster respiratory rate, and higher tidal volumes.
d. More pliable ribcage and paucity of type I muscle fibers render neonates more vulnerable to fatigue when increased respiratory effort is required.

C. TEMPERATURE AND FLUID LOSS

1. Neonates have high surface:volume ratios, increasing heat loss by radiation and convection.

13

PEDIATRIC ANESTHESIA

2. Higher respiratory rates lead to increased evaporative heat loss from the airway.
3. Premature infants are at risk for major evaporative losses through the skin.
4. Neonates are exquisitely sensitive to effects of hypothermia, as it is difficult for them to compensate for the increased oxygen demand needed for thermogenesis.

D. RENAL
1. Neonates have less renal blood flow and consequently a lower glomerular filtration rate than adults.
a. Range in neonates is 17 to 60 versus 89 to 165 mL/min/1.73 m^2 in adults.
b. Neonates have immature tubular cells with an impaired response to aldosterone.
2. Anesthetic implications.
a. Medications that are excreted in the urine may have prolonged effects in neonates as compared with adults.
b. Neonates have limited ability to reabsorb sodium and are susceptible to hyponatremia without adequate sodium provision.

E. HEMATOLOGIC
1. Neonatal Hb values are high relative to adults, with mean Hb = 16.5 g/dL in term neonates versus 14 and 15.5 g/dL in adult females and males, respectively.
a. Neonatal RBCs are relatively short lived and are composed primarily of fetal Hb.
2. Anesthetic implications.
a. Increased RBC turnover contributes to elevated unconjugated bilirubin levels in neonates.
   i. Drugs that displace bilirubin from serum albumin (e.g., ceftriaxone) have been associated with the development of kernicterus and should be avoided during the neonatal period when hyperbilirubinemia is present.
b. The O_2 dissociation curve is left-shifted for fetal Hb, although theoretically, less O_2 will be released to tissue during times of hypoxemia.
   i. This finding is of unclear clinical significance.
c. Fetal Hb does not possess a β chain.
   i. Therefore neonates with sickle cell disease and β thalassemia may be asymptomatic.

F. HEPATIC
1. Neonatal livers are immature and have impaired ability to catalyze phase II biotransformation reactions.
2. Anesthetic implications.

a. Impaired hepatic conjugation contributes to hyperbilirubinemia during the neonatal period.

b. Impaired conjugation affects the metabolism of many drugs and may result in increased or decreased activity of many drugs (e.g., decreased production of the active morphine metabolite morphine-6-glucuronide).

G. NEUROLOGIC

1. The neurologic system of neonates is immature.

a. The central respiratory centers default to fetal patterns in times of stress; therefore abnormal situations, including postanesthetic states, can result in apnea at as old as 60 wk postconceptional age in former premature infants.

   i. Healthy term infants can be discharged at 48 wk postconceptional age.

   ii. Former premature infants should be admitted postoperatively unless >60 postconceptional age.

b. Because of immature baroreceptors, the sympathetic nervous system provides limited support to the neonatal circulation.

2. Anesthetic implications.

a. Admit neonates and monitor for apnea postoperatively.

b. Neonates are vulnerable to bradycardia from increased parasympathetic activity due to succinylcholine or airway manipulation.

   i. Consideration should be given to administering a vagolytic drug prior to these procedures.

c. Neonates do not get reflex tachycardia in response to hypovolemia.

d. MAC changes with age, peaking at 3 to 6 mo of age.

e. Premature infants are susceptible to intraventricular hemorrhage.

H. ENDOCRINE

1. In utero, neonatal blood glucose levels are maintained by transplacental passage of glucose from the mother to the fetus.

2. After birth, neonates maintain euglycemia by the breakdown of glycogen.

3. Anesthetic implications.

a. Neonates have small glycogen stores and are prone to hypoglycemia without adequate glucose provision.

b. This problem is particularly common in infants of diabetic mothers, neonates who are small for gestational age, and premature neonates.

VIII. NEONATAL EMERGENCIES

A. ABDOMINAL

1. Omphalocele.

a. Herniation of abdominal contents into the base of the umbilical cord.

b. Incidence—1/6000 to 1/10,000 live births.

   c. Associated with other midline anomalies—malrotation, intestinal atresias, congenital heart disease (CHD), bladder exstrophy, craniofacial and trisomy 13 and 15, and Beckwith-Wiedemann syndrome.

   d. Anesthetic implications.

      i.   Increased fluid and heat loss from exposed bowel.

      ii. Attempts to close the abdomen may result in abdominal compartment syndrome; a silo might be necessary until bowel edema subsides and the bowel can fit into the abdominal cavity.

      iii. Postoperative mechanical ventilation is necessary owing to risks of postoperative apnea and to afford abdominal relaxation for closure of abdominal wall.

      iv. Implications related to associated anomalies, especially cardiac.

2. Gastroschisis.

   a. Defect in the abdominal wall lateral to the umbilicus.

   b. Incidence—1/30,000 live births.

   c. Bowel is always exposed and subject to chemical peritonitis, infection, edema, and heat and fluid losses.

   d. NOT associated with other anomalies.

   e. Anesthetic implications.

      i.   See "Anesthetic implications i-iv" above.

      ii. Under omphalocele; silo is usually necessary and abdominal compartment syndrome is more of a risk.

3. Necrotizing enterocolitis.

   a. Ischemic bowel injury from many possible causes; often followed by gram-negative endotoxemia; occurs primarily in premature infants.

   b. Incidence varies between centers.

   c. If no evidence of perforation, treatment is medical.

      i.   Once free air is discovered, treatment becomes operative and is emergent.

   d. Because of the systemic nature of the illness, expect respiratory and CV decompensation, bleeding diathesis, and renal insufficiency.

   e. Anesthetic implications

      i.   When possible, stabilize prior to giving anesthetic agents.

          • Volatile agents are poorly tolerated; narcotic-based anesthetic is recommended.

      ii. Vasopressors are often required.

      iii. MAJOR third-space fluid losses; blood products are usually required.

      iv. Postoperative (and usually preoperative) mechanical ventilation is required.

      v. If infant is stable, adjust FiO_2 to keep arterial oxygen tension at 50 to 70 mm Hg to minimize risks of retinopathy of prematurity.

4. Imperforate anus.

   a. Mild stenosis to complete atresia of the anus.

   b. Incidence is 1/5000 live births.

   c. Operative choices include anoplasty or colostomy.

d. Anesthetic implications.
   i. Associated anomalies, especially the VACTERL anomalies (**v**ertebral, **a**nal, **c**ardiac, **t**racheo**e**sophageal **f**istula, **r**enal, **l**imb).
   ii. Intraoperative third-space losses.
   iii. Postoperative mechanical ventilation needed because of postoperative apnea risks.
   iv. Anoplasty may require prone positioning.

5. **Intestinal obstruction.**
a. Duodenal atresia is associated with other congenital anomalies: trisomy 21, cystic fibrosis, renal anomalies, malrotation, imperforate anus.
b. Jejunal atresia is less frequently associated with other anomalies.
c. Meconium ileus is diagnostic of cystic fibrosis, but not all pts with cystic fibrosis have meconium ileus.
d. Malrotation and volvulus are associated with congenital diaphragmatic hernias, intestinal atresias, CHD, and urinary and anal anomalies.
   i. Volvulus is an absolute emergency that left untreated results in bowel strangulation.
e. Anesthetic implications.
   i. Full stomach/aspiration risk.
   ii. Abdominal compartment syndrome with cardiopulmonary and renal impairment.
   iii. Third-space losses and fluid resuscitation.
   iv. Associated anomalies.
   v. Postoperative mechanical ventilation for apnea risk.

B. CARDIAC

1. **Cyanotic CHD.**
a. Pulmonary or tricuspid atresia/stenosis, tetralogy of Fallot.
   i. Pulmonary blood flow may be dependent on flow through the patent ductus arteriosus (PDA).
   ii. Prostaglandin E1 (PGE1) might be needed to reopen a closing PDA.
   iii. Pulmonary blood flow is also dependent on PVR.
      • If PDA is wide open, therapies such as hyperventilation, increased oxygenation, and possibly, pulmonary vasodilator therapies are needed.
   iv. Balloon atrial septostomy or balloon pulmonary valvuloplasty procedures are performed in pts with inadequate pulmonary blood flow despite medical management.
   v. Pts who fail all of the above are taken to the OR for a shunting procedure, such as the Blalock-Taussig shunt.
   vi. Anesthetic implications.
      • Continue all previous support.
      • PGE1 therapy is associated with apnea.
      • Diagnostic catheterization requires that pts have stable FiO_2 and E_TCO_2 to calculate shunts.

13

PEDIATRIC ANESTHESIA

- Cath lab cases can be complicated by dysrhythmias or cardiac arrest.
b. Transposition of the great arteries (TGA).
  i. Survival depends on the presence of mixing at atrial septal defect, ventricular septal defect, or PDA.
  ii. Infants without adequate mixing need emergent PGE1 and possible balloon atrial septostomy—and if that fails, operative management (arterial switch).
  iii. Anesthetic implications.
    - See above ("Anesthetic implications vi.").

2. Pressure overload CHD.
a. Critical aortic stenosis or interrupted aortic arch.
  i. Ductal-dependent systemic blood flow.
  ii. Pts might present with profound shock due to marked reduction in systemic perfusion and myocardial strain or ischemia.
  iii. Therapies are directed at opening the PDA; decreasing SVR; increasing PVR, fluid, and renal resuscitation; and treatment of acidosis.
  iv. Infants are at higher risk of necrotizing enterocolitis.
  v. Anesthetic implications.
    - See above ("Anesthetic implications vi.").

C. THORACIC
1. Tracheoesophageal fistula (TEF) and esophageal atresia.
a. Five types of anomalies are described and shown in Fig. 13.3.
b. Incidence is 1/4000 live births.
c. Associated with VACTERL anomalies.
  i. Cardiac anomalies are present in 25%.
  ii. 25% are preterm infants.
  iii. Mortality depends on severity of underlying lung disease, associated anomalies, and degree of prematurity.
  iv. In most cases esophageal atresia and TEF occur together, and the most common is type C.
d. Anesthetic implications.
  i. Spontaneous breathing must be maintained; NMB is contraindicated until the fistula is ligated.
    - Positive-pressure ventilation (PPV) will result in distention of the stomach, inadequate pulmonary ventilation, and possibly, death due to inadequate oxygenation.
    - Assistance by gentle hand ventilation is acceptable to aid in oxygenation.
  ii. Endotracheal intubation is performed, either awake or under spontaneous breathing, with volatile anesthetics.
  iii. Positioning of the ETT depends on location of the fistula.
    - When the fistula is in the midtracheal position, the ETT can be advanced past the fistula, and PPV can sometimes be used.

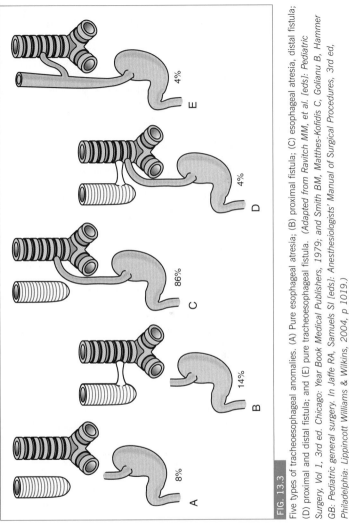

FIG. 13.3

Five types of tracheoesophageal anomalies. (A) Pure esophageal atresia; (B) proximal fistula; (C) esophageal atresia, distal fistula; (D) proximal and distal fistula; and (E) pure tracheoesophageal fistula. *(Adapted from Ravitch MM, et al. [eds]: Pediatric Surgery, Vol 1, 3rd ed. Chicago: Year Book Medical Publishers, 1979; and Smith BM, Matthes-Kofidis C, Golianu B, Hammer GB: Pediatric general surgery. In Jaffe RA, Samuels SI [eds]: Anesthesiologists' Manual of Surgical Procedures, 3rd ed, Philadelphia: Lippincott Williams & Wilkins, 2004, p 1019.)*

- When the fistula is low, near the carina, PPV is nearly always detrimental, as airflow preferentially fills the low-pressure stomach.
  iv. The infant is placed in the lateral position for thoracotomy.
    - Desaturation is expected at least until the fistula is ligated and PPV can be used.
    - ETT occlusion can occur from kinking or occlusion with blood.
  v. Arterial catheters are useful for monitoring of both BP and arterial blood gas.

2. Congenital diaphragmatic hernia.

a. The herniation of abdominal contents through a defect in the diaphragm into the thoracic cavity.
  i. The most common defect is a posterolateral defect in the left hemidiaphragm, known as a *foramen of Bochdalek hernia*.
  ii. The incidence ranges from 1/2000 to 1/5000 live births.
  iii. The most important associated defect is pulmonary hypoplasia.
  iv. Some infants have associated CHD.
  v. Most infants suffer from significant impairment of oxygenation.
  vi. Initial management includes endotracheal intubation WITHOUT bag/mask ventilation, decompression of the stomach, and gentle PPV.
    - Pneumothorax on the right side is common with aggressive ventilation.
    - Persistent pulmonary hypertension (PPHN) is common.
    - ECMO is often used to stabilize these infants until PPHN resolves.
    - When infants are nearly well enough to have ECMO discontinued, they are ready for diaphragmatic repair.
  vii. Anesthetic implications.
    - Continue previous medical management, including ECMO.
      - If still on ECMO, flows should be increased to decrease systemic heparinization.
      - Transport must be well orchestrated; moving pts on ECMO is dangerous.
    - Repair can be from a subdiaphragmatic approach or an intrathoracic approach.

3. Congenital lobar emphysema.

a. Hyperinflation and progressive air trapping of the affected lobe can cause significant respiratory distress, mediastinal shift, and impaired CO.
b. Infants who show rapid deterioration constitute a surgical emergency.
c. Anesthetic implications.
  i. Induction and securing of the airway are critical steps.
    - PPV must be avoided.
    - Crying and struggling can lead to more gas trapping.
    - A smooth inhalational induction is recommended; N_2O is avoided.
  ii. The surgeon must be in the room for induction.

- In case of CV collapse or inability to oxygenate, the treatment is emergent thoracotomy to allow the emphysematous lobe to herniate out the chest incision and relieve cardiopulmonary compression.

iii. As occlusion of the ETT with blood clots is possible, the anesthesiologist must always be ready to reintubate.

D. NEURAL TUBE DEFECTS

1. Meningomyelocele.

a. Failure of the neural tube to close at 28 days' gestation.

b. Usually not associated with anomalies of other body systems but is commonly associated with Arnold-Chiari malformation, hydrocephalus, and tethering of the spinal cord.

c. Closure is usually done in the first 1 to 2 days of life to minimize bacterial contamination of exposed neural tissue.

d. Anesthetic implications.

   i. Endotracheal intubation is performed either in the lateral position or with the meningocele defect placed into the center of a head ring.

   ii. The pt is then placed prone.

   iii. Some pts with large defects will need to remain intubated, relaxed, in the prone position to prevent dehiscence.

   iv. Latex avoidance is practiced because of the increased lifetime risk of latex allergy.

E. OTHER

1. Sacral teratoma.

a. Sacrococcygeal teratoma is a tumor that is usually benign, noted at birth.

b. The mass may be associated with underlying vertebral anomalies and may impair the function of the GI or urinary tracts.

c. The mass can be ruptured during delivery, causing hemorrhage.

d. Surgical excision is required—and emergent if hemorrhaging.

F. BLADDER EXSTROPHY

1. The word *exstrophy* is of Greek derivation and means *turned inside out*. A spectrum of disorders is associated, including classic exstrophy, cloacal exstrophy, and epispadias.

2. The incidence of classic exstrophy is 1/50,000, and cloacal exstrophy is 1/400,000.

3. Classic exstrophy is not associated with other anomalies.

a. Cloacal exstrophy includes spina bifida; anal, renal, and limb anomalies; and sometimes omphalocele.

4. Improved outcomes can be expected if successful surgery is performed in neonatal period.

13

PEDIATRIC ANESTHESIA

5. By definition, the symphysis pubis is separated; therefore repair includes repair of pubic diastasis, which might require pelvic osteotomies.

a. Osteotomies are sometimes not needed if symphysis pubis can be repaired in first days of life.

6. Anesthetic implications.

a. GA/ETT required; combined regional anesthetic recommended with tunneled caudal/epidural catheter for prolonged postoperative pain management.

b. Some infants require ≥24 hr of NMB to prevent dehiscence (especially if pelvic osteotomies are not done).

c. Osteotomies increase risk of blood loss and need for transfusion.

d. Latex avoidance is practiced because of the increased lifetime risk of latex allergy.

e. Central or PICC access recommended because of prolonged hospital stay.

IX. NONCARDIAC SURGERY FOR PTS WITH CONGENITAL HEART DISEASE

A. PREOPERATIVE EVALUATION

1. History.

a. In addition to usual preoperative questions, ask about occurrence of cyanotic episodes, diaphoresis, feeding difficulties, failure to gain weight, activity level, and stridor.

2. Airway assessment.

a. Pts with CHD may have other abnormalities and syndromes associated with difficult airway.

b. Vascular rings, dilated pulmonary arteries, or severely enlarged left atrium may cause extrinsic airway obstruction.

c. Pts with trisomy 21 often have large tongues and may have atlanto-occipital subluxation, for which flexion can result in neck instability. Subluxation may not be evident on neck radiographs during infancy and early childhood.

3. Recent visit with cardiologist.

a. It is important that cardiologist knows pt is having surgery.

b. Review most recent visit and echocardiogram.

B. INDUCTION OF ANESTHESIA

1. Ensure that IV fluids contain no bubbles.

2. Inhalational inductions are generally well tolerated by pts with stable CHD.

3. IV induction may be necessary for severe aortic stenosis and severe CHD with limited CV reserve.

a. Ketamine or etomidate are better tolerated in pts with potentially unstable hemodynamics or limited reserve.

4. Atropine may be administered prior to or during induction in infants.

a. CO is heart-rate dependent in neonates.

C. INTRACARDIAC SHUNTING
1. Right-to-left shunting.
a. Factors that increase PVR shift blood flow from the pulmonary vascular bed to the systemic bed and increase systemic BP.

b. Crying increases RV outflow tract obstruction and PVR, thus worsening the right-to-left shunt and cyanosis.

c. Use oxygen to avoid hypoxemia, and hyperventilate to promote pulmonary vasodilation in these pts.

d. Defects with right-to-left shunts are listed in Table 13.11.

e. Pts with severe polycythemia may require IV fluids during the NPO period to prevent thrombosis.

f. Hb > 12 g/dL should be maintained in pts with cyanotic lesions; these children require higher Hb for adequate oxygen delivery.

g. PGE1 maintains a PDA in pts with ductal-dependent lesions.

2. Left-to-right shunting.
a. Factors that decrease PVR shift blood toward the pulmonary bed and decrease systemic BP.

b. Avoid hyperventilation and use room air or lowest FiO_2 tolerated.

c. Defects with left-to-right shunts are listed in Table 13.12.

D. PTS WITH PRIOR CARDIAC SURGICAL PROCEDURES
1. Blalock-Taussig shunt.
a. Subclavian arterial flow is diverted to the pulmonary artery.

b. Usually right-sided shunt, but in small number of cases, may be left-sided.

c. Use opposite arm for BP cuff or arterial line.

2. Fontan procedure.
a. Pulmonary blood flow is passive and dependent on CVP.

b. Avoid increasing the intrathoracic pressure with high airway pressures or positive end-expiratory pressure during ventilation.

E. CARDIAC CATHETERIZATION FOR PTS WITH CHD
1. Diagnostic catheterization.
a. Maintain a physiologic state similar to the pt's awake state.

b. Preferably have pt on room air.

c. If mechanical ventilation is used, pressure measurement will be taken at end-expiration.

   i. Ventilation will be held for short time when pressure measurements are taken.

2. Interventional catheterization.
a. Abrupt hemodynamic changes may result, with balloon inflation or catheter obstruction of outflow tracts.

b. Balloon dilatation of a valve can be acutely painful and stimulating.

F. CONGENITAL LONG QT SYNDROME
1. Review cardiology evaluation preoperatively.

TABLE 13.11

CONGENITAL HEART DISEASE WITH RIGHT-TO-LEFT SHUNTS

Disease	Features	Specific Anesthesia Management	Surgical Management
TOF	Large VSD, aorta overriding the VSD, RVOT obstruction, RVH. Variants: pulmonary stenosis, pulmonary atresia, absent pulmonary valve.	Preoperative anxiolysis to avoid "tet" (cyanotic) spells. Prolonged spell can result in cerebral injury.	Palliative BT shunt connects subclavian artery to PA; infant not a candidate for complete repair.
	Severity of disease depends on degree of RVOT obstruction and its effect on SVR.	High airway pressure and PEEP may worsen already decreased pulmonary blood flow.	Complete repair: VSD closure, relief of RVOT obstruction.
TGA	D-transposition: RV → aorta and LV → PA. Mixing between the parallel pulmonary and systemic systems is essential for life via an ASD, VSD, or the great vessels. Large VSD may result in pulmonary hypertension. L-transposition: RA → anatomic LV (venous ventricle) → PA, and LA → anatomic RV (arterial ventricle) → aorta. Compatible with life if no other defects.		D-transposition: Atrial septostomy. PA banding to decrease pulmonary hyperperfusion. Atrial switch. Arterial switch.
Truncus arteriosus	Both the aorta and PA arise from a common outflow tract from both ventricles. Large VSD. Associated with truncal valve insufficiency or stenosis, PA stenosis, aortic arch anomalies.	PEEP is beneficial to counter the increased pulmonary blood flow.	PA banding palliation. Repair with VSD closure, truncus valve to LV, and RV-to-PA conduit.

TABLE 13.11

CONGENITAL HEART DISEASE WITH RIGHT-TO-LEFT SHUNTS—CONT'D

Disease	Features	Specific Anesthesia Management	Surgical Management
	Pulmonary and systemic circulations are completely dependent on each other's relative resistances, particularly if there is no PA stenosis.		
Tricuspid atresia	Associated with TGA, pulmonary atresia, pulmonary stenosis; ASD with right-to-left shunt required for survival. PDA or bronchial collaterals are required for survival if there is coexistent pulmonary atresia.	High airway pressure and PEEP may worsen already decreased pulmonary blood flow.	Modified BT shunt at birth; bidirectional Glenn shunt connects SVC to RPA at 3–6 mo; Fontan completion to fully separate the pulmonary and systemic circulations at 3–5 yr.
TAPVR	Pulmonary veins connect to the systemic venous system (RA, coronary sinus, IVC, portal vein, hepatic vein, ductus venosus).	PEEP is beneficial to counter the increased pulmonary blood flow.	Atrial septostomy may be necessary; surgical repair to redirect pulmonary venous return to the LA; may be a true surgical emergency if veins are obstructed.
Pulmonary atresia with intact ventricular septum	Pulmonary blood flow depends on a PDA. Systemic venous return flows from the RA to the LA via an ASD or PFO.	High airway pressure and PEEP may worsen already decreased pulmonary blood flow.	Treatment with PGE1 initially; may need atrial septostomy, then modified BT shunt. Eventually requires an RV-to-PA conduit unless valve can be opened.

ASD, Atrial septal defect; *BT*, Blalock-Taussig; *IVC*, inferior vena cava; *LA*, left atrium; *LV*, left ventricle; *PA*, pulmonary artery; *PDA*, patent ductus arteriosus; *PEEP*, positive end-expiratory pressure; *PFO*, patent foramen ovale; *PGE1*, prostaglandin E1; *RA*, right atrium; *RPA*, right pulmonary artery; *RV*, right ventricle; *RVH*, right ventricular hypertrophy; *RVOT*, right ventricular outflow tract; *SVC*, superior vena cava; *SVR*, systemic vascular resistance; *TAPVR*, total anomalous pulmonary venous return; *TGA*, transposition of the great arteries; *TOF*, Tetralogy of Fallot; *VSD*, ventricular septal defect. (Data from Qu JZ: Congenital heart diseases with right-to-left shunts. Int Anesthesiol Clin 2004;42:59–72.)

13

PEDIATRIC ANESTHESIA

CONGENITAL HEART DISEASE WITH LEFT-TO-RIGHT SHUNTS

Disease	Features	Surgical Management
ASD	Primum (often involves MV and TV); secundum (area of foramen ovale); sinus venosus (often involves right pulmonary veins).	Device closure possible for secundum ASD, otherwise surgical closure.
VSD	Large VSD results in pulmonary overcirculation, CHF, pulmonary hypertension, Eisenmenger syndrome (late), and may be associated with conduction defects. Aortic valve cusp may herniate through the VSD and cause aortic regurgitation and RVOT obstruction.	Usually surgical closure; some may be candidates for device closure.
PDA	Common in premature infants. Large PDA can result in pulmonary overcirculation, CHF, pulmonary hypertension, and atelectasis.	Usually surgical ligation; some may be candidates for device occlusion.
AV canal defect	ASD (primum), VSD, MV and TV clefts, elevated PVR. May have conduction abnormalities. Associated with Down syndrome.	ASD and VSD closure; valve reconstruction.

CHF, Congestive heart failure; *MV*, mitral valve; *PVR*, pulmonary vascular resistance; *TV*, tricuspid valve. (Data from Mann D, Qu JZ, Mehta V: Congenital heart diseases with left-to-right shunts. Int Anesthesiol Clin 2004;42:45–58.)

2. Prophylactic β blockers, left cardiac sympathetic denervation, pacemaker, or implantable defibrillator may be indicated in some cases.
3. Maintain normal electrolyte balance; temperature; and potassium, magnesium, and calcium levels.
4. Preoperative anxiolysis may be needed because anxiety can trigger dysrhythmias.
5. Cardiac defibrillator, pacing devices, and emergency drugs should be readily available.
6. Events that increase circulating catecholamines increase the risk of dysrhythmias.
a. Ensure deep anesthesia prior to laryngoscopy.
7. Continue ECG monitoring during the recovery period.

BOX 13.2

CONGENITAL SYNDROMES, ACQUIRED DISORDERS, AND MEDICATIONS ASSOCIATED WITH PROLONGED QT INTERVAL

CONGENITAL SYNDROMES ASSOCIATED WITH PROLONGED QT INTERVAL

Jervell and Lange-Nielsen syndrome	Romano-Ward syndrome

ACQUIRED DISORDERS ASSOCIATED WITH PROLONGED QT INTERVAL

Hypokalemia	Liquid protein diets
Hypomagnesemia	Hypothyroidism
Hypocalcemia	Bradyarrhythmias
Starvation	Sinus node dysfunction
Anorexia nervosa	AV block—second or third degree

MEDICATIONS THAT CAN PROLONG QT INTERVAL

Ranolazine
HIV protease inhibitors
Organophosphate insecticides
Probucol
Terodiline
Papaverine
Certain Chinese herbs
Antiarrhythmics
  Quinidine
  Procainamide or N-acetylprocainamide
  Disopyramide
  Amiodarone
  Sotalol
  Dofetilide, ibutilide, azimilide, sematilide
Antibiotics
  Erythromycin
  Clarithromycin
  Telithromycin
  Azithromycin (minor)
Antihistamines
  Terfenadine
  Astemizole

Antipsychotics
  Thioridazine
  Phenothiazines
  Tricyclic or tetracyclic
    antidepressants
  Haloperidol and other
    butyrophenones
  Selective serotonin reuptake
    inhibitors
  Risperidone
Anesthetic and Sedative-Related Drugs
  Methadone
  Droperidol
  Cocaine
  Chloral hydrate
Vasodilators
  Prenylamine
  Bepridil
  Mibefradil
Diuretics
  Via electrolyte changes
    (hypokalemia,
    hypomagnesemia)
Serotonin Antagonist
  Ketanserin
Motility Drugs
  Cisapride
  Domperidone

13

PEDIATRIC ANESTHESIA

TABLE 13.13

ADULT PTS WITH CONGENITAL HEART DISEASE

Disease	Features
Atrial septal defect	Mostly left-to-right shunting.
	Risk paradoxical emboli.
	Risk Eisenmenger syndrome if large defect not repaired.
Ventricular septal defect	Mostly left-to-right shunting.
	Risk Eisenmenger syndrome if large defect not repaired.
	Ventricular dysfunction or irreversible pulmonary hypertension results from delayed closure.
	Increased risk of aortic insufficiency.
	AV conduction defects after surgical repair.
Patent ductus arteriosus	Left-to-right shunt.
	End-stage pulmonary hypertension.
	Risk Eisenmenger syndrome if not repaired.
Aortic coarctation, repaired	Revision of childhood repairs common.
	Arterial monitoring is more accurate in the right arm.
D-transposition of the great arteries, repaired	Atrial dysrhythmias, sick sinus syndrome after atrial switch repair (Mustard, Senning).
	Progressive RV failure, tricuspid insufficiency.
L-transposition of the great arteries	Dysrhythmias, heart block common.
	Systemic (right) ventricular failure.
	Associated with VSD.
Ebstein anomaly	CHF or cyanosis, depending on RV output.
	Supraventricular tachycardias.
	Atrial dysrhythmias, AV block after tricuspid replacement.
Tetralogy of Fallot, repaired	Ventricular dysrhythmias, AV conduction defects after surgical repair.
	Pulmonary insufficiency or RV-to-PA conduit failure.
AV canal defect, repaired	Mitral regurgitation.
Truncus arteriosus, repaired	RV-to-PA conduit or truncal valve failure.
	Pulmonary hypertension, Eisenmenger syndrome.
Single-ventricle physiology	Systemic and pulmonary venous blood mixing if pre-Fontan completion.
	Post-Fontan: pulmonary blood flow depends on CVP. Positive-pressure ventilation decreases pulmonary blood flow and CO.
	Atrial dysrhythmias, sick sinus syndrome.

AV, Atrioventricular; *CHF*, congestive heart failure; *CO*, cardiac output; *CVP*, central venous pressure.

8. Congenital syndromes, acquired disease states, and medications associated with prolonged QT interval are listed in Box 13.2.
9. Anesthetic drugs that do not prolong the QT interval.
a. Propofol
b. Etomidate
c. Methohexital
d. Vecuronium
e. Atracurium
. Fentanyl
g. Alfentanil
h. Midazolam
. Phenylephrine

13

G. **CARDIAC FEATURES OF PTS WITH CORRECTED OR PALLIATED CHD ARE LISTED IN Table 13.13**

REFERENCES

Cravero JP, Kain ZN: Pediatric anesthesia. In Barash PG, Cullen BF, Stoelting RK: Clinical Anesthesia, 5th ed. Philadelphia: Lippincott Williams & Wilkins, 2006.

Johns Hopkins: The Harriet Lane Handbook: A Manual for Pediatric House Officers, 17th ed. Philadelphia: Mosby, 2005.

Mann D, Qu JZ, Mehta V: Congenital heart diseases with left-to-right shunts. Int Anesthesiol Clin 2004;42:45–58.

Poortmans G: Anaesthesia for children with congenital heart disease undergoing diagnostic and interventional procedures. Curr Opin Anaesthesiol 2004;17:335–338.

Qu JZ: Congenital heart diseases with right-to-left shunts. Int Anesthesiol Clin 2004;42:59–72.

Stayer SA, Andropoulos DB, Russell IA: Anesthetic management of the adult patient with congenital heart disease. Anesthesiology Clin N Am 2003;653–673.

Sumpelmann R, Osthaus WA: The pediatric cardiac patient presenting for noncardiac surgery. Curr Opin Anaesthesiol 2007;20:216–220.

Wisely NA, Shipton EA: Long QT syndrome and anaesthesia. Eur J Anaesthesiol 2002;19:853–859.

PEDIATRIC ANESTHESIA

Anesthesia for Remote Locations

Christopher McKee, DO
Edited by Deborah Schwengel, MD

GENERAL PRINCIPLES

- Standard of pt care does not change with location.
- Extra vigilance is required to overcome poor lighting, difficult access, or positioning and separation from the pt due to magnetic fields and ionizing radiation.
- Anesthesia monitors and equipment should be comparable to those found in conventional ORs.
- Back-up personnel, laboratory, and blood bank services may not be readily available.
- ASA guidelines recommend ensuring adequate primary and secondary oxygen sources, reliable suction, and immediate availability of emergency resuscitation equipment (http://www.asahq.org/publicationsAndServices/standards/14.pdf).
- Remote anesthetizing locations are often not designed with the needs of the anesthesia team in mind.
- Anesthesia team should inspect location and equipment thoroughly prior to proceeding with case.
- Emergency plans and two-way communication systems should be established so that the anesthesiologist can summon help quickly.
- Pt recovery facilities should be comparable to those in main ORs.

14

I. RADIOLOGY

A. OVERVIEW

1. Site that commonly requires anesthesia services.
2. Procedures are often painless but require pts to lie still and endure confined spaces or loud noises.
3. Interventional radiologists are now performing complicated procedures on sicker pts.

B. CONTRAST AGENTS (Table 14.1)

1. New contrast agents have good safety profile.
2. Fatal reactions occur in ~1 : 17,000 procedures.
3. Reactions to contrast agents (Table 14.2).
   a. Data are weak for the use of prophylaxis with newer non-ionic contrast agents.
   b. IV antihistamines and corticosteroids may have some benefit in pt with documented contrast reactions.
4. Protection from ionizing radiation.
   a. Three types of radiation exposure.

345

TABLE 14.1

CONTRAST AGENTS

	High Osmolality	Low Osmolality	Gadolinium-Containing
Ionic	Diatrizoate sodium (Hypaque) Iothalamate meglumine (Conray) Ioxitalamic acid (Telebrix) Amidotrizoic acid (Urografin)	Meglumine ioxaglate (Hexabrix)	Gadopentetate dimeglumine Gd-DTPA Gadobenate dimeglumine Gd-BOPTA Gadoxetic acid Gd-EOB-DTPA Gadofosveset Gd-DTPA
Non-ionic		Gadodiamide (Omniscan) Gadoteridol (ProHance) Iodixanol (Visipaque) Iopamidol (Isovue) Iopromide (Ultravist) Ioversol (Optiray) Iohexol (Omnipaque) Iopentol (Imagopaque) Ioxilan (Oxilan) Iomeprol (Iomeron) Iobitridol (Xenetix) Iopamidol (Iopamiro) Iotrolan (Isovist)	Gadodiamide Gd-DTPA-BMA Gadoteridol Gd-HP-DO3A Gadobutrol Gd-BT-DO3A Gadoterate meglumine Gd-DOTA

---

   i. Direct exposure to radiation from tube.
   ii. Leakage through collimator's shielding.
   iii. Scatter reflected from pt and areas surrounding imaged body part.
b. Direct exposure should be avoided by healthcare workers at all times.
c. CXR radiation exposure is high during fluoroscopy and even higher during digital-subtraction angiography.
d. All healthcare workers at risk for radiation exposure should wear lead aprons, thyroid shields, and radiation-exposure badges.
e. Movable leaded-glass shields should be available to further limit exposure.

C. ANGIOGRAPHY
1. Pulse-oximetry probe placed on toe of leg with femoral artery sheath may provide warning of vascular occlusion or distal thrombosis.
2. All lines and monitors should be positioned away from areas of interest to ensure unobstructed image.
3. Arms are often tucked at sides for angiography; adequate IV access should be obtained prior to start of procedure.

TABLE 14.2

CONTRAST REACTIONS

Complication	Description	Patients at Risk
Anaphylaxis	Hives, flushing, hypotension, bronchospasm	Previous allergic reaction, other significant allergic history, asthma
Delayed reactions	• Occur >30 min after the contrast is injected • Fever, chills, N/V, abdominal pain, fatigue, congestion • Renal injury	• More common with ionic agents • Renal injury in pts with preexisting renal insufficiency, multiple medical problems, or an underlying disease (e.g., cardiac disease, preexisting azotemia) • Treatment with nephrotoxic agents (e.g., aminoglycosides, nonsteroidal anti-inflammatory agents) • Advanced age
Dose-dependent	• Include N/V, metallic taste in mouth, generalized warmth or flushing • Usually non-life-threatening, self-limited problems • Renal failure	More common with high-osmolality agents
Host-dependent	Gadolinium-induced fibrosing dermatopathy	Severe renal failure
Extravasation	• Direct toxic effect of the agent • Compartment syndrome may occur	

High-risk patients are candidates for low-osmolar, non-ionic contrast agents, according to the American College of Radiology Guidelines.

14 ANESTHESIA FOR REMOTE LOCATIONS

4. Almost all pts who undergo angiography receive anticoagulation of some type.
5. "Roadmapping" consists of a bolus of contrast to outline vascular anatomy, providing a map onto which live images can be projected.
6. Procedures that will require roadmapping often require muscle relaxation to prevent pt movement and ensure correlation between roadmapped images and live shots.
7. Arteriovenous malformations, aneurysms, vascular fistulas, and tumors can be angiographically embolized.
8. Pts can experience severe pain with administration of some embolizing agents.

9. Embolizing materials can migrate and cause ischemia elsewhere in body.
10. Sclerosing agents, in particular ethyl alcohol, can cause transient pulmonary hypertension and, rarely, fatal acute lung injury.

D. NEURORADIOLOGY

1. A variety of CNS diseases can be diagnosed and treated with angiographic procedures.
2. Coilings and embolizations carry a greater risk of catastrophic complications when performed intracranially.
3. NMB is often preferred for these cases as an aid to prevent catheter migration and potential cerebral ischemia or hemorrhage.
4. Deliberate hypotension may help to identify potential watershed areas prior to embolization.
5. Manipulation of pt's BP may aid in catheter placement.
6. Continuous arterial BP monitoring should be employed in such cases.
7. Hypothermia has not been shown to be of benefit.
8. Hyperthermia should be avoided in pts undergoing intracranial procedures.
9. Pts may require a full neurologic exam post-procedure.
   a. In these cases, the anesthetic should be tailored to provide rapid emergence and recovery.
10. During super-selective functional examinations, the pt is awakened shortly after catheter placement and a neurologic exam is performed with the catheter in different locations.
11. Complications during intracranial procedures can be rapid and life threatening.
12. Rapid communication between the anesthesiologist and radiologists must occur to determine if the pathologic process is hemorrhagic or occlusive.
13. Hemorrhagic complications should be treated with reversal of anticoagulation.
14. Occlusive complications should be managed with BP augmentation and possible thrombolysis.
15. Bradycardia and extravasation of contrast on fluoroscopy may be the only signs of hemorrhage in the anesthetized pt.
16. Seizures have been reported as a reaction to intracranial contrast and transient ischemia.
17. A post-ictal pt may have prolonged emergence.

E. COMPUTED TOMOGRAPHY

1. CT is a rapid and painless imaging modality.
2. Most adults can tolerate CT imaging without sedation.
3. Children often experience fear and anxiety.

4. Induction of anesthesia or sedation can be performed away from the scanner to minimize anxiety.
5. Standard ASA monitors are required.
6. Scanning rooms are often cooled to keep machinery functioning properly.
7. Temperature monitoring is important for prolonged procedures.
8. Changes in gantry position may dislodge monitors or airway equipment during the scan.
9. Pts receiving oral contrast are considered to have full stomachs.
10. Stereotactic-guided needle placement for biopsies is performed using CT scanning.
a. Needle placement can cause discomfort.
b. Intracranial biopsies require a radiolucent frame to be bolted to pt's skull.

F. MAGNETIC RESONANCE IMAGING
1. Lack of ionizing radiation and superb image quality for soft tissues have increased the popularity of MRI.
2. MRI scans are painless.
3. Older children and adults usually remain awake throughout the scan, which lasts ~30 to 90 min. However, most children and some adult pts require sedation or GA because they cannot tolerate:
a. Confined spaces.
b. Loud noises.
c. Lying still or flat for the length of the scan.
4. Pts who are sedated or anesthetized must be deep enough not to move in response to a stimulus from the BP cuff or airway device (e.g., LMA).
5. Pt should always have earplugs while in the scanner (staff should also wear earplugs).

G. MRI SAFETY FACTS
1. The magnetic field is ALWAYS on.
2. Force of MRI field is 1.5 to 3.0 Tesla.
3. Force increases as one moves closer to the magnet.
4. The magnet will wipe clean any credit cards, ID badges, or other types of magnetized strips.
5. MRI technicians must check equipment brought into the scanning room and have the final say regarding all equipment.
6. Multiple cases of equipment being pulled into the bore have been reported.
7. Only non-magnetic metals and alloys are used to make MRI-compatible equipment.
8. Only MRI-compatible monitors should be placed on pt in magnetic field.
9. Traditional, non-MRI-compatible ECG leads and pulse oximeters can cause burns through radio-frequency pulsation.

10. MRI-compatible monitoring leads can cause burns if loops are created in the cables.
11. MRI safety ratings for medical devices can be viewed at http://www.mrisafety.com.
12. MRI technicians and radiologists have the final say regarding compatibility of implanted medical devices.
13. Prosthetic joints made from titanium alloys are non-ferromagnetic.
14. Stainless steel implants are weakly magnetic and tend to cause image artifact only.
15. Pts are not subject to irresistible magnetic force.
16. Implanted devices such as automated internal cardiac defibrillators, vagal nerve stimulators, and others are generally not MRI compatible.
17. Some cardiac pacemakers may be compatible.
18. Intravascular wires, such as those in pulmonary artery catheters, or other wire-reinforced catheters in body cavities, such as epidural catheters, can be subjected to radio-frequency pulsation.
19. Radio-frequency pulsation will generate heat and electrical current and may cause pt shock or catheter walls to melt.
20. Ventricular peritoneal shunts are usually compatible, but programmable shunts must be reprogrammed immediately after the scan. This must be arranged with neurosurgery prior to scan.
21. Pregnant staff should not remain in scanning room during scan.

H. MRI EMERGENCIES
1. Resuscitation: CPR and defibrillation should take place in a designated location outside of the scanning room.
a. Attempts to resuscitate the pt in the scanner should never be made.
2. Objects that can be pulled into scanner.
a. Oxygen canisters.
b. Laryngoscopes.
c. Stethoscopes.
d. Clipboards.
e. Chairs.
f. ID badges.
g. Infusion pumps.
h. Metal stretchers.
3. In the event that a missile traps a pt in the scanner, the magnetic field must be disabled.
4. Quench: **EVACUATE SCANNER IMMEDIATELY**.
a. MRI scanners are supercooled with inert gases (cryogens) such as helium.
b. Loss of supercooled cryogens over 5 to 15 sec is called a *quench*.
c. During a quench, cryogens flood into the scanning room, potentially resulting in frostbite and asphyxia to anyone trapped in the room.

d. Room may then become a fire hazard, as flammable liquid oxygen is formed with rapid drop in room temperature.

I. ENDOSCOPY

1. **Overview.**
   a. Invasive procedures are increasingly taking place in endoscopy suites.
   b. Pts are often very ill.
   c. Anesthesiologist must exercise judgment as to the appropriate location for procedure to take place.

2. **Upper GI procedures.**
   a. Esophagogastroduodenoscopy is a diagnostic tool for many complaints.
   b. Endoscopic retrograde cholangiopancreatography is a therapeutic and diagnostic modality for diseases of gallbladder and pancreas.
   c. These procedures carry a risk of aspiration, perforation, GI hemorrhage, and N/V.
   d. Often, topical anesthesia to pharynx and light sedation are all that is required.
   e. Pts are often positioned prone or in extreme lateral position.
   f. Emergent airway management can be compromised by pt positioning and the presence of the endoscope in the mouth.

3. **Lower GI procedures.**
   a. Colonoscopy, sigmoidoscopy, and proctoscopy are common procedures performed in the endoscopy suite.
   b. Pts are positioned laterally, facilitating a patent airway and the expulsion of vomitus.
   c. Often, light sedation is all that is required.

4. **Bronchoscopy.**
   a. Diagnostic and therapeutic bronchoscopic procedures are often performed in the endoscopy suite.
   b. Anesthesia providers are often consulted to assist with airway management and ventilation.
   c. Awake diagnostic bronchoscopy can be performed on selected pts with a mix of topical anesthesia and light sedation.
   d. GA with airway control via LMA or ETT may be required for more invasive procedures.
   e. Potentially disastrous complications such as tracheal or bronchial obstruction or disruption may occur with therapeutic procedures.

J. POSITRON EMISSION TOMOGRAPHY (PET) SCAN AND NUCLEAR MEDICINE

1. Scans are ordered to give functional or anatomic information.
2. A radioisotope is injected and often concentrated in the urine, so that gloves should be worn for changing diapers.
3. In PET scanning, isotopes are sometimes tagged to glucose for brain uptake.

a. In these cases, the use of glucose- or dextrose-containing IV fluids is contraindicated.

K. RADIATION THERAPY
1. Overview.
a. Several oncologic disorders are treated with external-beam radiation.
b. Sessions are often scheduled multiple times over a period of several weeks.
c. GA is required for pts who cannot remain motionless.
d. Because of the high levels of radiation, medical personnel cannot remain in the room.
e. Direct pt observation is not possible.
f. A closed-circuit camera system should be positioned so that pt and anesthesia equipment can be viewed simultaneously.
g. Telemetric monitoring is needed.
h. In case of pt emergency, the radiation treatment must be stopped immediately so that medical personnel can have access to pt.

2. Gamma knife.
a. Targets single intracranial lesions with a precise radiation beam.
b. It is used for certain tumors and vascular malformations.
c. Procedure requires placement of a cranial frame and performance of an MRI of the brain prior to therapeutic irradiation.
  i.   Pts with vascular malformations will also require angiography.
d. Many older children and adult pts can tolerate all of the procedures under sedation.
e. Young children require GA for entire process, which takes most of a day.

L. MISCELLANEOUS
1. The performance of many other procedures may require the care of an anesthesiologist, depending on the amount of time required, temperament and condition of the pt, and potential for pain during the procedure.
2. Some of these are performed in procedure rooms or other hospital locations, and protocols must follow the same rules as any other anesthetic, providing pt safety and comfort, success of the procedure, and safety of the staff.

REFERENCE
http://www.asahq.org/publicationsAndServices/standards/14.pdf.

Crisis Management and Resuscitation

Lyndsey Cox, MD, Kelly Gidusko, MD, Alex Paganegelou, MD,
Shreyas Bhavsar, MD, Polly-Anna Silver, MD, and Jennifer Seebach, MD
Edited by Robert Thomsen, MD

I. ACUTE CHANGES IN BLOOD PRESSURE

A. ACUTE HEMORRHAGE

1. Clinical signs.

a. Hypotension, tachycardia, decreased pulse pressure, reduced urine output.

b. Increased catecholamine output may normalize BP.

c. Tachycardia may be absent in certain situations (i.e., increased vagal tone, β-blocker therapy).

2. Treatment.

a. Crystalloid, colloid, or blood products.

3. Special intraoperative situations for acute hemorrhage.

a. Intracerebral hemorrhage (ICH).

    i.   Intraoperative ICH is a difficult diagnosis without neurologic exam or imaging.

    ii.   Clinical settings.

- Hemorrhagic conversion of an acute stroke.
- Hemorrhagic conversion of septic emboli (e.g., from endocarditis).
- Hemorrhage into tumor or metastasis.
- Primary ICH.

    iii. Expect ICP elevation with acute HTN and bradycardia (Cushing response).

    iv. Most recent guidelines for acute ICH.

- SBP ≤210 is not clearly related to hemorrhagic expansion or neurologic worsening.
- Previous recommendation was systolic BP ≤180 or MAP <130.

    iv. Expansion of ICH is associated with elevated systolic BP, but it is not clear whether this is due to ICP issues causing higher BP or whether the higher BP is the culprit.

    v.   Rapid reduction in BP during the acute phase was associated with increased mortality in one retrospective review.

    vi. Reduction of MAP by 15% does not result in reduction of CBF and thus should be a safe target when considering the potential of ischemic penumbra.

b. Mediastinoscopy.

    i.   Potential for massive hemorrhage.

    ii.   Pay attention to surgical field and communicate with surgeon.

    iii. May need to convert to open thoracotomy to achieve hemostasis.

15

      iv. Can get reflex bradycardia with aortic compression.
      v. Resuscitation may be lost into surgical field if SVC is injured.
        • Consider emergent lower-extremity access.
  c. Obstetric. The following situations often result in life-threatening hemorrhage and require hysterectomy for definitive management.
      i. Placental abruption.
        • Painful vaginal bleeding due to separation of placenta before delivery can cause disseminated intravascular coagulation.
        • Low threshold for C section.
      ii. Placenta previa.
        • Painless vaginal bleeding caused by low implantation of placenta. Hemorrhage often stops spontaneously.
      iii. Placenta accreta.
        • Placenta adherent to myometrium.
      iv. Placenta increta.
        • Placenta invades myometrium.
      v. Placenta percreta.
        • Placenta extends beyond myometrium.
  d. Ocular.
      i. Retrobulbar hemorrhage seen in 1 in 700 retrobulbar blocks.
      ii. If bleed is arterial, it can cause spike in intraocular pressure.
      iii. Increased intraocular pressure may cause the oculocardiac reflex.
  e. Cerebral aneurysm.
      i. Surgical management is aimed at securing aneurysm to minimize risk of rebleeding.
      ii. Clipping performed in acute setting (≤72 hr), or rarely, after 14 days to avoid period of vasospasm.
      iii. Avoid acute HTN; BP spike may cause fatal rebleeding.
      iv. Maintain high normal MAP to maintain cerebral perfusion.
      v. Maintain normovolemia.
      vi. Hyponatremia is common and most likely secondary to cerebral salt wasting (intravascular volume depletion).
        • Less likely secondary to SIADH (syndrome of inappropriate antidiuretic hormone) (normovolemic to slight hypervolemic state).

B. HEART FAILURE
1. Preoperative considerations.
a. Is there a history of heart failure or is this a new finding?
b. Is this a compensated heart or is it decompensated?
c. ACC/AHA Guidelines for elective noncardiac surgery in 2002.
      i. Decompensated heart failure is likely to lead to cancellation.
      ii. Compensated heart failure is an intermediate risk factor.
2. Preoperative testing.
a. ECG.
b. CXR.

. TTE (transthoracic and transesophageal color-flow Doppler echocardiography).
   i. In pts with poorly controlled failure, a TTE may not be necessary if prior testing revealed severely reduced function.
. Stress test.
   i. Consider if suspected ischemic cardiomyopathy.
. Coronary angiography.
   i. Consider if strong evidence of adverse outcome based on noninvasive testing.
3. **Intraoperative monitoring.**
. Routine ASA monitors.
. Arterial line.
. Consider CVP monitoring.
. No absolute indication for Swan-Ganz catheter, but may consider in pt with severe CHF undergoing high-risk surgery.
. Alternative to Swan-Ganz catheter is intraoperative TEE.
4. **Intraoperative considerations.**
. Look for signs of new or worsening heart failure.
   i.   Pulmonary congestion.
      • Wheezes and crackles.
      • SpO_2 may not drop when pt receives high FiO_2.
   ii. Hypotension.
      • Compensatory increased heart rate.
   iii. New onset dysrhythmia may worsen cardiac function or may be a sign of cardiac ischemia.
   iv. Cardiac ischemia.
      • Look for ECG changes.
b. Treatment of new or worsening failure.
   i.   Depends on severity and etiology of failure.
   ii.   Convert new-onset dysrhythmia (chemical or electrical).
   iii. Treat myocardial ischemia.
   iv.   Optimize cardiac preload.
      • Consider 10 mL/kg volume challenge.
   v.   Consider diuretic treatment if volume overload (excreting more free water than sodium).
   vi.   Consider phosphodiesterase inhibitor to increase inotropy and provide vasodilation.
      • Increasing inotropy alone will increase myocardial oxygen requirements, and vasodilation alone will decrease BP.
      • The combined effects may be most helpful.
   vii. Take caution with β blockers, as they can further reduce function.
   viii. Based on response, consider intraaortic balloon pump placement.

C. HYPERTENSION.
1. Etiology.
a. Preoperative HTN.

b. Drug error (inadvertent administration, incorrect dosage).
c. Surgical cause (stimulation, aortic crossclamping).
d. Light anesthesia (pain, awareness).
e. Hypoxia.
f. Hypercarbia.
g. Secondary causes (e.g., pheochromocytoma, hyperthyroidism).
h. Malignant hyperthermia (evidenced by elevated temperature, increasing CO_2 production).
i. Elevated ICP (expect Cushing response with concomitant bradycardia).
j. Fluid overload.
k. Acute stroke, ICH.
l. Myocardial ischemia.

2. Actions.

a. Simultaneously diagnose and treat.
b. Confirm that HTN is real.
   i.   Recheck BP.
   ii. Re-zero arterial line transducer.
c. Stop vasopressors, if applicable.
d. Scan other vital signs for clues (E_TCO_2, saturation, HR, ECG).
e. Confirm adequacy of ventilation ± ETT placement and patency.
f. Check machine and circuit for proper delivery of anesthetic vapor and oxygen.
g. Review drug administration.
h. Examine surgical field and discuss with surgeon.
i. Deepen anesthesia.
j. Consider opioids.
k. Consider antihypertensive therapy.
   i.   0.1 to 0.25 mg/kg labetalol.
   ii. 2.5 to 5 mg hydralazine q15 min.
   iii. 0.5 to 1 mcg/kg sodium nitroprusside, 0.1 to 10 mcg/kg/min.
l. 25 to 50 mcg nitroglycerin.
m. If pt is hypertensive preoperatively, consider possibility of altered autoregulatory systems when initiating antihypertensive therapy.

D. HYPOTENSION

1. Defined as a BP drop below 20% of baseline.
2. Severe if signs of end-organ damage (under anesthesia, this is mainly myocardial ischemia).
3. MAP <50 mm Hg often considered an absolute treatment threshold as this is the lower limit of autoregulation in normotensive individuals.
4. Simultaneously diagnose and treat.
5. Validate measurement (recycle cuff, assess arterial-line waveform, flush arterial line).
6. Confirm presence of a palpable pulse.
7. If pt is bradycardic, strongly consider vagolytic agent.

a. Hypotension may be secondary to severe bradycardia.

8. Check E_TCO_2.
a. Acute drop may indicate lack of perfusion to lungs (i.e., pulmonary embolism, low cardiac output).
9. Discuss with surgeon to identify cause that may be reversed or controlled.
a. Massive hemorrhage.
b. IVC compression (obstetric procedures, laparotomy/laparoscopy).
c. Tourniquet or vascular clamp release (i.e., aortic).
10. Likely causes.
a. Massive surgical hemorrhage.
b. Impaired venous return (surgical positioning, elevated airway pressure, pneumothorax, surgical technique).
c. Vasodilation (sympathectomy from neuraxial anesthesia; anesthetic agents, drug reactions, including anaphylaxis).
d. Embolism (air, CO_2, fat, venous).
e. Cardiac dysrhythmia.
f. Depressed myocardial function (baseline, anesthetic vapors, etc.).
g. Cardiac ischemia/infarction.
h. Drug error.
i. Rare causes (anaphylaxis, transfusion reaction, mitral valve rupture, pericardial tamponade, systemic inflammatory response syndrome/septic shock, adrenocortical insufficiency).
11. Remember ABCDs to help with diagnosis.
a. Check *a*irway pressure and minute ventilation.
b. Confirm adequate ventilation (oxygenation and CO_2 exchange)—*b*reathing.
c. Ensure adequate *c*irculation including volume.
   i. Confirm a perfusing rhythm and assess for signs of ischemia.
d. Check for *d*rug error, adverse reaction, or depth of anesthesia.
12. Management.
a. Volume resuscitation (crystalloid, colloid, blood products).
b. Lighten anesthesia.
c. Vasopressor, depending on severity, duration, and response of BP.
   i. 5 to 10 mg ephedrine.
   ii. 50 to 200 mcg phenylephrine, 0.15 to 0.75 mcg/kg/min.
   iii. 2 to 10 mcg bolus epinephrine, 0.01 to 0.03 mcg/kg/min infusion.

II. ACUTE CHANGES IN ECG
A. RHYTHM CHANGES
1. Ventricular fibrillation (VF) and pulseless ventricular tachycardia (VT).
a. Initiate CPR (30 compressions: 2 breaths).
   i. If airway is secure, place pt on ventilator, 8 to 10 breaths/min.
   ii. Do not hyperventilate.
   iii. CPR at the rate of 100 compressions/min.

15

CRISIS MANAGEMENT AND RESUSCITATION

    b. Defibrillate as soon as possible.
        i.   Manual biphasic—200 J.
        ii. Monophasic—360 J.
    c. Resume CPR.
    d. 1 mg epinephrine IV/IO q 3 to 5 min.
        i.   40 U vasopressin IV/IO can replace first or second dose of epi.
    e. Rhythm check q 2 min; if VF/VT, defibrillate as above.
    f. Consider antiarrhythmic.
        i.   300 mg amiodarone IV/IO; may repeat 150 mg once.
        ii. 1 to 1.5 mg/kg lidocaine; may repeat 0.5 to 0.75 mg, 3 mg/kg max.
    g. Consider 1 to 2 g magnesium IV/IO for torsades de pointes.

2. Asystole/pulseless electrical activity (PEA).

    a. Initiate CPR (30 compressions: 2 breaths).
        i.   If airway is secure, place pt on ventilator, 8 to 10 breaths/min.
        ii. Do not hyperventilate.
        iii. CPR at the rate of 100 compressions/min.
    b. 1 mg epi IV/IO q 3 to 5 min.
        i.   40 U vasopressin IV/IO can replace first or second dose of epi.
    c. 1 mg atropine IV/IO for asystole or slow PEA, q 3 to 5 min.
        i.   Up to three doses.
    d. PEA associated with the "Hs" and "Ts."
        i.   Hypovolemia.
        ii. Hypoxia.
        iii. Hydrogen (acidosis).
        iv. Hyperkalemia/hypokalemia.
        v. Hypoglycemia.
        vi. Hypothermia.
        vii. Toxins.
        viii. Tamponade (cardiac).
        ix. Tension pneumothorax.
        x. Thrombosis (cardiac and pulmonary).
        xi. Trauma.

3. Bradycardia.

    a. If there is concern for poor perfusion, action is required.
    b. If ECG reveals type II second-degree or third-degree block, prepare for transcutaneous pacing.
    c. Consider 0.5 to 1 mg atropine, based on severity of dysrhythmia.
        i.   May repeat, up to a total dose of 3 mg.
    d. Consider epinephrine, 2 to 10 mcg/min.
    e. Consider dopamine, 2 to 10 mcg/kg/min.
    f. Consider transvenous pacing with high-degree block.

4. Tachycardia.

    a. If there is concern for poor perfusion, action is required.
    b. With unstable tachycardia, immediate synchronized cardioversion is required. The sequence of shocks with a monophasic device is as follows:

i.   Atrial fibrillation: 100 to 200 J, 300 J, 360 J (100–120 J for synchronous biphasic devices, with escalation as needed).
ii. Stable monomorphic VT: 100 J, 200 J, 300 J, 360 J.
iii. Other SVT/atrial flutter: 50 J, 100 J, 200 J, 300 J, 360 J.

. With a stable tachycardia, assess available leads on monitor.

. Narrow complex regular tachycardia.
   i.   Attempt vagal maneuver.
   ii. Consider 6 mg adenosine.
        • If no conversion, give 12 mg rapid IV push.
        • May repeat 12 mg dose once.
   iii. If conversion, suspect reentry SVT.
        • Treat recurrence with adenosine or longer-acting AV nodal blocking agent (i.e., diltiazem, β blocker).
   iv. If no conversion, consider atrial flutter ectopic atrial tachycardia and junctional tachycardia.
        • Control rate (e.g, diltiazem, β blocker).

. Narrow complex irregular tachycardia.
   i.   Likely atrial fibrillation; less likely atrial flutter or multifocal atrial tachycardia.
   ii. Control rate with diltiazem or β blocker.

. Wide complex regular tachycardia.
   i.   Suspected VT or uncertain rhythm.
   ii. 150 mg amiodarone IV over 10 min.
        • Repeat to a max dose of 2.2 g/24 hr.
   iii. Consider elective synchronized cardioversion.
   iv. SVT with aberrancy.
        • Refer to narrow complex regular (see d above).

. Wide complex irregular tachycardia.
   i.   Atrial fibrillation with aberrancy.
   ii. Pre-excited atrial fibrillation (AF + Wolff-Parkinson-White syndrome).
        • Avoid AV nodal blocking agents.
        • Consider antiarrhythmic (i.e., amiodarone).
        • Torsades de pointes—1 to 2 g magnesium over 5 to 60 min, then continue an infusion.

B. ST DEPRESSION/ISCHEMIA
1. Preoperatively, may be diagnosed by symptoms.
2. Intraoperatively, diagnosis may be made by ECG, echocardiography, and/or hemodynamics.
3. ST depression >2 mm or elevation >1 mm should prompt intervention.
4. Management centers on maximizing myocardial oxygen supply and minimizing demand.
a. Demand—HR, contractility, systolic wall tension.
b. Supply—diastolic phase allowing for coronary blood flow, oxygen-carrying capacity, coronary artery tone/stenosis.

15

CRISIS MANAGEMENT AND RESUSCITATION

5. β blockade—controls HR, improves coronary blood flow.
6. Nitrates—vasodilators that decrease preload have direct effect on coronary blood flow.
a. Be careful not to compromise coronary perfusion pressure.
7. Optimize oxygenation and oxygen-carrying capacity.
8. Consider heparin—inhibition of thrombus formation.
9. Consider antiplatelet agents.
10. Consider intraaortic balloon pump placement.
11. In noncardiac surgery, consider case cancellation. Risk and benefit of continuing case should be carefully considered.

III. DESATURATION

A. ASPIRATION

1. Can occur anytime—on induction, during maintenance, and on emergence.
2. Risk factors.
a. Supine position.
b. Depression of airway protective reflexes (decreased gag reflex).
c. Gastroesophageal reflux disease.
d. Advanced age.
e. Decreased level of consciousness (intoxication, encephalopathy).
f. Neuromuscular disease.
g. Endotracheal intubation.
h. Mechanical ventilatory support.
i. Tracheostomy.
j. Delayed gastric emptying (diabetic gastroparesis, drug-induced motility disorder).
k. Elevated gastric residual volume.
l. Abnormal anatomy of pharynx or esophagus (hiatal hernia, Zenker diverticulum).
m. Scleroderma.
n. Pregnancy.
o. Obesity.
p. Recent oral intake.
q. Abdominal pathology (acute abdomen, peptic ulcer disease, obstruction, inflammation).
r. Pain.
s. Anxiety.
t. Opioids.
u. Increased intraabdominal pressure (pregnancy, laparoscopic surgery).
v. Trauma.
w. Difficult intubation, requiring periods of positive-pressure mask ventilation.
3. Pathophysiology of pulmonary aspiration.
a. Immediate airway obstruction from aspirated particulate debris, causing small airway blockage.

b. Chemically induced bronchoconstriction.
c. Alveolar necrosis from a chemical burn of the airway.
d. Intense inflammatory response with fluid loss into the injured area, and finally, lung infection.
e. Earliest physiologic change is intrapulmonary shunting, which results in hypoxia.

4. Clinical presentation.
a. Varies with volume of aspirate, pH of aspirate, presence of particulate matter.
b. Mild aspiration.
   i.   Transient coughing.
   ii. Minimal bronchospasm.
c. Severe aspiration.
   i.   Severe hypoxemia.
   ii. Tachycardia.
   iii. Tachypnea.
   iv. Severe bronchospasm.
   v. Pulmonary edema.
   vi. Pulmonary HTN.
   vii. Hypovolemia from pulmonary edema and alveolar fluid shift.
   viii. Decreased lung compliance.
   ix. Sepsis.
   x. Respiratory acidosis.
   xi. CXR findings of bilateral (right > left) infiltrates are often delayed.

5. Prevention.
a. Prevention is key—remember risk factors.
b. If pt has risk factors, use of LMA is contraindicated.
c. Gastric decompression whenever possible.
d. Adhere to NPO guidelines.
e. Agents that decrease gastric acid production:.
   i. H_2 receptor antagonists.
     • Decrease acid secretion and inhibit further acid production.
     • Both pH and gastric volume are affected.
     • Delayed onset of action as compared with antacids.
   ii. Proton pump inhibitors.
     • Increase gastric pH.
     • Generally as effective as H_2 blockers.
f. Agents that neutralize gastric pH.
   i.   Antacids.
   ii. Raise gastric fluid pH and alter the acidity of existing gastric contents.
   iii. Also raise intragastric volume.
   iv. Preference is for clear antacids (sodium citrate).
   v. Immediately effective.
g. Agents that promote gut motility.
   i.   Shorten gastric emptying time.

   ii. Increase lower esophageal sphincter tone.
   iii. Antiemetic.
   iv. No effect on gastric pH.
   v. In conjunction with H_2 blocker, make a good combination for most at-risk pts.
 h. No current role of anticholinergics.
   i. Decrease secretions of stomach only after large doses.
   ii. Lower esophageal sphincter tone.

6. Treatment for suspected aspiration.
 a. Immediate suction and removal of debris.
 b. Head-down position to prevent further flow of aspirate into bronchioles.
 c. Consider need for intubation and FOB with pulmonary lavage for severe aspiration.
 d. Addition of continuous positive airway pressure or positive end-expiratory pressure to facilitate oxygenation.
 e. Place NG tube to decompress and evacuate any remaining gastric contents.
 f. Deliver 100% FiO_2.
 g. Treat with bronchodilator for bronchospasm.
 h. Maintain normal volume status and normal perfusion.
 i. Vasoactive and inotropic support if necessary.
 j. Treatment of pneumonia with antibiotics only after positive results of culture and gram stain.
 k. Steroids show NO benefit.

7. Possible treatment approach for pt with significant risk factors for aspiration.
 a. Regional anesthesia with minimal sedation.
 b. Premedication with metoclopramide, H_2 blocker, and nonparticulate antacid.
 c. Evacuation of gastric contents with NG tube.
 d. Rapid-sequence induction.
 e. Cricoid pressure.
 f. Avoidance of positive-pressure ventilation.
 g. Awake extubation.

8. Notes on cricoid pressure.
 a. Also called the Sellick maneuver.
 b. Cricoid cartilage is the only complete tracheal ring that allows pressure to be transmitted through it to compress underlying tissue.
 c. Pressure directly on it causes esophageal collapse and prevents gastric content from reaching hypopharynx.
 d. Downward pressure required to adequately compress esophagus is between 8 and 9 pounds (very uncomfortable in an awake pt).
 e. Pressure must be maintained from the time pt loses protective airway reflex until ETT cuff is inflated and tube position is confirmed, even during difficult intubation or during multiple attempts.

Avoid ventilation between intubation attempts to prevent positive pressure from forcibly entering the stomach and leading to regurgitation/ aspiration.

No studies currently prove that cricoid pressure is truly beneficial.

. **BRONCHOSPASM**
. **Causes.**
. Asthma.
. Endobronchial intubation.
. Laryngoscopy.
. Potentially severe in lightly anesthetized pt with reactive airways disease.
. NSAIDS, aspirin, and acetaminophen.
. Pain.
. **Pathophysiology.**
. Transient increases in airway resistance due to increased bronchial smooth muscle tone.
. **Treatment.**
. Symptomatic.
. O_2.
. Bronchodilators (in order of effectiveness: β agonists, inhaled glucocorticoids, leukotriene blockers, theophyllines, and anticholinergics).
. Deepening anesthesia with IV or inhaled agents.
. Corticosteroids and antihistamines if immunologic cause.
. Severe bronchospasm can be treated with epinephrine (300 mcg SQ q 20 min, up to 3 doses).
. Theophylline—used only as an alternative, not as a preferred treatment medication. Serum levels must be monitored. May work by increasing intracellular concentration of cAMP.
. Consider ketamine.
. Adjust ventilation .
    i.   Ventilate at slow rates (6–10 breaths/min).
    ii. Use lower tidal volume (<10 mL/kg).
    iii. Increase exhalation time.
4. **Anesthetic considerations.**
a. Propofol may be induction agent of choice in pts prone to bronchospasm.
b. Bronchospasm may be blunted with pretreatment with anticholinergics, steroids, inhaled $β_2$ agonists, lidocaine, and narcotics.
c. Rule out other causes of wheezing—mechanical obstruction of ETT from kinking, clot, mucus, biting, foreign body, bevel against tracheal wall, active expiratory efforts, pulmonary edema.
d. Indications of possible bronchospasm.
    i.   Steep upward curve to the CO_2 waveform: severity of obstruction is generally inversely related to the rate of rise in E_TCO_2.

    ii. Increase in peak airway pressure.

    iii. Decreased E_TCO_2.

e. Minimize airway irritation and maintain adequate depth of anesthesia.

f. Depress airway reflexes to avoid bronchoconstriction during mechanical stimulation.

C. LARYNGOSPASM

1. Definition.

a. Involuntary muscular spasm (reflex closure) of the larynx via the stimulation of the superior laryngeal nerve.

b. Can occur in the immediate postoperative period or later in the PACU as pt wakes up.

2. Causes.

a. Pharyngeal secretions.

b. ETT passing through the cords during intubation or extubation.

c. Attempted extubation when pt is not fully awake and not deeply anesthetized (light planes of anesthesia).

d. Can occur at induction, emergence, or anytime in between.

3. Pathophysiology.

a. Reflex closure of the false cords and epiglottis body leads to glottic closure via inhaled agents, foreign bodies, or secretions.

b. The degree of laryngospasm determines airflow and vocal sounds.

    i. Mild laryngospasm—high-pitched squeaks and little air flow.

    ii. Severe laryngospasm—complete closure of the glottis with no sound and no air flow.

c. Stimulation of the superior laryngeal nerve leads to apnea via inhibition of the respiratory center in the medulla and decreased phrenic nerve activity.

d. Laryngospasm can cease spontaneously as severe hypoxemia and hypercarbia develop and decrease brainstem output to superior laryngeal nerve.

4. Prevention.

a. Deep extubations.

b. Fully awake pt prior to extubations.

c. Sometimes unpreventable.

5. Risk factors.

a. Recent upper respiratory tract infection.

b. Exposure to second-hand smoke.

c. Some authors suggest ketamine use and consequent increased secretions.

d. Hypocalcemia.

e. LMA use.

f. Recent thyroid surgery.

6. Treatment.

a. 100% O_2 via gentle positive pressure, using a bag valve mask in attempt to pass air through adducted vocal cords.

    i. The use of high positive pressure to break laryngospasm outweighs the risk of pulmonary barotrauma.
    ii. However, caution is advised regarding distention of the stomach, as some ventilation is passively directed into esophagus.
b. Jaw thrust.
c. IV lidocaine (adult, 1–1.5 mg/kg).
d. Sedative.
    i. Propofol (adult, 40 mg IV, repeated prn).
    ii. Versed (adult, 1–2 mg IV).
e. If hypoxemia develops:
    i. Succinylcholine (adult).
       • 0.25 to 1 mg/kg IV.
       • 4 to 6 mg/kg IM.
    ii. Start with smaller dose to help relax laryngeal muscles and allow ventilation.
    iii. Also, rocuronium (adult, 0.4 mg/kg IV).
    iv. Intubation.

7. A particular postanesthetic complication in the pediatric population.
a. Highest risk: infants 1 to 3 mo old.
b. Position children in lateral recumbent position to avoid secretions pooling around vocal cords.

8. Complication.
a. Negative-pressure pulmonary edema from the large, negative intrathoracic pressure generated against a closed glottis.
b. Can occur even in normal, healthy adults.
c. Prolonged hypoxemia.

D. PULMONARY EDEMA
1. Pathophysiology.
a. Transudation of fluid from the pulmonary capillary into the pleural interstitium and then from the interstitium into the alveoli.
b. Normally, interstitial fluid is removed by pulmonary lymphatics and returned to the central venous system.
c. Mechanisms.
    i. Cardiogenic.
       • Increase in the net hydrostatic pressure across the capillary.
       • Wedge pressure >18 mm Hg.
       • Pleural fluid with low protein content.
    ii. Noncardiogenic.
       • Increase in the permeability of the alveolar capillary membrane (i.e., ARDS).
       • Wedge pressure normal.
       • Pleural fluid with high protein content.
       • Loss of protective plasma oncotic pressure as protein leaks into interstitium.

2. Causes.
a. Cardiogenic.
    i.   LV failure.
    ii. CHF.
    iii. Mitral stenosis.
b. Noncardiogenic.
    i.   Breathing against a closed glottic opening (negative-pressure pulmonary edema).
    ii. ARDS.
    iii. Reexpansion of a collapsed lung.
    iv. High altitude.
    v. Hypervolemia.
    vi. Sepsis.
    vii. Trauma.
    viii. Aspiration.

3. Treatment.
a. Cardiogenic pulmonary edema.
    i. O_2.
- Depending on degree of congestion.
- BiPAP in severe cases.
- Intubation for severe hypoxemia, impending respiratory failure, and change in mental status.

    ii. Preload reduction relieves pulmonary congestion.
- Diuretics.
- Morphine.
- Nitrates.
- ACE inhibitors.
- Nesiritide.

    iii. Inotropes.
- Dobutamine.
- Afterload reduction improves cardiac output.
- ACE inhibitors.

b. Noncardiogenic pulmonary edema.
    i.   Focus treatment on reversible causes.
    ii. O_2.
- Mild cases can be treated with CPAP.
- Most require intubation.
- Avoid high peak inflation pressures (>35 cm H_2O).
- Avoid high tidal volumes (>8–10 mL/kg).
- Avoid high FiO_2 (>0.5).
- Improve oxygenation with:
  - PEEP.
  - Nitric oxide.
  - Inhaled prostacyclin or prostaglandin.

PULMONARY EMBOLISM (PE)

Etiology.

Entry of blood clot, fat, tumor cells, air, amniotic fluid, or foreign material into the venous system.

Clots usually originate from the lower extremities (nearly always above the knee) and pelvic veins.

Can occur intraoperatively in normal individuals undergoing any procedures.

Risk factors.

Lower extremity fracture.

Postpartum state.

Prolonged bed rest.

Cancer.

Heart failure.

Obesity.

Surgery duration >30 min.

Hypercoagulability.

Antithrombin III deficiency.

Protein C deficiency.

Protein S deficiency.

Venous stasis.

Pathophysiology

Clot in the pulmonary circulation increases dead space, and this increase should theoretically increase $PaCO_2$.

PVR increases by decreasing cross-sectional area of pulmonary vasculature, which increases shunting and subsequently causes hypoxemia.

RV failure can develop with sustained RV afterload.

Clinical manifestations.

Often, symptoms are absent, mild, and nonspecific.

Difficult to diagnose in OR; however, always part of differential.

Clinical manifestations of pulmonary embolism include sudden tachypnea, dyspnea, chest pain, or hemoptysis.

Wheezing may be present.

ABG reveals mild hypoxemia with respiratory alkalosis.

CXR commonly normal but may show atelectasis with elevated diaphragm, oligemia, asymmetric enlarged pulmonary artery, or a wedge-shaped density that is consistent with infarction.

Tachycardia and wide fixed split of S2.

Hypotension with elevated CVP indicative of massive PE with RV failure.

ECG.

    i. Often nonspecific.

    ii. Tachycardia.

    iii. Right bundle-branch block.

    iv. Right axis deviation.

    v. S1Q3T3 (deep S wave in V1, Q waves and inverted T in V3).

15

CRISIS MANAGEMENT AND RESUSCITATION

5. Diagnosis.

a. Diagnosis requires a high index of suspicion.

b. Gold standard for diagnosis is pulmonary angiography.

c. Other modalities.

   i.   V/Q scan.
- Uses gamma-emitting radionuclide.
- Normal scan indicates very low chance of PE (basically negative).
- Use pretest probability for any result other than normal.
- Diagnostic if perfusion defects are present in areas with normal ventilation.

   ii. Helical CT more commonly used.
- Requires IV contrast.

d. Intraoperative diagnosis of PE.

   i.   May have been present preoperatively or developed during procedure.

   ii. Risk increased during long procedures.

   iii. Surgical manipulation or change in pt position may dislodge clot.

   iv. Intraoperative presentation.
- Unexplained sudden hypotension.
- Hypoxemia.
- Bronchospasm.
- Decrease in E_TCO_2 concentration.
- Invasive monitoring may reveal elevated CVP.
- Elevated pulmonary arterial pressures.

   v. Intraoperative treatment.
- If air embolism in right atrium.
  - Emergent central vein cannulation and aspiration of air.
- All other emboli.
  - Supportive treatment.
  - IV fluids.
  - Inotropes.

6. Treatment.

a. Prevention is key.

b Prophylaxis.

   i.   5000 U heparin SQ q 12 hr begun preoperatively or immediately postoperatively.

   ii. TEDs and sequential compression devices decrease incidence of DVT in lower extremity but not in pelvis.

c. Systemic anticoagulation.

   i.   Prevents new clot formation.

   ii. Prevents extension of existing clot.

   iii. Heparin.
- Goal aPTT—1.5 to 2.4 times normal.
- Given IV.

   iv. LMWH.
- As effective as heparin, weight based.

- Given SQ.
- Requires no lab monitoring.
- More expensive than heparin, but overall cost effective.

v. Warfarin therapy.
- Started concomitantly with heparin.
- Continued for 3 to 12 mo.

vi. Thrombolytic therapy.
- Indicated for massive PE or circulatory collapse.

d. Pulmonary embolectomy.

i. Indicated for pts in whom thrombolytic therapy is contraindicated and with massive PE.

7. Anesthetic considerations.

a. For pts already with diagnosis of PE and unrelated surgery.

i. Risk of interrupting anticoagulant treatment perioperatively is unknown.

ii. With diagnosis >1 yr and normal baseline pulmonary function, risk of stopping anticoagulant treatment perioperatively is small.

iii. Perioperative goal is to minimize development of new clot.

b. Pts who present for pulmonary embolectomy.

i. Tolerate positive-pressure ventilation poorly.

ii. Require inotropic support until clot is removed.

iii. Tolerate all anesthetic agents poorly.
- Opioids, etomidate, or ketamine may be used, but the latter can increase pulmonary artery pressures.

iv. Require CPB.

c. Consider regional anesthesia whenever possible.

i. For some procedures (e.g., hip surgery), it decreases the incidence of postoperative DVT and PE.

ii. Contraindicated in pts with residual anticoagulation or a prolonged bleeding time.

iii. Neuraxial anesthesia may reduce thromboembolic complications.
- Sympathectomy.
  - Increases lower-extremity venous blood flow.
  - Attenuates postoperative increases in factor VIII and vWF.
  - Attenuates postoperative decreases in antithrombin III.
  - Alters stress hormone release.
- LA (IV lidocaine).
  - Decreases platelet aggregation and reactivity.
  - Enhances fibrinolysis.

F. UNPLANNED EXTUBATIONS

1. Signs/symptoms.

a. Loss of E_TCO_2.

b. Low minute ventilation.

c. Air leak.

15

CRISIS MANAGEMENT AND RESUSCITATION

    d. Hypoxemia.

    e. Low O_2 saturation.

2. Causes.

a. Inappropriate positioning of ETT (too high above carina).

b. Positioning/repositioning of pt.

    i.   Caution in children.

- Head movement (especially neck extension) or coughing can cause ETT dislodgment.
- Weight of tubing and monitors attached to ETT can dislodge tube from proper position.

c. Surgical manipulation.

IV. HYPERCARBIA

A. E_TCO_2 AND $PaCO_2$ DISCREPANCY

1. Capnograph types.

a. Mainstream (flow through).

b. Sidestream (aspiration).

2. High aspiration rates (250 mL/min) and low dead space sampling tubing increases sensitivity and decreases lag time.

a. With low tidal volumes (pediatric pts), high aspiration rates may entrain fresh gas from the circuit, diluting E_TCO_2 measurements.

b. Low aspiration rates (<50 mL/min) may diminish E_TCO_2 measurements during rapid respiratory rates.

3. Sampling tube and aspiration unit cell are prone to obstruction by water precipitation.

4. Gradient between E_TCO_2 and $PaCO_2$ (typically, 2–5 mm Hg) reflects alveolar dead space.

a. Significant reductions in lung perfusion increase alveolar dead space and decrease E_TCO_2.

b. Conditions that increase alveolar dead space.

    i.   Pulmonary and air embolism.

    ii.   Upright positions.

    iii.   Neck extension.

    iv.   Decreased cardiac output.

    v.   Hypotension.

    vi.   Emphysema.

    vii.   Age.

    viii. Anticholinergic drugs.

    ix.   Positive-pressure ventilation.

    x.   Endobronchial intubation.

B. HIGH EXPIRED CO_2

1. Often a reflection of increased sympathetic activity.

a. Inadequate level of anesthesia.

b. Malignant hyperthermia.

c. Thyroid storm.

Pheochromocytoma.
Carcinoid.
Hypoglycemia.
Drugs (pancuronium, ketamine, ephedrine).

HIGH INSPIRED CO_2
. **Unidirectional valve malfunction.**
Increases dead space and allows rebreathing of expired CO_2.
. **Soda lime exhaustion.**
. Absorbent should be replaced when 50% to 70% color change is present.
   i. Exhausted granules may revert to their original color, but no absorptive capacity remains.
. **Failure to close absorbent bypass valve.**

V. METABOLIC

ACID-BASE ABNORMALITIES
. **Metabolic acidosis.**
. Diagnosed by a primary decrease in serum bicarbonate levels on serum electrolyte tests or ABG.
. May or may not be associated with a corresponding acidemia or serum pH < 7.35.
. **Etiology.**
. Typically classified into anion gap and non-anion gap acidosis.
   i. Anion gap = $[Na+] - ([Cl^-] + [HCO_3^-])$.
   ii. Normal value is 7 to 12 mEq/L.
   iii. Anion gap >12 mEq/L considered to be a "gap" acidosis.
. Decreased gap acidosis.
   i. Lithium toxicity.
   ii. Hypercalcemia.
   iii. Hypermagnesemia.
   iv. Hyperkalemia.
   v. Hypoalbuminemia.
. Increased gap acidosis.
   i. Lactic acid.
   ii. Ketoacids.
   iii. Ethylene glycol.
   iv. Methanol.
   v. Paraldehyde.
   vi. Aspirin.
   vii. Renal failure.
. Normal gap acidosis.
   i. Diarrhea.
   ii. Renal tubular acidosis/renal failure.
   iii. Ureteral diversions.
   iv. Acetazolamide.

e. Suspect non-gap if massive fluid resuscitation has been performed wit a bicarbonate-free IV fluid such as normal or half-normal saline.

3. Clinical manifestations.

a. Acidosis of any etiology can increase the effects of many drugs.

   i. Sedatives and inhaled anesthetics can cause increased sedation.

   ii. Opioids have increased CNS penetration, resulting in increased sedation.

4. Treatment.

a. Acidosis of any cause should be identified, its etiology determined, anc appropriate therapy instituted prior to induction.

b. Specific therapies include:

   i. Concomitant respiratory acidosis should be corrected by hyperventilation.

   ii. Severe acidemia (pH < 7.20).

     • Administration of sodium bicarbonate solution (should only be considered if effective ventilation is maintained).

   iii. Non-gap should be treated separately, and the cause corrected.

   iv. Gap acidosis from lactate should be treated with sodium bicarbonate (1 mEq/L or 1 amp), with frequent monitoring.

   v. Metabolic acidosis from diabetic ketoacidosis should be corrected with IV fluid resuscitation and institution of insulin therapy.

B. GLUCOSE ABNORMALITIES

1. Hyperglycemia.

a. Normal serum glucose is 80 to120 mg/dL.

b. Diagnosed if serum glucose is >120 mg/dL.

c. Etiologies.

   i. Diabetes mellitus type 1 or 2.

   ii. Corticosteroids.

   iii. Surgical stress response.

d. Clinical manifestations.

   i. Immediate effects include polyuria and hyperosmolarity, with significantly elevated blood glucose.

   ii. Long-term effects include decreased wound healing, increased infection rate, and poorer neurologic outcomes.

e. Treatment.

   i. Begin regular insulin drip (normal concentration, 1 unit/mL), using a sliding scale.

     • Infusion rate in units per hour can be estimated by dividing the plasma glucose level (mg/dL) by 150.

     • Check serum glucose every 30 to 60 min until a steady state is obtained.

   ii. Consider tighter glycemic control in both cardiac and neurosurgical cases.

   iii. Strong evidence exists for tight glucose control in critically ill pts, but the perioperative period has not been studied.

    iv.   Iatrogenic hypoglycemia and neuroglycopenia may be difficult to detect under anesthesia and can result is severe morbidity and mortality.

2. **Hypoglycemia.**

a. Normal serum glucose is 80 to 120 mg/dL.

b. Diagnosed if serum glucose is <80 mg/dL.

c. Etiology.

    i.   Iatrogenic.
- Overcorrection of hyperglycemia with insulin.
- Withdrawal from TPN.
- Inadequate stress dose steroids in adrenally suppressed pts.

d. Clinical manifestations.

    i.   Intraoperative.
- Tachycardia.
- Diaphoresis.
- Slow awakening.

    ii.   Postoperative.
- Weakness.
- Trembling.
- Nervousness.
- Confusion.
- Difficulty speaking.
- Sweating.
- Palpitations.

e. Treatment.

    i.   Administer 1 amp D50 and recheck glucose in 30 min.

    ii.   If persistent hypoglycemia, start D5 or D10 drip at maintenance IV fluid rate and recheck every hour.

    iii.   The most important treatment is prevention.
- Give half of the pt's normal insulin dose preoperatively.
- Hold all insulin normally given with meals.
- Hold all oral hypoglycemics on the morning of surgery.

C. HYPERKALEMIA

1. **Normal potassium concentrations.**

a. Normal intracellular potassium is estimated to be 140 mEq/L.

b. Normal extracellular potassium is estimated to be 4 mEq/L.

2. **Hyperkalemia is defined as plasma [K^+] >5.5 mEq/L.**

3. **Four primary etiologies for hyperkalemia.**

a. Shift from intracellular to extracellular.

    i.   Acidosis.

    ii.   Hyperthermia.

    iii.   Succinylcholine administration can cause an increase of serum potassium by 0.7 mEq/L after a single dose.

    iv.   Rhabdomyolysis.

b. Renal disturbance, resulting in decreased urinary excretion.

15

CRISIS MANAGEMENT AND RESUSCITATION

      i.   A very low GFR will predispose to elevated potassium.

      ii.   Hypoaldosteronism.

      iii. Defect in distal nephron secretion.

      iv. ACE inhibitor therapy.

c. Increased potassium intake.

      i.   Massive transfusion (up to 70 mEq/L in older units of packed RBCs).

      ii.   Hemolytic transfusion reaction.

      iii. Medications such as potassium-containing antibiotics or TPN.

d. Spurious—due to release in laboratory specimen.

      i.   RBC hemolysis.

      ii.   If WBC count is >70,000 or platelet count is >1 million, in vitro release of potassium is possible, giving a false elevation.

4. Clinical manifestations.

a. Cardiac muscle changes occur generally as [K+] >7 mEq/L.

      i.   Delayed depolarization, then ECG changes.

         • Narrowing of the QT interval.

         • Peaking T waves.

         • Widening of QRS complex.

         • Prolongation of PR interval.

         • Loss of P and R waves.

         • ST depression (resultant ECG resembles a sine wave).

b. Skeletal muscle changes are seen if [K$^+$] >8 mEq/L.

      i.   Sustained spontaneous depolarization and inactivation of sodium channels, leading to an ascending paralysis.

5. Treatment.

a. Primary treatment is aimed at stabilizing cardiomyocytes.

      i.   1 amp of calcium gluconate if peripheral access.

      ii.   1 amp of calcium chloride if central access.

b. Secondary treatment is aimed at lowering plasma potassium.

      i.   Stop exogenous administration of potassium via IV fluids or TPN.

      ii.   1 amp sodium bicarbonate.

      iii. 10 units regular insulin via IV route given with 1 amp of D50.

      iv. Furosemide can be given to promote renal excretion.

      v.   If hypoaldosteronism is suspected, can give mineralocorticoids.

      vi. Refractory hyperkalemia should receive hemodialysis or continuous venovenous dialysis.

D. SODIUM ABNORMALITIES

1. Hyponatremia.

a. Diagnosed with serum [Na$^+$] <135 mEq/L.

b. Etiologies.

      i.   Typically discussed relative to volume status.

c. Clinical manifestations

      i.   Typically seen only when serum [Na$^+$] drops acutely to <125 mEq/L.

     ii.   Wide range of manifestations from confusion, cramping, and lethargy to seizures and coma.

d. Treatment.

     i.   Treatment of hyponatremia is based solely on etiology, unless seizures or severe effects are seen.

     ii.   Generally, aim to correct serum $[Na^+]$ by 0.5 mEq/L per hr.

     iii.   Hypovolemic hyponatremia.
* Give NS slowly to correct deficit.

     iv.   Normovolemic hyponatremia.
* Restrict fluids if pt is drinking.
* During surgery, can attempt slow infusion of hypertonic saline, with frequent monitoring.

     v.   Hypervolemic hyponatremia.
* Restrict fluids if pt is drinking.
* Treatment with diuretics during surgery.

e. Aggressive correction of hyponatremia may result in central pontine myelinolysis and permanent neurologic injury.

2. Hypernatremia.

a. Diagnosed if serum sodium is >145 mEq/L.

b. Etiologies.

     i.   Usually from inability to obtain water.

     ii.   Total body water can be low, normal, or high.

$$\text{Free water deficit} = [\text{body weight}(kg) \times 0.6] \times [(\text{current serum }[Na^+] - \text{normal serum }[Na^+])/140]$$

     iii.   Hypervolemic hypernatremia.
* Iatrogenic from hypertonic saline (2% or 3%) or sodium bicarbonate infusions.
* Mineralocorticoid excess.

     iv.   Normovolemic hypernatremia.
* Typically from diabetes insipidus (occasionally seen with transsphenoidal hypophysectomy).

     v.   Hypovolemic hypernatremia.
* Diarrhea, vomiting, or osmotic diuresis.

c. Clinical manifestations.

     i.   Wide range of manifestations, ranging from weakness and neuromuscular irritability to seizures and/or neurologic damage (typically seen if $[Na^+]$ is >158 mEq/L).

d. Treatment.

     i.   Hypervolemic hypernatremia.
* Diuresis—either IV diuretic or dialysis if necessary, then replacement of the free water deficit with D5W.

     ii.   Normovolemic hypernatremia.
* Typically, a correction of the etiology, then of the total body water deficit and plasma osmolality, should occur prior to giving a hypotonic solution.

    iii.   Hypovolemic hypernatremia.
- Replace volume loss with resuscitation fluids such as 0.9% NS o LR.
- Recalculate the free water deficit after hemodynamic instability (if any) has been corrected; then replace remaining deficit using hypotonic solution as needed.

    iv.   Correction of all types should be slow to avoid seizures, brain edema, and neurologic damage.

E. MALIGNANT HYPERTHERMIA
1. Pathophysiology.
a. Occurs with exposure to succinylcholine or a halogenated anesthetic agent in a genetically susceptible individual.

b. Involves uncontrolled release of intracellular calcium from skeletal muscle.

c. Leads to uncontrolled ATP activation.

2. Clinical manifestations.
a. Hypermetabolic state.

    i.   Lactic acidosis.

    ii.   Hypercarbia.

    iii.   Hyperthermia.

    iv.   Hyperkalemia.

b. All of the above can result in VF and death within 15 min.

3. Prevention.
a. Always inquire as to family history of problems with anesthesia.

b. Always inquire as to family history of muscle or neuromuscular disorder.

c. Avoid the use of triggering agents in pts with central core disease and multi-minicore disease.

4. Treat promptly and aggressively.
a. Stop all potential triggers immediately.

b. Place pt on 100% O_2 and change to new breathing circuit, bag, and soda lime as soon as possible to remove residual anesthetics.

c. 2.5 mg/kg dantrolene IV q 5 min until symptoms stop (maximum dose 10 mg/kg).

d. Use cooling blankets, ice packs, and ice lavage of body cavities to reduce temperature.

e. Sodium bicarbonate to correct lactic acidosis.

f. Use vasopressors as needed.

g. Calcium-channel blockers should be avoided after dantrolene administration.

h. Contact the Malignant Hyperthermia Association of the United States (MHAUS) immediately, for support and to report case if malignant hyperthermia is suspected. 1-800-MH-HYPER (1-800-644-9737); www.mhaus.org.

VI. RENAL

A. INTRAOPERATIVE OLIGURIA/ANURIA

1. Definition.

a. <0.5 mL/kg/hr urine output.

2. Differential diagnosis.

a. Prerenal.

    i. Most common intraoperative etiology.

    ii. Decreased intravascular volume, causing decreased renal blood flow.

    iii. Tubular function intact.

    iv. Urine low in sodium (still able to concentrate).

    v. Decreased renal blood flow can also be caused by sepsis, liver failure, and CHF.

b. Intrinsic renal.

    i. Most commonly caused by acute tubular necrosis, which is the result of prolonged ischemia to renal tubule cells.

    ii. Manifested by inability to concentrate urine.

    iii. Urine has high sodium content.

c. Postrenal.

    i. Mechanical obstruction in ureters, bladder, or urethra.

       • Blood clot.

       • Edema.

       • Surgical ligation.

       • Calculi.

    ii. Obstruction of Foley catheter.

3. Treatment goal is to limit duration and magnitude of inadequate renal blood flow.

a. Carefully assess volume status.

    i. Use estimated blood loss, preoperative deficit, fluid replacement, insensible losses, and hemodynamics to assess likely fluid requirement.

b. Consider pt risk factors for possible cause of low cardiac output.

    i. Consider placement of pulmonary artery catheter.

    ii. Consider inotropes—dobutamine, dopamine, epinephrine.

    iii. Consider loop diuretics or mannitol.

c. Administer fluid challenge of 10 mL/kg rapidly and monitor for response.

    i. If urine output increases, it is most likely of prerenal etiology, due to hypovolemia.

    ii. If no increase, etiologies could be inadequate volume of fluid administered or low cardiac-output state, causing decreased renal blood flow.

d. If etiology is unclear or pt has no known risk factors:

    i. Send basic metabolic panel, ABG, and urine studies (sodium and osmolarity).

    ii.   Prerenal—urine sodium is <40 and osmolarity is >400.

    iii.   Renal—urine sodium is >40 and osmolarity is <400.

e. If decreased urine output continues, monitor for dialysis indications.

    i.   Acidosis.

    ii.   Electrolyte abnormalities, especially hyperkalemia.

    iii.   Fluid volume overload.

B. HEMATURIA

1. Definition.

a. Blood in urine.

2. Differential.

a. Trauma to urinary system.

b. Surgical disruption.

c. Coagulopathy.

d. Neoplasm.

3. Response.

a. Attempt to determine cause.

b. Notify surgeon.

c. Transfuse blood products as needed.

d. Assess for coagulopathy; send blood sample for platelets PT, PTT, INR.

e. Maintain adequate urine output.

f. Consider input from urology if bleeding continues.

VII. EQUIPMENT

A. AIRWAY LEAKS

1. Identifying a leak.

a. Failure of the ventilator bellows to return to the preset level.

    i.   A closed-circuit anesthetic is an exception, in which case the rate of gas absorption is greater than the rate of fresh gas in-flow.

b. Ascending (standing) bellows facilitate detection of a leak, while descending (hanging) bellows may obscure it.

c. Threshold pressure alarm.

    i.   Alarms if the peak inspiratory pressure in the breathing circuit does not reach the preset threshold limit.

    ii.   The threshold limit should be set to within 5 cm of the current peak inspiratory pressures to reliably detect a complete or partial circuit disconnection.

d. Respiratory volume alarm.

    i.   Alarms if exhaled tidal volume and minute volume fall below predetermined levels.

e. CO_2 monitor.

    i.   A dramatic drop or disappearance of E_TCO_2 may represent a disconnection.

2. Leak locations.

a. Disconnections occur most commonly between the right angle elbow and the ETT.

b. Leaks occur most commonly at the CO_2 absorber canisters.

c. Any additional devices added to the circuit (e.g., antibacterial filter) or attempts to utilize tubing not intended by the manufacturer for a particular purpose represent a source of potential misconnections and leaks.

d. Inappropriately sized uncuffed ETTs or cuffed ETTs, the cuff of which is damaged or deflated, may cause leaks.

e. Cracked flow meter tubes, loose vaporizer caps, cracked oxygen analyzer, improperly adjusted scavenging devices, and detachment of pressure monitor tubing may all cause leaks.

3. Leak tests

a. Low-pressure circuit leak test checks the integrity of the system downstream from all safety devices, except the oxygen analyzer.

   i. Leaks here can result in hypoxia and pt awareness.

b. Older machines can be tested with a traditional positive-pressure test.

   i. Close pop-off valve, occlude the Y-piece, build pressure to 30 cm H_2O, and hold for 10 sec.

   ii. In these machines, a positive-pressure test checks the integrity of the entire low-pressure system.

c. Newer machines (i.e., most Datex-Omeda products) have a one-way check valve placed near the common gas outlet.

   i. In these machines, a positive-pressure test checks only the integrity of the breathing circuit downstream from the check valve (i.e., flow meter cracks, loose vaporizer caps can still be present).

   ii. For these machines, a negative-pressure test (aka FDA universal low-pressure circuit test) must be performed.

     • Turn off the master switch, vaporizers, and flow valves.

     • Attach a suction bulb to the common gas outlet.

     • Squeeze several times until bulb is deflated.

     • Bulb must stay deflated for at least 10 sec; otherwise, a leak is present.

     • Each vaporizer must be turned on sequentially to test for internal vaporizer leaks.

d. Even newer machines have an automatic self-test.

   i. However, internal vaporizer leaks still can only be detected with vaporizers turned on one at a time.

4. Discovering a leak intraoperatively.

a. Check for gross disconnections.

   i. At the elbow connector and ETT.

   ii. All along the circuit, i.e., loose-fitting bag, additional filters, etc.

   iii. Ensure that flow meters are turned on.

b. Rule out pipeline supply failure.

   i. Check the pipeline gauge; it should read ~55 PSI.

15

CRISIS MANAGEMENT AND RESUSCITATION

   c. Check ETT cuff and listen to breath sounds.
      i. May need extra air in cuff.
   d. Try to readjust CO_2 absorber canisters.
   e. Quantify the leak.
      i. Increase flows until the bellows return to the preset level with every expiration.
      ii. If able to compensate easily with just a small increase in flows and the case is near completion, may be able to complete the case; however, machine must be serviced or exchanged before the next case.
   f. Can attempt to occlude the fresh gas outflow tubing briefly.
      i. Creates a back pressure, which normally would cause flow meter bobbins to drop down and briskly return to previous position after obstruction is relieved.
      ii. If this does not happen, a substantial leak is present.
   g. Use backup ventilation system and maintain anesthesia via IV route.
   h. When significant leak is present, machine generally must be taken out of service for maintenance.

B. PIPELINE FAILURE

1. Pipeline source is the main supply of gases for the anesthesia machine, unless working in a remote or office location.
2. Most hospitals use a centralized piping system for medical gases and various safety devices (e.g., gas-specific pipeline-inlet fittings) to minimize risks of wrong gas delivery to the pt.
3. Pipeline gas is usually delivered to the anesthesia machine at a pressure of 50 psig.
4. Fail-safe valve within the high-pressure circuit of the anesthesia machine will shut off or decrease flow of all other gases if oxygen pressure drops below a certain preset limit, such as 30 psig.
   a. However, in older machines, which lack a proportioning system, this will not prevent delivery of a hypoxic mixture.
5. 2000 ASTM standard requires a medium-priority alarm to be activated within 5 sec when the oxygen pressure drops below certain factory preset limits.
6. Despite multiple precautionary measures, central supply sources may deliver variable pressures, fail entirely, or in worst case scenarios, result in a crossover of oxygen and nitrous oxide pipelines.
7. Deaths attributed to pipeline crossover have been reported as recently as 2002 in the US.
8. It is crucial, therefore, to routinely check for adequate oxygen supply in the backup oxygen tanks to prevent a rare but potentially fatal consequence of pipeline failure/crossover.
9. If oxygen pipeline failure or crossover is suspected intraoperatively:
   a. Turn on the backup oxygen cylinder.
   b. Turn off the wall supply source.

    i.   Especially important in case of crossover, as the machine will preferentially use the higher (50 psig) wall gas source instead of the lower (45 psig) tank source.

c. Estimate the amount of time based on the amount of oxygen available in the tank.

    i.   For a gas that exists solely in gaseous state under pressure (e.g., oxygen, air, helium), the volume of gas in the tank will decline in proportion to a decrease in pressure.

    ii. Full oxygen tank: ~2000 psig = 660 L

                    ~1000 psig = 330 L, etc.

    iii. Time can be estimated by dividing the volume of gas remaining by the anticipated flow rate (e.g., for a full tank at 2 L/min: 660 L ÷ 2 L/min = 330 min.)

d. Backup cylinders should be kept turned off at all times, except during machine check, to avoid silent depletion of cylinder oxygen supply.

    i.   Silent tank leak will occur whenever oxygen pressure within the machine decreases to <45 psig, such as during oxygen valve flashing.

C. VENTILATOR FAILURE

1. Definition.

a. Inability to obtain set tidal volume or pressure set on ventilator.

2. Differential.

a. Circuit leak.

b. Poor lung compliance.

c. Bellows stuck.

d. Fresh gas flow failure.

e. Power failure.

f. Circuit assembled incorrectly.

3. Recognize ventilator failure early.

a. Absent chest movement.

b. Decreased or absent breath sounds.

c. Capnograph shows little or no E_TCO_2.

d. Spirometry shows little or no tidal volume.

e. Apnea alarm.

f. Low-pressure alarm.

g. Hypoxemia.

h. Pt may attempt respiration as $PaCO_2$ rises.

4. Treatment.

a. Call for help.

b. Attempt manual ventilation with anesthesia circuit.

c. If unable to fill the reservoir bag with the flush valve:

    i.   Use backup ventilation system.

d. If able to fill bag, but cannot ventilate:

    i.   Check inspiratory limb for obstruction.

    ii. If no obstruction is found, use backup ventilation.

15

CRISIS MANAGEMENT AND RESUSCITATION

   e. If unable to ventilate with backup system:
      i.   Check pt for kinked ETT, pneumothorax, bronchospasm.
   f. While completing the above steps:
      i.   Maintain anesthesia with IV agents.
      ii. Check all hoses and gas flowmeters.
   g. Power failure.
      i.   Ensure that machine is plugged into emergency outlet (uninterruptible power supply).
   h. If unable to identify problem, machine must be taken out of service.

D. VAPORIZER FAILURE

1. Definition.
a. Incorrect amount of anesthetic gas administered by vaporizer.

2. Differential.
a. Vaporizer malfunction.
b. Wrong agent in vaporizer.
c. Vaporizer tilted.
d. Barometric pressure changes (high altitude).

3. Overdose.
a. Hypotension, bradycardia, dysrhythmias, or cardiac arrest.
b. High concentration of agent as measured by gas analyzer.
c. Call for help.
d. Discontinue all volatile agents.
e. Ensure adequate oxygenation and ventilation.
f. Ventilate with 100% FiO_2.
g. Monitor vitals frequently.
h. Flush circuit with O_2.
   i.   Concentration of agent should decrease once discontinued and pt is ventilated with 100% at high flows.
   ii. If no change in concentration after flush:
      • May indicate a leak inside the machine.
      • Use backup ventilation system.
i. Care is supportive.
   i.   If CV compromise:
      • Support with fluids, inotropes, and vasopressors.
   ii. If cardiac arrest:
      • Follow ACLS protocol.
j. Surgery should be aborted if pt has severe hemodynamic compromise.

4. Underdose.
a. Unexplained tachycardia, HTN, sweating, tearing, tachypnea, or movement.
b. Check agent analyzer.
c. Rule out other causes for increased hemodynamics.
   i.   History of poorly controlled HTN.
   ii. Hyperthyroid.
   iii. Preoperative drug use (cocaine).

1. If light anesthesia is suspected:
   i.   Deepen anesthesia with volatile or IV agents and consider administration of benzodiazepines.
   ii. Consider switching to IV technique or replacing machine.
2. In either situation, an equipment specialist should be notified of the problem, and the machine should have a complete inspection prior to returning to service.

E. BLS ALGORITHM
1. Check for unresponsiveness and activate emergency alert system.
2. ABC.
a. Open airway with head tilt and chin lift or jaw thrust.
b. Look, listen, and feel for breathing, 10 sec.
   i.   If victim is breathing, assume recovery position.
   ii. If victim is not breathing, give two rescue breaths.
       • Do not hyperventilate.
c. Check for pulse, 10 sec (adults and children, carotid; infant, brachial).
   i.   If victim has a pulse but is not breathing, resume rescue breaths.
       • 1 breath q 5 sec for adults.
       • 1 breath q 3 to 5 sec for infant or child.
       • Check for pulse after each 2 min interval.
   ii. If victim has no pulse, commence chest compressions at a rate of 100/min.
       • In adults, 30 compressions followed by two rescue breaths for one- and two-rescuer technique.
       • In infants and children, the ratio is 30:2 for single rescuer and 15:2 for two rescuers.
   iii. An infant with pulse <60 requires chest compressions.
d. Chest-compression depth.
   i.   Adults, 1.5 to 2 inches.
   ii. Children and infants, 1/3 to 1/2 depth of the chest.
3. Defibrillator or AED arrives.
a. Place pads in appropriate position.
b. Begin ACLS algorithm.

F. ACLS ALGORITHM
1. Pulseless arrest
a. BLS algorithm/CPR initiated until defibrillator arrives.
b. Assess rhythm.
   i.   VF/VT.
       • Shock.
           - Biphasic device—200 J.
           - Monophasic device—360 J.
           - AED—specific to device.

- Immediately resume CPR (5 cycles), then assess rhythm.
  - Shock if indicated.
- Establish IV/IO access.
  - 1 mg epinephrine q 3 to 5 min.
  - 40 units of vasopressin may be used in place of the first or second dose of epinephrine but should not be repeated.
- Administer antiarrhythmics.
  - 300 mg amiodarone, followed by an additional 150 mg if needed.
  - 1 to 1.5 mg/kg lidocaine, followed by 0.5 to 0.75 mg/kg (max 3 mg/kg) if needed.
  - 1 to 2 g magnesium for torsades de pointes.

ii. Asystole/PEA.
  - Resume CPR.
  - Establish IV/IO access.
    - 1 mg/kg epinephrine q 3 to 5 min.
    - 40 units of vasopressin may be used in place of the first or second dose of epinephrine but should not be repeated.
    - 1 mg atropine may be given for asystole or slow PEA every 3 to 5 min.

c. Check for possible etiologies (6 Hs and 6 Ts).
  i.   Hypoxia, hypovolemia, hydrogen ions, hypokalemia and hyperkalemia, hypoglycemia, hypothermia.
  ii. Toxins, cardiac tamponade, tension pneumothorax, coronary thrombosis, pulmonary thrombosis, trauma.
  iii. Perform physical exam, send labs, and check pt history.

2. Bradycardia.

a. Provide oxygen, check vital signs, IV access, and ECG.
b. Consider transcutaneous pacing for type II second-degree AV block, third-degree AV block, or in pts with signs of poor perfusion.
c. Administer 0.5 mg atropine (max 3 mg) while awaiting pacer.
d. Consider 2 to 10 mcg/min epinephrine or 2 to 10 mcg/kg/min dopamine.

3. Tachycardia

a. Provide oxygen, check vital signs, IV access, and ECG.
b. If pt is unstable, perform immediate synchronized cardioversion.
c. If the pt is stable, evaluate the QRS complex.
  i.   Regular narrow QRS.
    - Vagal maneuvers and/or 6 mg adenosine, followed by 12 mg; max 30 mg.
  ii. Irregular narrow QRS.
    - Atrial fibrillation, atrial flutter, or multifocal atrial tachycardia.
    - Rate control with β blocker or calcium-channel blocker and expert consultation.
  iii. Regular wide QRS.

- SVT with aberrancy.
  - Adenosine.
- VT.
  - 150 mg amiodarone infusion over 10 min, repeat to max dose of 2.2 g/24 hr.
  - Elective synchronized cardioversion.
    iv. Irregular wide QRS.
- Atrial fibrillation with aberrancy.
  - Treat as above.
- Pre-excitation atrial fibrillation (Wolff-Parkinson-White).
  - Expert consultation.
  - Avoid AV nodal blocking agents (adenosine, diltiazem, verapamil, digoxin).
  - Consider amiodarone.
- Torsades de pointes.
  - Magnesium.

G. PALS ALGORITHM
1. Pulseless arrest.
a. Initiate BLS algorithm/CPR until defibrillator arrives.
b. Assess rhythm.
   i. VF/VT.
- Shock 2 J/kg.
- Resume CPR, 5 cycles.
  - If repeat shock is indicated, give 4 J/kg and resume CPR.
  - All subsequent shocks are 4 J/kg.
- Once IV/IO access is obtained, give 0.01 m/kg epinephrine and repeat q 3 to 5 min.
- Epinephrine may be given via ETT if IV/IO access is not yet established.
  - Dose—0.1 mg/kg.
- Consider antiarrhythmics.
  - 5 mg/kg amiodarone.
  - 1 mg/kg lidocaine.
  - 25 to 50 mg/kg magnesium (max 2 g) for torsades de pointes.
   ii. Asystole/PEA.
- Resume CPR.
- Give 0.01 mg/kg epinephrine q 3 to 5 min.
c. Remember to assess pt for possible etiologies (see ACLS protocol).
2. Bradycardia.
a. Provide oxygen and attach monitors.
b. Perform CPR for HR <60 and signs of poor perfusion.
c. Give 0.01 mg/kg epinephrine.
   i. Repeat q 3 to 5 min.

   d. Consider 0.02 mg/kg atropine.
      i.   Repeat as necessary (max 1 mg).
   e. Consider pacing.
3. Tachycardia.
a. Narrow QRS.
   i.   Sinus tachycardia.
        • Search for etiology and treat.
   ii. SVT.
        • Vagal maneuvers.
        • 0.1 mg/kg adenosine (max 6 mg).
           - Repeat by doubling first dose (max 12 mg).
        • Consider synchronized cardioversion.
           - 0.5 to 1 J/kg, increase to 2 J/kg.
b. Wide QRS.
   i.   VT.
        • Consider synchronized cardioversion.
           - 0.5 to 1 J/kg, increase to 2 J/kg.
        • Expert consultation.
        • Consider 5 mg/kg amiodarone *OR* 15 mg/kg procainamide, each
          over 30 to 60 min.

REFERENCES

American Heart Association. ALCS Provider Manual, 2006.

American Heart Association, PALS Provider Manual, 2006.

Barash PG, Cullen BF, Stoelting RK (eds): Clinical Anesthesia, 5th ed.
   Philadelphia: Lippincott Williams & Wilkins, 2005.

Brockwell RC, Andrews JJ: Delivery systems for inhaled anesthetics. In:
   Barash PG, Cullen BF, Stoelting RK (eds): Clinical Anesthesia, 5th ed,
   Philadelphia: Lippincott Williams & Wilkins, 2006, pp 582–586.

Broderick J, Connolly S, Feldmann E, et al: Guidelines for management of
   spontaneous intracerebral hemorrhage in adults, 2007 update. A
   Guideline from the American Heart Association, American Stroke
   Association Stroke Council, High Blood Pressure Research Council, and
   the Quality of Care and Outcomes in Research Interdisciplinary Working
   Group. Stroke 2007;38(6):2001–2023.

Eagle KA, Berger PB, Calkins H, et al: ACC/AHA Guideline Update for
   Perioperative Cardiovascular Evaluation for Noncardiac Surgery—
   Executive Summary. A report of the American College of Cardiology/
   American Heart Association Task Force on Practice Guidelines
   (Committee to Update the 1996 Guidelines on Perioperative
   Cardiovascular Evaluation for Noncardiac Surgery). Anesth Analg
   2002;94:1052–1064.

Effective Management of Anaesthetic Crises. http://www.anaesthesia.org.
   au/emac/cardio/hypotension.html.

Faust RJ, Cucchiara RF: Anesthesiology Review, 3rd ed. Philadelphia:
   Churchill Livingstone, 2001.

Gaba DM, Fish KJ, Howard SK: Equipment Failure. In: Gaba DM, Fish KJ, Howard SK: Crisis Management in Anesthesia. Philadelphia: Churchill Livingstone, 1994.

Hurford WE: Clinical Anesthesia Procedures of the Massachusetts General Hospital, Philadelphia: Lippincott Williams & Wilkins, 2002, pp 42–45.

Miller RD (ed): Miller's Anesthesia, 6th ed, vol 2. Philadelphia: Elsevier, 2005.

Morgan GE, Mikhail MS, Murray MJ: Clinical Anesthesiology, 3rd ed, New York: McGraw-Hill, 2002, pp 604–610, 612–619, 653–655, 737–740.

O'Hara JF, Cywinski JB, Monk TG: The Renal System and Anesthesia for Urologic Surgery. In: Barash PG, Cullen BF, Stoelting RK (eds): Clinical Anesthesia, 5th ed, Philadelphia: Lippincott Williams & Wilkins, 2006, pp 1017–1023.

Paix AD, Runciman WB, Horan BF, et al: Crisis management during anaesthesia: Hypertension. Qual Saf Health Care 2005;14:e12.

Stoelting RK, Miller RD: Renal disease. In: Stoelting RK, Miller RD: Basics of Anesthesia, 5th ed, Philadelphia: Churchill Livingstone, 2006, pp 300–304.

15

CRISIS MANAGEMENT AND RESUSCITATION

Postoperative Issues, Complications, and Home Readiness

Tina Tran, MD, and Shireen Gujral, MD
Edited by Tracey Stierer, MD

I. AWARENESS AND RECALL DURING GENERAL ANESTHESIA

A. RISK
1. Risk of any type of awareness is 0.1% (1 per 1000) of all general anesthetics.
2. Auditory awareness is most common (48%); pt hears music and/or voices.
3. Awareness with pain: 3 per 10,000.
4. Increased risk: OB, cardiac, trauma, bronchoscopy, total IV anesthesia.

B. ETIOLOGY
1. 70% technique.
2. 20% equipment failure or misuse.
3. 10% unknown.

C. PREVENTION
1. Amnestic drugs.
2. Volatile anesthetics in minimum alveolar concentration (MAC) doses.
3. Avoidance of full paralysis if possible (maintain two twitches).
4. Bispectral index monitoring may be of value in prevention of recall in pts receiving total IV anesthesia.

D. POSTOPERATIVE QUESTIONS TO DETECT AWARENESS
1. What is the last thing you remember before going to sleep?
2. What is the first thing you remembered when you woke up?
3. Do you remember anything in between?
4. Did you dream during anesthesia?

E. RESPONSE TO PT REPORT OF AWARENESS AFTER GA
1. Believe the pt.
2. Notify the attending anesthesiologist.
3. Report episode of awareness as an adverse event to be investigated.
4. Determine the possible cause for the awareness and discuss with pt.
5. Obtain psychiatric counseling if doctor or pt feels it is necessary.

II. CORNEAL ABRASIONS AND OTHER EYE INJURIES

A. CORNEA
1. Anatomy.
a. Anterior portion of the outer coat of the eyeball.

b. Avascular

c. Protected by a film of precorneal tears.

2. Changes during anesthesia.

a. Tear production is decreased.

b. Bell phenomenon (upward turning of the eyes during sleep) is abolished.

c. Blink reflex is abolished.

B. MECHANISMS OF INJURY TO THE CORNEA DURING GA

1. Direct trauma.

2. Chemical injury.

3. Lagophthalmos or failure to properly close the eyelid, leading to corneal drying.

C. CORNEAL ABRASION

1. The most common ocular complication of GA.

2. Eye pain with a sensation of foreign body; the eye pain can be severe and is often worse than the pain associated with the surgical procedure.

3. Associated with tearing, photophobia, conjunctivitis.

4. Can be seen clinically as a nonreflective area of cornea or with a positive fluorescein-staining test result.

5. Increased risk with pts in the lateral or prone position and long duration of head and neck surgeries.

6. Can occur at any time in the perioperative period.

7. Caused by disruption in the epithelial layer of the cornea.

D. STRATEGIES TO PROTECT THE EYES

1. No one strategy has been shown to be superior to another.

2. Manually close eyelids and tape them closed.

3. Ointments—paraffin-based (Lacri-Lube, Duratears) or water-based (methylcellulose drops).

a. Pts who have had paraffin-based ointments placed intraoperatively complain of blurry vision and sensation of foreign body in the eye.

4. Hydrophilic contact lens.

a. Can lead to corneal injury if not placed properly.

5. Suture eyelids closed when taping is in the surgical field.

E. RESPONDING TO POSTOPERATIVE EYE PAIN

1. Listen to the pt.

2. Examine the pt immediately.

3. Consult ophthalmologist.

4. Usual course of treatment includes application of antibiotic ointment and a patch to the affected eye.

F. OTHER MECHANISMS OF PERIOPERATIVE VISION CHANGES (Figure 16.1)

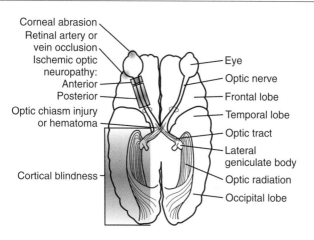

Corneal abrasion
Retinal artery or
vein occlusion
Ischemic optic
neuropathy:
Anterior
Posterior
Optic chiasm injury
or hematoma

Cortical blindness

Eye
Optic nerve
Frontal lobe
Temporal lobe
Optic tract
Lateral
geniculate body
Optic radiation
Occipital lobe

FIG. 16.1

Causes of perioperative eye complications are depicted. Corneal abrasions are most common. Swelling or pressure can lead to retinal vein or artery occlusion. Ischemic optic neuropathy is caused by infarction of the optic nerve. Injuries to the optic chiasm can occur during pituitary surgery, and cortical blindness can occur after some cardiac and neurosurgical procedures. *(Adapted from Williams EL, Hart WM, Tempelhoff R: Postoperative ischemic optic neuropathy. Anesth Analg 1995;80:1018–1029.)*

16

POSTOPERATIVE ISSUES

III. EMERGENCE DELIRIUM

A. OCCURRENCE

1. When pts awaken from anesthesia, they can become disoriented, agitated, and inconsolable.
2. Common in the pediatric population when children wake up in pain, nauseous, and in a strange environment separated from their parents.
a. Associated more with use of sevoflurane and with eye, ear, and throat procedures but can be seen with all anesthetics.
3. Also seen in the elderly population who have other comorbidities, undergo major operations, and may have underlying cognitive dysfunction.
4. When considering delirium, rule out life-threatening causes such as hypoxia, hypercarbia, intracranial process, and acidosis.
5. The reported incidence of emergence delirium in the PACU averages 3%, whereas delirium during the postoperative period can range from 15% to 45%.

B. DIAGNOSTIC CRITERIA FOR DELIRIUM
1. Rapid onset—hours to days.
2. Disturbed consciousness.
3. Fluctuating mental status changes throughout the day.
4. Cognitive changes and/or perceptual disturbances.
5. Evidence of a causal condition or substance intoxication or withdrawal.

C. ETIOLOGY
1. No mechanism of delirium has been established.
a. Multiple neurotransmitter abnormalities may be involved, including:
   i.   Reduction in cholinergic function.
   ii. Excess of dopamine, norepinephrine, and glutamine.
   iii. Changes in serotonergic and GABA activity.

D. COMMON CAUSES OF EMERGENCE DELIRIUM
1. ETT.
2. Pain.
3. Anxiety.
4. Urgent need to urinate.
5. Residual NMB.

E. PREOPERATIVE RISK FACTORS FOR POSTOPERATIVE DELIRIUM
   (Box 16.1)

BOX 16.1

PREOPERATIVE RISK FACTORS FOR POSTOPERATIVE DELIRIUM

Functional impairment
Cognitive impairment
Sleep deprivation
Immobility or poor physical condition
Visual impairment
Hearing impairment
Dehydration
Advanced age
Low serum albumin level
Alcohol abuse
Abnormal preoperative serum sodium, potassium, or glucose level
Comorbidity, ASA class III or IV
Anticholinergic drugs
Depression
High-risk surgery per AHA guidelines

F. TREATMENT

1. Adequate pain control.
2. Avoid benzodiazepines in pts with known cognitive disorders.
3. Correct hypoxia, hypercarbia, acidosis.
4. Frequently reorient pt to environment and situation.
5. Correct metabolic and electrolyte disorders.
6. Continue medical treatment for neuropsychiatric disorders.
7. Medically and/or physically protect pt from harm to self and others.
8. Prevent the known causes of delirium in hospitalized pts.

IV. HOME DISCHARGE CRITERIA

An increasing number of surgical procedures are being performed on an outpatient basis. The PACU is a vitally important area where the pt is monitored in the immediate postoperative period and where it is decided that the pt may safely be discharged. Before the day of outpatient surgery, it is important to evaluate the pt's appropriateness for same-day discharge (Table 16.1).

A. ANESTHESIOLOGIST'S RESPONSIBILITIES

1. After the pt is transported from the OR to the PACU, the anesthesiologist is responsible for:
a. Giving a report of intraoperative management.

TABLE 16.1

MODIFIED POSTANESTHESIA DISCHARGE SCORING SYSTEM

VITAL SIGNS	
2	Within 20% of the preoperative value
1	20%–40% of the preoperative value
0	40% of the preoperative value
AMBULATION	
2	Steady gait; no dizziness
1	With assistance
0	No ambulation; dizziness
NAUSEA AND VOMITING	
2	Minimal
1	Moderate
0	Severe
PAIN	
2	Minimal
1	Moderate
0	Severe
SURGICAL BLEEDING	
2	Minimal
1	Moderate
0	Severe

Adapted from Chung F, Chan VW, Ong D: A post-anesthetic discharge scoring system for home readiness after ambulatory surgery. J Clin Anesth 1995;7:500.

16

POSTOPERATIVE ISSUES

b. Responding to any abnormalities in symptoms, vital signs, or physical exam findings.

c. Addressing issues with pain and nausea.

d. Addressing any pt-related concerns of the PACU staff.

B. THREE STAGES OF RECOVERY

1. Early.

a. Pt emerges from anesthesia, recovers control of protective reflexes, and recovers early motor activity.

   i. Usually done in the OR and in the PACU.

2. Intermediate.

a. Progressive care toward discharge; includes sitting in a chair, ambulating, drinking, voiding, etc.

   i. This stage is longer in females, the elderly, those who underwent long operations or in whom muscle relaxant or spinal anesthesia was used, and those with large fluid or blood requirements, large opioid requirements, postoperative pain, and N/V.

3. Late.

a. Recovery at home until return to functional status.

C. CRITERIA FOR DISCHARGE

1. On day of surgery, a responsible adult should accompany pt at discharge from the facility and remain with pt for several hours.

2. Level of consciousness.

a. Pt's mental status and level of consciousness should be at baseline.

b. Often, being accompanied by someone familiar helps to more quickly reorient pt to surroundings.

3. Mobility as appropriate per procedure.

a. Pt who was ambulating and fully independent should be able to walk with very minimal assistance.

b. If pt's movement is limited as a result of the surgical procedure, instructions should clarify to the PACU staff the requirements for discharge.

c. Adult pt who has undergone an intraabdominal or urologic procedure should exhibit ability to void before discharge.

d. Pt who has received neuraxial regional anesthesia should be assessed for return of motor and sensory function.

4. Vital signs should be within normal range.

a. BP— taken when pt is not anxious or in pain—should be within 20% of baseline, taken over a period of time to show a stable trend.

b. Heart rate and rhythm at baseline.

   i. Deviations in heart rate or rhythm or pt complaint of chest pain, discomfort, or difficulty breathing should be evaluated with a 12-lead ECG.

c. Respiratory rate.

   i. Should be within normal range for pt's age.

d. Oxygen saturation.
   i. Room air oxygen saturation should be >93% or at baseline.
   ii. Pt should be encouraged to cough, take deep breaths, and ambulate.
   iii. Consider CXR if exam reveals auscultatory abnormalities.
e. Pain.
   i. Often the cause of abnormalities in vital signs.
   ii. Pt's pain should be scored with a standardized system.
   iii. A pain scale of 1 to 10 or the visual assessment of pain scale is frequently used.
   iv. Pt who has chronic pain may have high tolerance to pain. It is important to determine pt's baseline pain score and whether pt can "tolerate" the increase in pain from the surgical procedure.

5. Enteral intake.
a. PONV can delay or prohibit discharge from the facility.
b. Moderate-to-high-risk pts should receive prophylactic treatment, and pts who experience PONV should be treated promptly.
c. It is not necessary for a pt to exhibit ability to tolerate food or liquids.
   i. However, attempts to feed the pt should be made only when pt is fully awake and alert and showing signs of ability to swallow and clear secretions.

6. Dressings and drains.
a. Pt's surgical sites should be evaluated and have minimal bleeding and drainage. The surgeons should be notified of any concerns.

D. CARE INSTRUCTIONS
1. Postoperative care instructions should be given to the family member or accompanying adult and should include what to expect during the recovery period, possible complications, and the correct person to contact with questions or concerns.

E. PTS WHO ARE NOT READY TO BE DISCHARGED
1. The PACU nursing staff is responsible for monitoring the pt and alerting physicians should any changes occur.
2. If there are any concerns regarding a pt's ability to be safely discharged to home, the pt should be admitted for monitoring in the hospital.
a. An algorithm and resources for admitting pts should be in place.
b. A well-organized outpatient facility has an unexpected admissions rate of <1%, with rates being higher for larger populations of young children, elderly, or pts who are ASA class III or higher.
3. Common reasons for unexpected admissions are pain, bleeding, intractable vomiting, surgical misadventures, more extensive surgery than planned, urinary retention, or lack of an escort, with the most common reason being bleeding at the surgical site.
a. Most pts who come to the ED are treated and discharged home.

16

POSTOPERATIVE ISSUES

4. After discharge, the pt and family members or friends should receive discharge information, including contact numbers and when to call 911 or bring the pt directly to the ED.
5. Likewise, the PACU should obtain contact information for the pt.

V. POSTOPERATIVE HYPOXIA

A. CAUSES OF HYPOXIA ON EMERGENCE

1. Residual effects from inhaled agents, opioids, or benzodiazepines.
2. Postextubation, pt may lose the respiratory drive that the "irritation" of endotracheal intubation may have caused.
3. If nitrous oxide is used during the case, pt may develop diffusion hypoxia, as nitrous oxide can displace oxygen and dilute alveolar carbon dioxide, thus decreasing respiratory drive and ventilation.
a. It is important to give pt 100% oxygen immediately after emergence from anesthesia and slowly wean the oxygen requirement to oxygen saturation and respiratory status.

B. CAUSES OF PERIOPERATIVE HYPOXIA

1. Acute upper airway obstruction manifested as stridor.
a. Can be caused by soft-tissue obstruction, laryngospasm, laryngeal edema, or cord paralysis.
b. Initial intervention includes 100% oxygen with CPAP through a tight-fitting face mask, jaw thrust, and chin tilt to open the airway.
c. Insertion of an oral or nasal airway can keep the soft tissue from falling back into the posterior pharynx.
d. Oral secretions should be suctioned to keep them from irritating the vocal cords and to prevent aspiration.
e. Treatment with inhaled racemic epinephrine can help, but the definitive treatment is intubation.
2. Atelectasis.
a. Defined as collapse of alveoli after a prolonged period of breathing with small tidal volumes.
b. During GA with controlled ventilation via an ETT, it is possible to deliver large tidal volumes to a pt.
c. If an LMA or green mask is used with GA, pt's respirations are more rapid and shallow, thus worsening atelectasis.
   i. In the PACU, pt should be encouraged to take deep breaths, cough, and use incentive spirometry.
d. Pt should be positioned with the head of the bed elevated, thus allowing gravity to expand lung volume.
3. Hypoventilation.
a. Defined as $PaCO_2$ >45 mm Hg in pts with normal pulmonary function.
b. Hypercarbia may become apparent when the $PaCO_2$ is >60 mm Hg or arterial blood pH is <7.25.
c. Decrease in respiratory drive can be caused by sedation due to benzodiazepines or narcotics, residual muscle blockage, and altered mental status, leading to hypoxia, hypercarbia, and acidosis.

d. Opioid-induced respiratory depression manifests as a slow respiratory rate.

e. If overdose of benzodiazepines or narcotics is suspected, consider administration of flumazenil or naloxone.

f. An additional dose of NMB may be warranted if pt exhibits signs of weakness.

4. Bronchospasm.

a. Caused by aspiration, histamine release from medications, allergic response, exacerbation of chronic obstructive pulmonary disease, or asthma.

   i. As the bronchodilatory effects of inhaled agents dissipate, tracheal irritation can trigger constriction of the bronchial smooth muscle.

5. Negative-pressure pulmonary edema.

a. If pt is struggling to breathe against an obstruction (e.g., closed glottis from laryngospasm, soft-tissue obstruction, biting on ETT), negative-pressure pulmonary edema can develop.

   i. May appear clinically as pink, frothy oral secretions and rales.

b. High risk in otherwise healthy and muscular men who can generate a large negative pressure.

6. Chemical pneumonitis.

a. Pt can silently aspirate if somnolent and not able to swallow secretions.

b. Factors that increase risk for morbidity and mortality include volume of vomitus, acidity of vomitus, and particulate matter in vomitus.

c. In pts who have a history of acid reflux, nausea, difficulties swallowing, or obesity, prophylactic measures should be considered to decrease risk of aspiration.

d. Preinduction administration of an oral nonparticulate (sodium citrate) or IV antacid may be useful in preventing complications from potential aspiration.

VI. POSTOPERATIVE NAUSEA AND VOMITING

A. PT-SPECIFIC RISK FACTORS

1. Female gender.
2. Nonsmoking status.
3. History of PONV or motion sickness.

B. ANESTHETIC RISK FACTORS

1. Use of volatile anesthetics.
2. Nitrous oxide.
3. Use of intraoperative and postoperative opioids.

C. SURGICAL RISK FACTORS

1. Duration of surgery (each 30 min increase in duration increases PONV risk by 60%, so that a baseline risk of 10% is increased by 16% after 30 min).
2. Type of surgery (laparoscopy; laparotomy; breast surgery; strabismus surgery; plastic surgery; maxillofacial, abdominal, gynecologic, neurologic, ophthalmologic, or urologic surgery).

TABLE 16.2

ANTIEMETIC DOSES AND TIMING FOR PREVENTION OF POSTOPERATIVE
NAUSEA AND VOMITING IN ADULTS

Drug	Dose	Timing
Dexamethasone	4–8 mg IV	At induction
Dimenhydrinate	1 mg/kg IV	
Dolasetron	12.5 mg IV	End of surgery (timing may not affect efficacy)
Droperidol*	0.625–1.25 mg IV	End of surgery
Ephedrine	0.5 mg/kg IM	End of surgery
Granisetron	0.35–1.5 mg IV	End of surgery
Haloperidol	0.5–2 mg IM/IV	
Prochlorperazine	5–10 mg IM/IV	End of surgery
Promethazine†	6.25–25 mg IV	At induction
Ondansetron	4 mg IV	End of surgery
Scopolamine transdermal patch		Prior evening or 4 hr before surgery
Tropisetron	2 mg IV RCT	End of surgery

*See FDA "black box" warning.
†FDA Alert: Should not be used in children <2 years old.
These recommendations are evidence-based, and not all the drugs have an FDA indication for
PONV. (Adapted from Gan TJ, Meyer TA, Apfel CC, et al: Ambul Anesth 2007;105:1615–1628.)

TABLE 16.3

ANTIEMETIC DOSES FOR PROPHYLAXIS OF POSTOPERATIVE VOMITING
IN CHILDREN

Drug	Dose
Dexamethasone	150 mcg/kg up to 5 mg
Dimenhydrinate	0.5 mg/kg up to 25 mg
Dolasetron	350 mcg/kg up to 12.5 mg
Droperidol*	10–15 mcg/kg up to 1.25 mg
Granisetron	40 mcg/kg up to 0.6 mg
Ondansetron†	50–100 mcg/kg up to 4 mg
Perphenazine‡	70 mcg/kg up to 5 mg
Tropisetron	0.1 mg/kg up to 2 mg

*See FDA "black box" warning. Recommended doses 10–15 mcg/kg.
†Approved for PONV in pediatric pts aged 1 month or older.
‡IV formulation of perphenazine is no longer available in the United States; only oral formulation is
available.
These recommendations are evidence-based, and not all the drugs have an FDA indication for
PONV. (Adapted from Gan TJ, Meyer TA, Apfel CC, et al: Ambul Anesth 2007;105:1615–1628.)

D. STRATEGIES TO REDUCE RISK OF PONV

1. Avoidance of GA by the use of regional anesthesia.
2. Use of propofol for induction and maintenance of anesthesia.
3. Avoidance of nitrous oxide.
4. Avoidance of volatile anesthetics.
5. Minimization of intraoperative and postoperative opioids.

6. Minimization of neostigmine.
7. Adequate hydration.

E.   TREATMENT OF PONV
1. Antiemetic treatment for adults (Table 16.2).
2. Antiemetic treatment for children (Table 16.3).

REFERENCES

American Psychiatric Association: Diagnostic and Statistical Manual of Mental Disorders, 4th ed. Arlington: American Psychiatric Publishing, 2000.

Chung F, Chan VW, Ong D: A post-anesthetic discharge scoring system for home readiness after ambulatory surgery. J Clin Anesth 1995;7: 500–506.

Davidson AJ, Huang GH, Czarnecki C, et al: Awareness during anesthesia in children: A prospective cohort study. Anesth Analg 2005;100:653–661.

Gan TJ, Meyer TA, Apfel CC, et al: Society for Ambulatory Anesthesia guidelines for the management of postoperative nausea and vomiting. Anesth Analg 2007;105:1615–1628.

Lepouse C, Lautner CA, Liu P, et al: Emergence delirium in adults in the post-anaesthesia care unit. Br J Anaesth 2006;96:747–753.

Miller RD (ed): Miller's Anesthesia, 6th ed. Philadelphia: Churchill Livingstone, 2004.

Morgan GE, Mikhail MS, Murray MJ: Clinical Anesthesiology, 3rd ed. New York: McGraw-Hill/Appleton & Lange, 2002.

Sebel PS, Bowdle TA, Ghoneim MM, et al: The incidence of awareness during anesthesia: A multicenter United States study. Anesth Analg 2004;99:833–939.

White E, Crosse M: The aetiology and prevention of peri-operative corneal abrasions. Anaesthesia 1998;53:157–161.

16

POSTOPERATIVE ISSUES

Acute Pain

Jay H. Patel, DO, and Aaron Rea, MD
Edited by Marie N. Hanna, MD

I. ADULT ACUTE POSTOPERATIVE PAIN

A. PAIN IS FIFTH VITAL SIGN (0 TO 10 VERBAL ANALOG SCALE)

1. Produced by injury of skin, deep somatic structures, visceral structures.

a. A-δ fibers (rapid conduction) conduct somatic pain (skin, muscle, peritoneum)—sharp, stabbing, well-localized.

b. C fibers (slow conduction) conduct visceral pain (caused by distention of hollow viscus or internal organ surgery)—dull, aching, poorly localized.

c. Interaction between ascending excitatory pain pathways and descending inhibitory pain pathways has been reported.

B. MULTIMODAL ANALGESIA

1. Most effective.

a. Opioids, LA via epidural or peripheral nerve catheters, NSAIDs, acetaminophen.

C. COMMON IV ANALGESICS USED IN THE IMMEDIATE POSTOPERATIVE PERIOD (Table 17.1)

D. COMMON ORAL OPIOIDS USED IN THE POSTOPERATIVE PERIOD (Table 17.2)

E. COMMON ORAL ANALGESICS (NONOPIOIDS) USED IN THE POSTOPERATIVE PERIOD

1. 650 mg acetaminophen PO q 6 hr.

a. Should not exceed 4 g daily.

b. Should not be used in pts with liver disease.

2. 600 mg ibuprofen PO q 6 hr.

a. Should not exceed 2400 mg daily.

b. Should not be used in pts with renal disease, GI bleeding, or platelet dysfunction or in pts at risk for bleeding.

c. Has peripheral antiinflammatory properties and centrally mediated analgesic effects.

d. Has an opioid-sparing effect and improves quality of postoperative analgesia.

3. 50 mg tramadol PO q 4–6 hr.

a. Should not exceed 300 mg daily.

4. Other oral agents to consider.

a. Muscle relaxants (cyclobenzaprine, tizanidine, baclofen).

b. Anxiolytics (midazolam, alprazolam, lorazepam, diazepam).

c. Anticonvulsants (gabapentin, pregabalin).

17

TABLE 17.1

COMMON IV ANALGESICS USED IN THE IMMEDIATE POSTOPERATIVE PERIOD

Agent	Dose	Route	Frequency	Onset	Duration
Fentanyl	25–50 mcg	IV	5–10 min	30 sec	30–60 min
Hydromorphone	0.2–0.4 mg	IV	5–10 min	1–5 min	2–4 hr
Morphine	0.5–2 mg	IV	5–20 min	<1 min	2–7 hr
Sufentanil	10–30 mcg	IV	5–10 min	1–3 min	20–45 min
Ketorolac*	15–30 mg	IV	6 hr	1 min	3–7 hr

*Contraindicated in pts with history of peptic ulcer disease, GI bleeding, renal impairment, or cerebrovascular bleeding and in pts with high risk of bleeding. Therapy should not exceed 5 continuous days.

TABLE 17.2

COMMON ORAL OPIOIDS USED IN THE POSTOPERATIVE PERIOD (OPIOID CONVERSION CHART)

Agent	IV Dose (mg)	PO Dose (mg)	IV Duration (hr)	PO Duration (hr)
Morphine*	10	30	2–7	4–7
Fentanyl	0.1	—	0.5–1	—
Hydromorphone	1.5	7.5	2–7	4–6
Oxycodone	—	5–10	—	4–5
Hydrocodone	—	30	—	4–5
Methadone	10	20	4–5	4–8

*Doses are given as equivalent to 10 mg of IV morphine over 4 hr. Conversions are approximate and should be adjusted based on clinical response.

II. IV PATIENT-CONTROLLED ANALGESIA (PCA)

A. GENERAL

1. A method of pain management involving the pt's participation that employs an infusion device with a locked medication cassette.
2. Pump can be programmed to deliver boluses, basal rate (continuous) infusion, or both of pain medication via the IV catheter as ordered by the physician.

B. OPIOIDS COMMONLY USED

1. Morphine (most commonly studied; the gold standard).
a. Delay in penetration of morphine across the BBB results in delayed expression of the analgesic and ventilatory depressant effects.
b. Metabolized via conjugation with glucuronic acid in hepatic cells to produce morphine-3-glucuronide (inactive) and morphine-6-glucuronide (active; produces opioid effects at μ receptors.
   i. Has greater potency and duration than morphine itself.
   ii. Elimination of this substrate is dependent on kidney function.
c. Not recommended when serum creatinine >2 mg/dL.
d. May cause histamine release.
2. Fentanyl.

TABLE 17.3

ROUTES AND SUGGESTED INITIAL SETTINGS OF COMMONLY USED IV PCAS

Drug	Demand Dose	Lockout (min)	Loading Dose
Morphine	0.6–2 mg	5–10	2–5 mg
Fentanyl	5–20 mcg	5–8	25 mcg
Hydromorphone	0.1–0.3 mg	5–10	0.4 mg

a. High lipid solubility (unlike morphine), which facilitates transfer across the BBB, providing a quicker onset and 75 to 100 times more potency than morphine.
b. Rapid onset makes this drug well suited for IV PCA.
c. Rapid distribution to inactive tissues (fat, skeletal muscle), resulting in a short duration of action.
d. Metabolized in the liver to norfentanyl, which is excreted by the kidneys.

3. Hydromorphone.
a. Morphine derivative.
b. Metabolized and excreted primarily as an inactive glucuronide metabolite.
c. Six to eight times as potent as morphine.
d. Suitable alternative for morphine-intolerant pts or those with altered renal function.

4. Others: meperidine, sufentanil, remifentanil, alfentanil, butorphanol, nalbuphine, pentazocine, buprenorphine, dezocine.

C. ROUTES AND THEIR SUGGESTED INITIAL SETTINGS (Table 17.3)
1. For opioid-tolerant pts.
a. Pt's 24 hr PO medication requirements are calculated, and the appropriate conversion per opioid conversion chart (PO to IV) is made and converted to mg/hr.
b. The PCA basal rate is started at one half to two thirds of calculated requirement.
  i. Example: Pt on 40 mg oxycodone PO tid will require ~3 mg/hr of IV morphine.
  ii. The basal rate is 1.5 to 2 mg/hr.

D. PCA SIDE EFFECTS
1. N/V—most common side effect.
a. Risk factors for development (female, history of N/V, nonsmoker, type of surgery) should be considered.
b. Single-drug prophylaxis with a serotonin antagonist (e.g., 4 mg ondansetron IV q 4 hr × two doses) for pts with mild-to-moderate risk (defined as one or two risk factors present).

c. Combination prophylaxis with dexamethasone plus serotonin antagonist for moderate- to high-risk pts (three or four risk factors present).

d. Other considerations—transdermal scopolamine, promethazine, metoclopramide, droperidol.

e. Even though droperidol is the only antiemetic that has been extensively studied when given concomitantly with PCA, its use in the United States has been extremely limited secondary to severe side effects (QT prolongation, life-threatening dysrhythmias).

2. Pruritus.

a. Consider 25 mg diphenhydramine IV push q 6 hr.

b. If itching is unrelieved after 1 hr, diphenhydramine is continued and 1 mg naloxone in 1000 mL 0.9% NS IV is given at 20 mL/hr.

3. Respiratory depression.

a. Risk factors include advanced age, head injury, sleep apnea syndrome, obesity, respiratory failure, concurrent use of sedative medications, hypovolemia, renal failure.

b. Seen commonly with the use of background infusion rates.

c. When RR is <8/min or sedation level is <4:

   i. Stop PCA infusion.

   ii. Check oxygen saturation.

   iii. Administer oxygen 10 L/min via face mask (in pts with chronic obstructive pulmonary disease, administer oxygen 4 L/min via nasal cannula).

   iv. Recheck oxygen saturation.

d. If oxygen saturation is <95% and RR is <8/min:

   i. Dilute 1 mL naloxone (0.4 mg/mL) in 9 mL of NS, for a total volume of 10 mL (0.04 mg/mL).

   ii. Administer 2 mL IV push q 2 min until RR is >8/min.

4. Sedation and confusion.

5. Urinary retention.

III. NEURAXIAL OPIOIDS

A. HYDROPHILIC OPIOIDS (MORPHINE, HYDROMORPHONE)

1. Slow onset of analgesia (30 to 90 min).

2. Longer duration of analgesia (6 to 24 hr).

3. Extensive CSF spread (delayed respiratory depression).

4. Dosing.

a. Spinal—0.1 to 0.5 mg as bolus.

b. Epidural—2 to 4 mg as bolus (begin at 0.3 mg/hr as infusion).

c. Decrease dose with age and with pregnancy.

5. Lumbar site may require slightly higher dose (20%).

B. LIPOPHILIC OPIOIDS (FENTANYL, SUFENTANIL)

1. Rapid onset (5 to 15 min).

2. Shorter duration of analgesia (2 to 4 hr).

3. Minimal CSF spread.
4. Dosing.
a. Spinal—10 to 25 mcg as bolus.
b. Epidural—50 to 100 mcg as bolus, continuous infusion (20 to 100 mcg/hr).
5. Owing to its lipophilicity, after 24 hr of continuous infusion, epidural fentanyl produces analgesic serum levels equivalent to those produced by IV infusion.
6. Administering fentanyl alone via epidural (regardless of catheter site) achieves no clinical advantage; neuraxial fentanyl should always be given with an LA.

C. INDICATIONS FOR USE
1. Used as sole agent to avoid side effects of LA (e.g., hypotension).
2. Lumbar epidural placement for thoracic surgery.
3. Pt-controlled epidural analgesia (PCEA) solutions in combination with LA and opioids produce synergistic effects.

D. SIDE EFFECTS
1. N/V (incidence, 30% to 50%).
2. Urinary retention (incidence, 10% to 50%).
3. Pruritus (incidence, 40% to 75%).
4. Respiratory depression (rostral spread of opioids).
a. No evidence that incidence of respiratory depression is higher with neuraxial opioids than with IV PCA opioids.
b. Respiratory depression may occur within 1 hr with morphine and within minutes with fentanyl.
c. Respiratory depression is preceded by increased level of sedation.
d. Usually occurs within 6 to 12 hr after epidural morphine administration.
e. Respiratory depression is potentiated by concomitant administration of sedatives or systemic opioids.
f. Other risk factors for respiratory depression—sleep, older age, coexisting pulmonary disease, opioid-naïve state.

IV. EPIDURAL PCA (PCEA)
A. GENERAL
1. Usually a combination of a low concentration of long-acting LA (e.g., bupivacaine) and a lipid-soluble opioid (e.g., fentanyl).

B. KNOWN BENEFITS
1. Superior analgesia.
2. Improved pulmonary function.
3. Better graft survival after lower-limb vascular procedures.
4. Increased bowel mobility (associated with shorter hospital stay).

17

ACUTE PAIN

5. Fewer cardiac ischemic events.
6. Shorter recuperation after joint surgery (associated with early aggressive mobilization).

C. CONTRAINDICATIONS

1. Pt refusal.
2. Coagulopathy.
3. Platelet abnormalities.
4. Bacteremia.
5. Presence of infection or tumor at the site of puncture.
6. Any pt started on Coumadin, IV heparin, LMWH, or clopidogrel bisulfate (Plavix) should have epidural pulled before the drug reaches therapeutic levels.

D. PCEA MANAGEMENT

1. All PCEA is managed by the Acute Pain Service (APS).
2. Evaluate pt before initiation of PCEA.
   a. Pain is fifth vital sign (0 to 10 verbal analog scale).
   b. Confirm sensory level, motor function, and vital signs.
3. Confirm patency of epidural catheter.
4. Aspirate for CSF or blood.
5. Consider giving test dose.
6. Assess sensory level and motor block.
7. If pt is in pain and there is no sensory level, give an adequate amount of LA before deciding whether a catheter is working.
8. May start PCEA with motor block, but recovery of motor function must be evident before pt leaves PACU.
9. Consider replacing epidural catheters that are not functioning; otherwise, start IV PCA and remove catheter.
10. Must give adequate amount of LA and adequate time before deciding whether an epidural catheter is not functioning.
11. Administer 7 to 10 mL (lumbar) or 3 to 7 mL (thoracic) of 1.5% to 2% lidocaine with 1:200,000 epinephrine in divided doses and in a monitored setting (diluted concentration may be considered in hypotensive pt and smaller boluses for older patients).
12. Monitor pt for at least 30 min after last bolus.
13. Communicate to the nurse and/or other members of the healthcare team that a bolus was given so that the pt receives appropriate monitoring.

E. EPIDURAL CATHETER COMPLICATIONS

1. Medication related.
   a. N/V.
   b. Pruritus.

. Respiratory depression.
. Hypotension.
. Intravascular migration.
4. Epidural hematoma.
. Severe back pain, progressive motor and sensory deficit.
5. Epidural abscess.

ANATOMIC CONSIDERATIONS
1. Placement of epidural catheter at site of surgical incision is best guarantee of providing superior analgesia with minimal side effects.
a. Thoracic surgery—T_4 to T_7.
b. Upper abdominal surgery (Whipple, gastrectomy, hepatic)—T_6 to T_7.
c. Midabdominal surgery (genitourinary)—T_7 to T_{10}.
d. Lower abdominal surgery (total abdominal hysterectomy, anterior-posterior resection, colectomy)—T_9 to T_{10}.

ADVANTAGES OF THORACIC EPIDURAL PLACEMENT
1. Decreased dose requirements (up to 30% less).
2. Segmental analgesia (sparing of lumbar-sacral segments).
3. Potentially less urinary retention.
4. Less motor block—earlier ambulation.
5. Limited sympathectomy—less hypotension.
6. May allow more intense block of thoracic segments (use of higher concentration of LA if needed).
7. Preservation of postoperative pulmonary function.

H. REASONS APS WILL BE CALLED
1. If RR is <8/min or if evidence of airway obstruction is present.
2. Sedation level <4.
3. Pain intensity level >4 on a 0 to 10 scale.
4. Hypotension.
5. Changes in mental status.
6. Signs or symptoms of LA toxicity (confusion, metallic taste, numbness about the mouth, irregular HR).
7. Signs or symptoms of epidural or spinal hematoma.
a. Sensory deficits—numbness and/or paresthesias.
b. Motor deficits—leg weakness and/or paralysis, bowel or bladder dysfunction.
c. Pain at insertion site.
d. Severe lower back pain.
8. Wet dressing.
9. Catheter break or dislodgement (remove catheter).
10. Signs of catheter-site infection, meningitis, or sepsis.
11. N/V or itching unrelieved by medication.
12. Urinary retention.

17

ACUTE PAIN

V. PERIPHERAL NERVE CATHETERS

A. **USED FOR INTRAOPERATIVE ANESTHESIA AND POSTOPERATIVE ANALGESIA**

B. **INDICATIONS**
1. Continuous femoral nerve block for anterior thigh and knee surgery.
2. Continuous sciatic nerve block for tibia, ankle, foot surgery.
3. Continuous lumbar plexus block for hip, anterior thigh, and knee surgery.
4. Continuous posterior cervical block for major shoulder, elbow, wrist surgery.
5. Continuous interscalene brachial plexus block for shoulder, arm, elbow surgery.
6. Continuous infraclavicular brachial plexus block for elbow, forearm, and hand surgery.

C. **PREMEDICATION—HELPS TO REDUCE PT DISCOMFORT AND ANXIETY**
1. 0.5 to 5 mg midazolam IV—titrated to desired level of sedation.
2. 25 to 100 mcg fentanyl IV—titrated to desired level of sedation.
3. Deeper level of sedation is not advantageous, depending on the level of pt cooperation.

D. **POSTOPERATIVE MANAGEMENT**
1. PCA via peripheral nerve catheter.
a. Initial bolus—15 to 20 mL of LA (ropivacaine 0.5%).
b. PCA settings—ropivacaine 0.2%.
c. Continuous—6 to 8 mL/hr.
d. Demand—4 to 6 mL.
e. Lock-out—20 min.

E. **SITE-SPECIFIC COMPLICATIONS**
1. Artery puncture.
a. Stop and apply firm, constant pressure to area for 2 to 3 min.
2. Site infection.
a. Check puncture site daily for redness or tenderness.

REFERENCES

de Leon-Casasola OA, Lema MJ: Postoperative epidural opioid analgesia: What are the choices? Anesth Analg 1996;83:867–875.

Grass JA: Patient-controlled analgesia. Anesth Analg 2005;101:S44-S61.

Lubenow TR, Ivankovich AD, Barkin RL: Management of acute postoperative pain. In Barash PG, Cullen BF, Stoelting RK (eds): Clinical Anesthesia, 5th ed. Philadelphia: Lippincott Williams & Wilkins, 2006.

McMahon S, Koltzenburg M: Wall and Melzack's Textbook of Pain, 5th ed. Philadelphia: Churchill Livingstone, 2005.

Momeni M, Crucitti M, De Kock M: Patient-controlled analgesia in the management of postoperative pain. Drugs 2006;66:2321–2337.

New York School of Regional Anesthesia Web sites: http://www.nysora.com. Assessed March 3, 2008.

Omoigui S: Sota Omoigui's Anesthesia Drugs Handbook, 3rd ed. Hawthorne, CA: State-of-the-Art Technologies, 1999.

Regional Anesthesia Study Center of Iowa Web site. Available at: www.anesth.uiowa.edu/rasci/movies.html. Accessed March 3, 2008.

Chronic Pain

Adam J. Carinci, MD, Matthew Crooks, MD, Brandon Lenox, MD, and
Danesh Mazloomdoost, MD
Edited by Paul J. Christo, MD, MBA

DEFINITIONS

Allodynia—condition in which ordinarily nonpainful stimuli (light touch) evoke pain.

Analgesia—pain relief.

Arthralgia—joint pain.

Breakthrough pain—pain that overcomes the analgesia produced by long-acting medical therapy.

Central pain—pain that originates in the CNS; may also be known as thalamic pain syndrome.

Central sensitization—a hypersensitive CNS state in response to chronic painful stimulation that incorporates NMDA activation and gene induction.

Chronic pain—pain that generally lasts longer than 3 mo.

Deafferentation pain—pain that develops from a lack of sensory input to the CNS.

Dysesthesia—a condition in which an unpleasant sensation is produced by ordinary stimuli.

Hyperalgesia—an exaggerated painful response to a painful stimulus (e.g., enhanced pain to a pinprick).

Hyperesthesia—increased sensitivity to stimulation.

Hyperpathia—increased pain after repetitive stimulation.

Hypesthesia—decreased sensitivity to stimulation.

Myofascial pain—pain that originates from the muscles.

Neuralgia—pain that radiates along the course of one or more nerves.

Neuraxis—the brain and spinal cord.

Neuropathic pain—pain that is caused by a primary lesion in the central or peripheral nervous system or both; may include lesions from disease processes, radiation, trauma, or chemicals.

Neuropathy—an abnormal and usually degenerative state of the nervous system or specific nerves.

Opioid—a substance that activates opioid receptors and includes drugs or endogenous compounds (e.g., endorphins).

Pain—an unpleasant sensory and emotional experience associated with actual or potential tissue damage.

Paresthesia—an abnormal sensation (e.g., pins and needles) that is not necessarily considered unpleasant.

Peripheral neuropathy—a disease or degenerative state of the peripheral nerves in which motor, sensory, or vasomotor nerve fibers may be affected.

18

Radicular pain—pain that is distributed along a dermatome and that results from inflammation or other irritation of the nerve root, ganglia, or spinal nerve.

Radiculopathy—a pathologic condition in which an individual nerve root or multiple nerve roots are affected, causing sensory and motor changes along the affected nerve distribution; condition includes a focal neuralgic deficit.

Referred pain—a painful sensation sensed at a site distinct from the actual location of trauma or disease; occurs because of similar convergence of nerve supply in the CNS.

Somatic pain—pain that results from nerve activation in the skin, muscles, bones, ligaments, and joints.

Spondylolisthesis—the displacement of a vertebra or the vertebral column in relation to the vertebra below.

Spondylolysis—a defect in the pars interarticularis of a vertebra.

Spondylosis—spinal degeneration and vertebral joint deformity often associated with disk herniation, osteophyte formation, and nerve root compression.

Trigger point—focal area of pain within a muscle, often referred to distal locations.

Visceral pain—pain resulting from stretching of nerve endings located in organs.

Wind-up phenomenon—a condition that results from overstimulation of the dorsal horn of the spinal cord from chronic C-fiber and NMDA activation.

II. EVALUATION OF THE PAIN PATIENT

A. HISTORY
1. Identify chief complaint.
2. Document and characterize pain.
3. Time of pain onset.
4. Context of pain onset.
a. Traumatic versus atraumatic.
5. Severity.
a. Use the visual analog scale (Figure 18.1).
6. Character.
a. Dull, sharp, achy, knifelike, gnawing, burning, numbing, etc.
7. Location.
a. Use a pain diagram (Figure 18.2).
8. Aggravating and alleviating factors.
9. Associated factors.
a. Symptoms associated with other organ systems, neurologic symptoms, weakness, numbness, or motor deficits.
10. Exclude life-threatening conditions such as cauda equina syndrome, tumors, fractures, and infections.

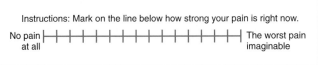

FIG. 18.1

Visual analog scale for pain.

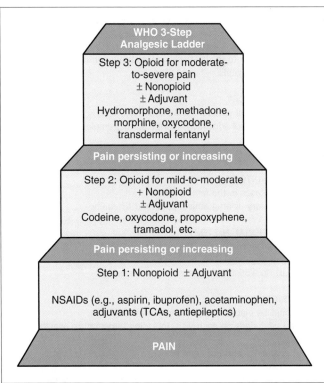

FIG. 18.2

WHO Three-Step Analgesic Ladder with examples of analgesics. *(Adapted from Agency for Health Care Policy and Research [AHCPR]: Management of Cancer Pain. Clinical Practice Guideline, No. 9. AHCPR Pub. No. 94-0592. Rockville, MD: AHCPR, Public Health Service, U.S. Department of Health and Human Services, 1994.)*

11. Review prior workups, tests, and treatments, including invasive, noninvasive, and physical therapy.
12. Assess functional loss that affects activities of daily living.
13. Assess use of assistive devices.

B. MEDICAL HISTORY
1. Conduct complete review of systems.
2. Review past medical and psychosocial history.
3. Review past surgical history, noting any association between prior surgery and current pain syndrome.
4. Obtain complete drug history, including prescription, over-the-counter, and alternative medications, as well as illegal substance use.
a. Include current medications and previous pain medications.
5. Identify allergies to medications, radiographic contrast, and environmental agents.

C. SOCIAL HISTORY
1. Assess pt's social structure and support systems.
2. Determine level of education, marital status, employment status, and lifestyle.
3. Assess tobacco and alcohol use.

D. FAMILY HISTORY
1. Review diseases in the family.
2. Identify history of drug abuse, pain, and disability.

E. OCCUPATIONAL HISTORY
1. Current and previous jobs, full time or part time.
2. History of litigation?
3. Is the pt on worker's compensation or disability?

F. PHYSICAL EXAM
1. Pt should be placed in a gown for examination.
2. Record vital signs on each visit, including temperature, weight, and height.
3. Note grooming, nutrition, and presence of assistive devices.
4. Inspection.
a. Visually inspect the pt and specific painful areas for structural abnormalities.
b. Inspect the skin of the affected area, noting color, temperature, and changes in skin texture, nails, and hair.
c. Evaluate muscle bulk and structural asymmetry and posture.
5. Palpation and range of motion.
a. Assess both the bony and soft-tissue structures of the painful area.
b. Palpate pulses.

. Determine both active and passive range of motion of affected areas and compare with contralateral side.

. **Gait.**

. Assess gait for functional strength, neurologic changes, and symmetry.

. **Motor strength and deep tendon reflexes.**

. Assess muscle strength in all applicable muscle groups.

   i.   Muscle strength grading.

- 5—normal power.
- 4—active movement against gravity and resistance.
- 3—active movement against gravity only.
- 2—active movement with gravity eliminated.
- 1—flicker or trace of contraction.
- 0—no contraction.

. Hyperreflexia indicates upper motor neuron injury, whereas hyporeflexia is consistent with nerve root compression.

   i.   Frequently tested deep tendon reflexes.

- Biceps reflex—C5 to C6.
- Brachioradialis reflex—C5 to C6.
- Triceps reflex—C6 to C7.
- Patellar reflex—L2 to L4.
- Achilles reflex—S1 to S2.

8. Sensation.

. Assess response to light touch (A-β fibers), pinprick (A-δ fibers), and hot/cold stimuli (A-δ and C fibers).

   i.   Neuropathic pain conditions may elicit specific sensory disturbances.

- Allodynia.
- Hyperalgesia.
- Dysesthesia.
- Hyperesthesia.
- Hypoalgesia.
- Hypoesthesia.

9. Mental status exam.

a. Assess orientation, mood, affect, thought content, level of consciousness, and speech.

G. SPECIAL TESTS

1. Straight leg raising.

a. Assesses the presence of lumbar disk herniation and radicular pain beyond the knee.

b. Typically performed with leg elevation between 30 and 60 degrees, with neck in flexion to increase dural sac tension.

2. Sacroiliac (SI) tests.

a. Assesses pain in the buttock by causing ligamentous strain in the SI joint and/or intraarticular pressure in the hip joint.

18

CHRONIC PAIN

b. Patrick or FABER test.

   i. With pt supine, *F*lex, *ab*duct, and *e*xternally *r*otate the hip while placing pressure on the contralateral anterior superior iliac spine.

c. Gaenslen test.

   i. Pt lies on unaffected side with hip flexed and affected hip hyperextended.

3. Facet joint test (lumbar spine).

a. Assesses pain associated with facet joint disease by direct pressure or by inducing lumbar hyperextension to load facet joints.

b. Direct pressure.

   i. Apply force lateral to the spinous process and over the facet joints.

c. Sphinx.

   i. Pt lies prone and rests on elbows.

d. Quadrant.

   i. With pt in standing position, examiner leans pt backward and toward the side of pain.

4. Piriformis test.

a. Assesses the presence of buttock pain associated with piriformis syndrome. These tests either stretch the sciatic nerve against the piriformis muscle or contract the piriformis muscle.

b. Freiberg test.

   i. Extend the hip and internally rotate.

c. Beatty maneuver.

   i. Pt lies with affected side up, hip is flexed, and knee is lifted a few inches above the exam table.

d. FADIR.

   i. *F*lex, *ad*duct, and *i*nternally *r*otate hip.

5. Cervical compression test.

a. Used to detect neuroforaminal narrowing, facet joint pressure, or muscle spasm.

b. With the pt supine, examiner applies downward pressure over the vertex of the skull.

c. Any pain in the cervical spine or upper extremity may reflect disk disease or facet irritation.

6. Adson test.

a. Used to detect subclavian artery compression, e.g., by a cervical rib or hypertrophied anterior scalene muscle.

b. Pt's radial pulse is continually taken at the wrist while the arm is abducted, extended, and externally rotated.

c. Pt then takes a deep breath and turns the head toward the tested arm.

d. Any drop or absence in the radial pulse suggests subclavian artery compression.

7. Valsalva test.

a. Increases intrathecal pressure.

b. If a tumor, disk, or abscess is present in the cervical spinal canal, this test can help to identify its presence and its location if dermatomal referral patterns are reproduced.

8. Hoover test.

a. Pt lies on the examination table with heels held in the examiner's hands.

b. Pt is then asked to lift one leg.

c. The expected response is to push down with the opposite heel into the examiner's hand.

d. If pt does not push down, malingering is suggested.

9. Tinel sign.

a. Percussion over a nerve that produces distal paresthesias.

b. Percussion over the carpal, tarsal, or cubital tunnels that causes paresthesias may suggest nerve entrapment.

10. Waddell signs.

a. A group of physical signs that may indicate nonorganic or psychologic components to complaints of chronic lower back pain (LBP).

b. Three or more are positively correlated with a nonorganic cause:

   i. Tenderness—generalized or does not follow any anatomic pattern, for instance, light touch causes widespread pain.

   ii. Pain on simulated rotation—pt reports pain in the lumbar region while examiner rotates the shoulders (sham rotation of the spine); or pt reports shoulder pain during the straight-leg-raise maneuver.

   iii. Distraction—pt complains of pain during straight-leg-raise test while lying down but does not report pain when the test is performed while sitting.

   iv. Regional sensory change—stocking sensory loss that does not follow a dermatomal pattern, or sensory loss in an entire extremity or side of the body.

   v. Regional weakness—weakness that is jerky, with intermittent resistance such as cogwheeling or catching.

     • Organic weakness can be overpowered smoothly.

   vi. Overreaction—exaggerated painful response to a stimulus that is not reproduced when the same stimulus is applied later.

     • May see excessive grabbing of the painful area or grimacing and sighing.

III. DIAGNOSTIC IMAGING FOR THE PAIN PATIENT

A. PLAIN RADIOGRAPHY

1. Displays skeletal anatomy.

2. Primarily used to assess bony structures.

3. Produces two-dimensional images.

4. Four basic densities or shades are visible on plain films.

a. Air, fat, water (blood and soft tissue), and bone.

b. Air appears black or very dark, fat appears generally gray and darker than muscle or blood, and bone and calcium appear almost white.

18

CHRONIC PAIN

5. Plain x-ray films are often the initial imaging modality for many conditions.
6. They are inexpensive and rapid.
7. Screening tool for spine fractures, vertebral misalignment, spondylolisthesis, and spondylolysis.
8. Flexion and extension views provide information about the integrity of fusion surgery and the presence of spondylolisthesis.

B. FLUOROSCOPY
1. Fluoroscopic images have similar principles to those of plain films.
2. Images are viewed on a screen, and the pt's body is imaged in real time.
3. They are used for diagnostic and therapeutic interventional pain procedures.

C. CT
1. Provides superior bone detail.
2. Can be used in pts with ferromagnetic devices (e.g., spinal cord stimulators, cardiac pacemakers).
3. Images have the potential to be reconstructed into three-dimensional images.
4. Because CT displays soft tissues reasonably well, it is used for soft-tissue evaluation if MRI is contraindicated or not available.
5. Useful in diagnosing spinal bone trauma, disk herniation, spinal stenosis, and nerve root impingement.
6. Scans are presented as a series of cross-sectional images.
7. Images are displayed as if the viewer is viewing the pt from the foot of the bed.
8. Numerous structures are visualized simultaneously.
9. Compared with plain x-ray films, CT uses ~10 to 100 times more radiation.
10. The basic four densities on CT images are similar to those in plain x-ray films.

D. MRI
1. Provides exceptional images of the CNS and stationary soft tissues.
2. MRI is noninvasive and uses no radiation.
3. Calcium and bone are difficult to visualize.
4. Generates images by applying a varying magnetic field to the body.
5. Two basic types of images: T1-weighted and T2-weighted.
a. T1-weighted.
   i. Displays fat as a white or a bright signal and water as dark.
   ii. Highlights end-plate changes, osteophytic narrowing, lateral disk herniation, spondylolisthesis.
b. T2-weighted.
   i. Displays fat as dark; blood, edema, and CSF appear white.
   ii. Highlights infection and inflammation.

. Equal to CT in evaluating disk herniation and spinal stenosis.

. More sensitive and specific in detecting osteomyelitis, diskitis, or malignancy.

. Helpful in evaluating arachnoiditis.

. Best technique to assess spinal cord compression and damage.

0. Disadvantages.

. Artifacts caused by pt motion.

. Inability to use in pts with ferromagnetic objects (e.g., aneurysm clips, cochlear implants, cardiac pacemakers).

. Cost.

MYELOGRAPHY

. Intrathecal injection of radiographic contrast followed by plain film or CT imaging.

. Provides information about structural changes affecting spinal nerves.

. Can help to diagnose structural spine disease when CT or MRI fails to provide sufficient information or produces artifact.

. Postmyelographic CT is highly sensitive for detecting osteophytic impingement, cervical radiculopathy, disk herniation, and subtle posterolateral nerve impingement from disk herniation missed by MRI.

. Useful in identifying subarachnoid tumor spread and arachnoiditis.

. Disadvantages.

. Invasive.

. Can cause postdural puncture headaches (PDPHs).

. Uses radiation.

DISKOGRAPHY

1. Injection of radiographic contrast into the nucleus pulposus of the intervertebral disk under fluoroscopic guidance.

2. Contrast accumulation inside the disk and the pt's response to a given volume of injectate provide structural and subjective evidence of whether a specific disk is pain sensitive.

3. Provoking the disk with contrast provides information about whether a disk is the source of axial or radicular pain in the cervical, thoracic, and lumbar spine.

4. CT scanning may follow diskography for further structural disk analysis.

5. Specific treatment recommendations (e.g., noninvasive modalities or surgery) are made following the outcome of the procedure.

IV. PHARMACOLOGIC APPROACHES TO CHRONIC PAIN TREATMENT (NONOPIOID)

A. ACETAMINOPHEN

1. Short-acting analgesic (plasma half-life 2 to 3 hr).

2. Effective analgesic, antipyretic agent.

3. Poor antiinflammatory drug.

4. Controls pain primarily through the spinal cord and cerebral cortex and produces weak central inhibition of prostaglandin synthase.

18

CHRONIC PAIN

5. Consider for initial therapy of osteoarthritis.
6. Metabolized by the hepatic microsomal enzyme system.
7. Often combined with opioids (e.g., oxycodone, hydrocodone).
8. Dose—325 to 650 mg orally q 4–6 hr.
9. Maximum daily dose—3 to 4 g.

B. TRAMADOL
1. Synthetic derivative of codeine but not a scheduled, controlled drug.
2. Low risk of abuse liability, psychologic dependence, and respiratory depression.
3. Weak μ-receptor agonist that inhibits reuptake of serotonin and norepinephrine.
a. Facilitates serotonin release.
b. Indirectly activates postsynaptic α_2 receptors.
4. Indications.
a. Osteoarthritic pain.
b. LBP.
c. Neuropathic pain.
d. Surgical pain.
e. Breakthrough pain.
5. Available as immediate-release, controlled-release, and combination products.
6. Immediate-release dose.
a. 50 to 100 mg orally 3 to 4 times daily, with maximum dose of 400 mg/day.
7. Controlled-release dose.
a. 100 mg, 200 mg, 300 mg daily.
8. Combination product with acetaminophen.
a. Ultracet: 325 mg acetaminophen and 37.5 mg tramadol; 1 to 2 tabs PO q 4–6 hr.
b. Max dose—8 tabs/day.
9. Metabolized by the liver.
10. Adjust dosage in the elderly and pts with liver or renal disease.
11. Typical adverse effects.
a. Nausea.
b. Emesis.
c. Dizziness.
d. Vertigo.
e. Constipation.
f. Somnolence.
g. Headache.
12. Possible elevated risk of seizures and serotonin syndrome with concurrent use of selective serotonin reuptake inhibitors, selective monoamine oxidase inhibitors, or tricyclic antidepressants (TCAs).

C. NSAIDS

1. Produce peripheral and CNS analgesic effects.
2. Useful analgesic, antiinflammatory, and antipyretic agents for mild-to-moderate pain that is often musculoskeletal in origin (e.g., osteoarthritis and rheumatoid arthritis).
3. Extensively metabolized by the liver.
4. Mechanism of action.
   a. Inhibit cyclooxygenase (COX)-1 and COX-2 enzymes and prostaglandin production, with direct action on spinal nociceptive processing.
5. Analgesic, antiinflammatory, antipyretic effects principally mediated by COX-2 inhibition.
6. Highly protein bound (e.g., albumin); therefore drug displacement occurs when drug is combined with other highly protein-bound drugs (e.g., lithium).
7. NSAID medicines may increase the chance of a heart attack or stroke that can lead to death.
   a. This chance increases:
      i. With longer use of NSAID medicines.
      ii. In people who have heart disease.
8. Risks and side effects.
   a. Contraindicated in pts with the syndrome of asthma, nasal polyps, and urticaria.
   b. COX-1 inhibition can produce:
      i. Gastric or intestinal ulceration.
      ii. Decreased platelet function.
      iii. Renal dysfunction: sodium and water retention, hyperkalemia.
9. COX-2 selective drugs are as effective as nonselective agents with less risk of GI damage and bleeding.
10. Commonly used agents for pain:
    a. Diflunisal (Dolobid)—250 to 500 mg PO q 8–12 hr.
    b. Ibuprofen (Motrin, Advil)—200 to 400 mg PO q 4–6 hr.
    c. Etodolac (Lodine)—200 to 400 mg PO 3 or 4 times/day.
       i. Some COX-2 selectivity.
    d. Ketorolac (Toradol)—15 to 30 mg IV/IM q 6 hr, or 10 mg PO q 4–6 hr.
       i. Duration not to exceed 5 days.
    e. Naproxen (Naprosyn)—250 mg PO 4 times/day or 500 mg PO bid.
    f. Oxaprozin (Daypro)—600 to 1800 mg PO daily.
       i. Slow onset of action—not appropriate for acute pain.
    g. Meloxicam (Mobic)—7.5 to 15 mg PO daily.
       i. Some COX-2 selectivity, especially at lower doses.
    h. Nabumetone (Relafen)—500 to 1000 mg 1 or 2 times PO daily.
    i. Celecoxib (Celebrex)—100 to 200 mg PO daily.
       i. COX-2-selective inhibitor.

18

CHRONIC PAIN

D. **ASPIRIN**
1. Effective for common headaches and short-term mild pain.
2. Irreversible inhibitor of COX-1 and COX-2 and therefore prostaglandin production.
3. Side effects and risks.
a. Anaphylaxis in pts with asthma, nasal polyps, and urticaria.
4. Not to be given to children <2 yr of age with cold, flu, or chicken pox owing to risk of Reye syndrome (e.g., encephalopathy, liver dysfunction, fatty infiltration of liver and viscera).
5. Inhibits platelet aggregation for 8 to 12 days (platelet turnover time).
6. Dose—325 to 650 mg PO q 4–6 hr.

E. **TCAS**
1. Mechanism of action is primarily mediated by the blockade of reuptake of norepinephrine and serotonin.
2. Increased levels of norepinephrine and serotonin enhance the activation of descending inhibitory neurons and therefore facilitate pain relief.
3. Other secondary mechanisms of action include interaction with opioid receptors and inhibition of NMDA receptors.
4. Antidepressants are typically classified by their specific neurotransmitter reuptake inhibition.
5. Those antidepressants that have a greater inhibition of norepinephrine reuptake are associated with better analgesic effect.
6. Relevant contraindications include cardiac dysrhythmias, recent heart attack, epilepsy, narrow-angle glaucoma, heart block, hyperthyroidism, urinary obstruction, and monoamine oxidase inhibitors.
7. Typical TCAs: amitriptyline, imipramine, nortriptyline, desipramine.
a. Initial dose.
   i. 10 mg or 25 mg PO every evening.
b. Titration.
   i. Increase by 10 or 25 mg q 7 days to maximum dose of 150 mg nightly.
8. TCAs are most effective in relieving neuropathic pain and headache syndromes.
9. Specific indications for TCAs.
a. Amitriptyline (Elavil)—central pain, painful diabetic neuropathy, headache, and postherpetic neuralgia.
b. Nortriptyline (Pamelor)—central pain.
c. Desipramine (Norpramin)—peripheral neuropathy.

F. **ANTICONVULSANTS**
1. Most commonly used medication for neuropathic pain.
2. All have different mechanisms of action, although all thought to act as membrane stabilizers.

. Primarily used to treat neuralgias, peripheral neuropathy (e.g., alcohol, HIV, diabetes mellitus), posttraumatic neuralgia, painful diabetic neuropathy, postherpetic neuralgia, central pain conditions (e.g., post-stroke pain), and lumbar and cervical radiculopathy.

. Gabapentin (Neurontin).

. GABA analog that binds to $\alpha_2\delta$ calcium channel and decreases neurotransmitter release, but exact mechanism is unknown.

   i. It does not interact with GABA receptors.

. Typical dosage.

   i. 300 mg nightly, titrated by 300 mg q 3–5 days as tolerated, to maximum dose of 1200 mg tid.

. Pt should receive up to 1800 mg/day before treatment is considered a failure.

. Relatively good side-effect profile and lacks drug interactions.

. Very little metabolism of drug; renally excreted.

  Often a first-choice anticonvulsant for treating chronic, neuropathic pain.

. Common adverse effects.

   i. Dizziness, somnolence, fatigue, and pedal edema.

. FDA approved for postherpetic neuralgia.

. Carbamazepine (Tegretol).

. Related chemically and pharmacologically to the TCAs.

. Inhibits norepinephrine reuptake and blocks sodium ionic conductance.

. Moderately protein bound.

. Hepatic metabolism and renal excretion.

. Typical dosage.

   i. 200 mg/day, titrated up by 200 mg q 1–3 days, to a maximum dose of 1500 mg/day.

  Common side effects include somnolence, dizziness, GI irritation, ataxia, vertigo.

. Thrombocytopenia, aplastic anemia, pancytopenia, and agranulocytosis can occur.

. Baseline CBC and liver function tests critical.

. FDA approved for trigeminal neuralgia.

5. Lamotrigine (Lamictal).

a. Phenyltriazene derivative.

b. Blocks sodium channels and inhibits glutamine release.

   i. May modulate potassium and calcium channels.

c. Metabolized by the liver.

d. Drug-drug interactions with carbamazepine, valproic acid, and phenobarbital.

e. Typical starting dose is 25 mg bid.

   i. Slow weekly titration is important because of increased risk of rash.

   ii. Increase by 25 mg/week until 100 mg bid.

   iii. Maximum dosage is 250 mg bid.

f. Side effects include rash (9% to 10% risk) that can progress to Stevens-Johnson syndrome (0.3% risk in adults), headache, somnolence, dizziness, ataxia, GI disturbance, and blurred vision.
    i. Discontinue medication if rash develops.
    ii. Taper over a 2-wk period.
g. Effective for complex regional pain syndrome (CRPS), spinal cord injury pain, trigeminal neuralgia, multiple sclerosis, central pain (e.g., after stroke).

7. Pregabalin (Lyrica).

a. Acts at the $\alpha_2\delta$ subunit of calcium channels; exact mechanism is unknown.
b. Increases GABA concentrations.
c. Undergoes very little metabolism and is excreted via kidneys.
d. Typical dose.
    i. 75 mg PO bid for 1 week; then increase to 150 mg PO bid.
e. Common side effects.
    i. Somnolence, dizziness, headache.
f. FDA approved for postherpetic neuralgia, painful diabetic neuropathy, and fibromyalgia.

8. Topiramate (Topamax).

a. Blocks sodium channels and calcium channels, facilitates GABA-A receptors, and inhibits glutamate activity.
b. Undergoes very little metabolism and is renally excreted.
c. Typical dose.
    i. 25 mg PO daily; increase by 25 or 50 mg/wk to maximum dose of 200 mg PO bid.
d. Common side effects.
    i. Renal stones (1.5% risk), dizziness, somnolence, visual changes, ataxia, nervousness, weight loss, memory and concentration difficulty, paresthesias, possible taste perversions.
e. May be more effective in spinal cord injury pain and painful diabetic neuropathy.

9. Oxcarbazepine (Trileptal).

a. Carbamazepine analog.
b. Binds to sodium channels, increases potassium flow, modifies calcium channels.
c. Extensively metabolized.
d. Typical dose.
    i. 150 mg PO bid, increased by 150 mg/day each wk until maximum dose of 600 to 1200 mg daily.
e. Common side effects.
    i. Fatigue, dizziness, somnolence, ataxia, nausea, visual changes.
    ii. Because hyponatremia is possible, serum sodium levels should be monitored.
f. Preferred drug for treating trigeminal neuralgia owing to favorable adverse effect profile.

G. MUSCLE RELAXANTS
1. Antispasmotics (muscle relaxants) are used to treat chronic pain conditions with associated muscle tension and spasms.
2. Baclofen (Lioresal).
a. Used for treatment of spasticity associated with spinal cord injury, multiple sclerosis, or spinal cord lesions.
b. Useful for neuropathic pain and trigeminal neuralgia.
c. Mechanism of action.
   i. Thought to be secondary to GABA-B agonist activity at the spinal level.
d. Anecdotal evidence that it has intrinsic analgesic properties.
e. Typical starting dose.
   i. 5 mg PO tid, escalating by 5 mg q 3–4 days, to a maximum dose of 80 mg/day.
f. Adverse effects.
   i. Fatigue, sedation, orthostatic hypotension, hypotonia, ataxia, urinary frequency.
3. Cyclobenzaprine (Flexeril).
a. Structurally similar to TCAs.
b. Useful for peripheral muscle spasms and painful musculoskeletal conditions.
c. Mechanism of action probably related to its effect on polysynaptic reflexes and descending pain-facilitatory pathways.
d. Not effective for spasticity due to CNS disease.
e. Typical dose.
   i. 5 to 10 mg PO tid, with a maximum dose of 40 mg/day in divided doses.
f. Adverse effects.
   i. Sedation, xerostomia, dizziness.
g. Contraindicated with monoamine oxidase inhibitors, and in pts with cardiac dysrhythmias, urinary obstruction, and hyperthyroidism.
4. Tizanidine (Zanaflex).
a. Centrally acting α_2-adrenergic agonist.
b. Decreases spasticity by increasing presynaptic inhibition of motor neurons and decreases sympathetic nervous system activity at the dorsal horn.
c. Structurally similar to clonidine.
d. Indicated for spasticity associated with spinal cord injury, multiple sclerosis, sympathetically maintained pain, and neuropathic pain (burning, electrical, lancinating).
e. Possible intrinsic analgesic activity resulting from α-adrenergic agonism.
f. Adverse effects.
   i. Sedation.
   ii. Dizziness.
   iii. Weakness.
   iv. Xerostomia.

18

CHRONIC PAIN

g. Typical dose.
  i. 2 mg nightly or tid, increased to 8 mg q 6–8 hr.

5. Metaxalone (Skelaxin) and methocarbamol (Robaxin).

a. Centrally acting skeletal-muscle relaxants.

b. Useful for muscle spasms and musculoskeletal pain.

c. Careful use in pts with severe hepatic or renal disease.

d. Long-term use of metaxalone requires monitoring of liver function tests, and methocarbamol is contraindicated in epilepsy.

e. Adverse effects.
  i. Sedation.

f. Typical dosing.
  i. Metaxalone—800 mg PO q 6–8 hr.
  ii. Methocarbamol—750 mg PO q 4 hr.

6. Carisoprodol (Soma).

a. Skeletal-muscle relaxant.

b. Mild analgesic effect in pts with musculoskeletal pain.

c. Enhances analgesic effects of other drugs.

d. Active metabolite is meprobamate, a sedative-hypnotic that is an anxiolytic agent with properties similar to those of the benzodiazepines.

e. Both carisoprodol and meprobamate have abuse potential.

f. Adverse effects.
  i. Drowsiness, ataxia.

g. Typical dose.
  i. 350 mg PO 3 or 4 times/day.

7. Topical agents.

a. Lidocaine patch (Lidoderm).
  i. Produces analgesia without causing local anesthesia.
  ii. Blocks sodium channels in small, sensitized pain fibers.
  iii. Useful for postherpetic neuralgia, myofascial pain, and peripheral neuropathy.
  iv. Typical dose.
    • Lidoderm 5%, one to three patches at a time for 12 hr.
  v. Adverse effects.
    • Rash, LA toxicity.

b. Capsaicin.
  i. Extract of hot chili peppers.
  ii. Depletes substance P and neuropeptides from nociceptive fibers, causing analgesia.
  iii. Useful for postherpetic neuralgia.
  iv. Adverse effects.
    • Burning sensation on application.
  v. Typical dose.
    • 0.025% or 0.075% cream or lotion applied three to five times per day.

V. LOW BACK PAIN

A. GENERAL

1. Defined as pain arising from the spinal or paraspinal structures of the lumbosacral region.
2. Extends from the iliac crest to the coccyx.
3. Some predictors of chronic LBP.
   - Decreased activity level.
   - Preexisting psychosocial disorders, including depression and anxiety.
   - Radicular symptoms.
   - Poor heath status.
   - Poor support system and coping strategies.
   - Decreased flexibility of the back.
4. Chronic LBP syndrome is characterized by pain with psychosocial and medical comorbidities.
5. Pain may derive from disks, vertebral bodies, spinal cord, facets, ligaments, muscles, or SI joints.
6. The differential diagnosis of LBP is divided into mechanical and nonmechanical causes.
7. Most pts have mechanical LBP.

B. COMMON MECHANICAL CAUSES

1. Fractures.
2. Osteoporosis with compression fracture.
3. Herniated disk.
4. Degenerative changes or disease of the disks, facet joints, or bony structures of the spine.
5. Spinal stenosis.
6. Facet joint disease.
7. Spondylolysis or spondylolisthesis.
8. Scoliosis.
9. Paget disease.

C. COMMON NONMECHANICAL CAUSES

1. Inflammatory arthritis.
2. Infection: diskitis, osteomyelitis, endocarditis.
3. Neoplasia: spinal cord tumors, metastatic carcinoma, multiple myeloma.
4. Visceral disease (prostatitis, endometriosis, nephrolithiasis, abdominal aortic aneurysm, pancreatitis, perforated bowel).

D. HISTORY

1. A thorough H&P is imperative to proper diagnosis and treatment.
2. In pts with acute LBP with no signs of neurologic deficit or trauma, imaging studies are not warranted.

18

CHRONIC PAIN

3. LBP described as excruciating may indicate recent fracture, infection or metastatic disease.

E. IMAGING
1. Delay imaging for 1 mo in pts <50 yr of age with acute LBP and without history of neurologic deficits, systemic disease, or trauma.
2. Imaging is appropriate in pts >50 yr of age with greater likelihood of spinal stenosis, degenerative changes, and compression fractures.
3. Indicated for those displaying "red flag" conditions (trauma, fever, IV drug use, pain worse at night, unexplained weight loss).
4. Initial image is usually plain film in anteroposterior and lateral views.
5. If pt has a prior fusion or if instability is suspected, obtain flexion, extension, and lateral oblique films.
6. MRI is best imaging modality for evaluating lumbar spine.

F. IMAGING TYPES
1. MRI.
a. Demonstrates details of the spinal cord, disks, and paraspinal soft tissue.
b. Poor for bony anatomy.
2. CT.
a. Shows bony and joint pathology well; shows lateral disk herniation, stenosis.
3. Plain films.
a. Demonstrate fractures, osteophytes, tumors, infection, stenosis, lumbar alignment.
b. Do not show disk herniations, bulges, neuraxial masses, or small paraspinal lesions.

G. DISTRIBUTION OF PAIN AND WEAKNESS FOR LUMBAR RADICULOPATHIES
1. L2 to L3.
a. Pain—anterior thigh.
b. Weakness—hip flexion.
2. L3 to L4.
a. Pain—anterolateral thigh, anteromedial calf.
b. Weakness—quadriceps, knee extension.
3. L4 to L5.
a. Pain—lateral thigh, anterolateral calf.
b. Weakness—dorsiflexion of foot.
4. L5 to S1.
a. Pain—gluteal region, posterior thigh, posterolateral calf, plantar surface of foot.
b. Weakness—plantar flexion of foot.

H. TREATMENT

1. Acute LBP (persisting no longer than 3 mo) usually resolves within 6 wk.
2. Noninterventional treatment for LBP.

a. Relief of pain and return of function are the primary goals.
b. Encourage pt to maintain normal activity level with light aerobic exercise (walking, swimming, stationary bicycle).
c. Pt should avoid strenuous exercise until symptoms have resolved.
d. Physical therapy.
e. Pt should avoid bed rest.
f. NSAIDs and acetaminophen are the first-line agents for acute LBP.
g. Muscle relaxants may be beneficial for muscle spasms or sleep disturbance.
h. Opioids indicated only in pts with pain not controlled by first-line therapies.
i. Adjuvant therapies, including antidepressants and anticonvulsants, may be beneficial in pts with chronic LBP.

3. Interventional treatment for LBP.

a. Epidural steroid injections.
   i. Most effective for symptomatic relief of nerve root compression that causes lumbosacral radicular pain.
   ii. Improvement correlates with a decrease in nerve-root inflammation.
   iii. Little benefit in the absence of radicular pain.
   iv. The two most commonly used steroids are methylprednisolone (60 to 120 mg) and triamcinolone (50 to 75 mg).
   v. Steroid preparations typically produce suppression of the hypothalamic-pituitary axis for 1 to 3 wk; therefore, space injections at >1 mo intervals.
b. Conventional therapies.
   i. May consider acupuncture, transcutaneous electrical nerve stimulation, traction.
c. Surgery.
   i. Surgery indicated in only 1% of pts with LBP.
   ii. Lumbar spine surgery corrects spinal instability and nerve-root compression.
   iii. Immediate surgery indicated for incapacitating pain, cauda equina syndrome, severe infection or tumor, progressive neurologic deficits, or bowel or bladder dysfunction.
   iv. If LBP is mechanical and acute, strongly consider nonsurgical treatment for a month before operative therapies.
d. Facet joint injection and denervation.
   i. Indicated for degenerative changes in the zygapophysial (facet) joint that are causing chronic LBP.
   ii. Pain is lateral to midline in the lumbar region and often radiates to the ipsilateral buttock, posterior thigh, and knee.

18

CHRONIC PAIN

   iii. Axial loading tends to exacerbate the pain.

   iv. Confirmed by pain relief from fluoroscopically guided LA injection into intraarticular facet joints or, more commonly, blockade of the lumbar medial branch nerves.

   v. >50% pain relief from LA injection is considered diagnostic.

   vi. Medial branch rhizotomy (denervation) can provide longer-term relief via radiofrequency ablation, 4% phenol, or cryogenic nerve block.

e. Trigger-point injections.

   i. Used to treat myofascial pain associated with LBP.

   ii. Often uncover tenderness or pain related to nodular hardening in a muscle called a "trigger point."

   iii. Dry needling can be performed or needle insertion with injection of LA.

   iv. For best results, needle (25 G, 1.5 in) inserted into the trigger point should elicit a twitch response.

   v. Combine needling with manual or physical therapy.

   vi. Lidocaine 1% commonly used, and 0.1 mL or 0.2 mL can inactivate a trigger point.

   vii. Procaine 0.5% recommended because it is the least myotoxic and very short-acting, in case a nerve is inadvertently blocked.

f. SI joint injection.

   i. Pain felt in the lumbar spine, buttock, groin, thigh, or foot.

   ii. Pain can be worsened by trunk flexion, extensive sitting, weight bearing on the affected extremity, and Valsalva maneuver.

   iii. Numerous nondefinitive diagnostic tests can be performed.
- Patrick test.
- Gaenslen test.
- Lateral compression test.
- Distraction test.
- Fortin finger test.

   iv. Fluoroscopically guided SI joint injection with 22-G, 3.5-in needle directed toward the inferior and posterior joint.
- First, 0.2 to 0.5 mL of contrast is injected to confirm intraarticular placement.
- Then 1 mL of LA and 2 mL of steroid are injected.

   v. Fluoroscopically guided SI joint denervation can be performed for more sustained relief.

VI. CERVICAL PAIN

A. GENERAL

1. Acute neck pain usually resolves spontaneously within 1 mo.
2. Nearly all pts improve within 3 mo.
3. Chronic cervical pain that persists for >6 mo has little chance of spontaneous improvement.

Acute neck syndromes in the absence of neurologic deficits often develop from inflammation of ligaments and muscles.

Cervical spine acceleration-deceleration injuries can cause painful sequelae.

COMMON CAUSES OF NECK PAIN

. Acute soft-tissue injury (muscular and ligamentous).
. Cervical disk herniation.
. Cervical spondylosis.
. Rheumatologic disease.
. Infection.
. Tumor.
. Nerve-root or spinal cord compression.
. Fracture.
. Facet joint disease and facet capsular injury.

DIAGNOSIS

. A thorough H&P is imperative to proper diagnosis and treatment.
. Physical exam is critical to determine neurologic status of pt.
. Assess deep tendon reflexes, strength, and sensation in the upper and lower extremities.
. Findings related to individual nerve roots suggest radiculopathy (radiating pain, weakness, loss of deep tendon reflexes, and sensory changes in a segmental distribution).
. Symptoms in multiple nerve distributions of the shoulder, arm, and hand indicate brachial plexus injury.
. Hyperreflexia, spasticity, gait disturbance (weakness), sensory loss, bowel or bladder dysfunction, Hoffmann sign (when pt flicks end of third finger, flexion of the end of the thumb indicates upper motor neuron dysfunction) may all suggest myelopathy.
. Myelopathy does not cause pain.

IMAGING AND TESTING

. Imaging studies are not warranted in pts with acute cervical pain and no signs of neurologic deficit, trauma, or infection.
a. Imaging studies are often normal.
2. Imaging is necessary in cases of trauma, tumor, infection.
3. Start with plain films in AP, lateral, oblique, odontoid, and flexion-extension views.
4. MRI is best for soft tissue.
5. CT is best for bony anomalies.
5. Electromyography helps to confirm radicular findings and polyneuropathy syndromes.
7. Diagnostic blocks of the facet joints, cervical nerve roots, and cervical disks may reveal correctible spinal abnormalities and may aid in controlling acute and chronic pain conditions.

E. TREATMENT OF ACUTE CERVICAL PAIN
1. If no "red flag" conditions, wait 1 mo before imaging neck and considering surgery.
2. Most pts recover within 3 mo with symptomatic treatment.
3. Passive physical therapy is recommended.
4. Pt should avoid strenuous activity.
5. Prescribe soft cervical collar for neck support and restriction of range of motion.
6. Maintain normal functional activities after short-term restriction.
7. NSAIDs and acetaminophen are the first-line agents for relief of acute cervical pain.
8. Muscle relaxants may be useful for muscle spasms.
9. Opioids are indicated only when pain is not controlled with first-line therapy.
10. Adjuvant therapies, including antidepressants and anticonvulsants, are typically considered when cervical pain becomes chronic.
11. If cervical pain persists after 3 mo, consider diagnostic facet blocks
12. >50% pain relief from LA blockade is considered diagnostic.
13. Medial branch denervation may provide long-term relief via radiofrequency ablation, 4% phenol, or cryogenic nerve block.
14. Acute cervical radicular pain may respond to cervical epidural steroid injections.
15. Consider surgical intervention if pt complains of intractable pain or significant neurologic deficits or if failure to improve within 3 mo of onset substantially disrupts lifestyle.
a. Surgery is indicated only for nerve root compression, spinal cord compression, or instability.

VII. COMPLEX REGIONAL PAIN SYNDROME
A. GENERAL
1. Involves abnormal activation of pain pathways, altered neuromodulation, nerve hyperexcitability, and central sensitization.
2. Two subtypes.
a. CRPS type I.
   i. Termed "reflex sympathetic dystrophy."
   ii. Occurs without a definable nerve lesion, and pain is not limited to single-nerve distribution.
   iii. May be caused by undetected neural injury.
   iv. Represents ~90% of clinical cases.
b. CRPS type II.
   i. Previously known as "causalgia."
   ii. Results from a specific nerve lesion.
3. Both types of CRPS can be subdivided into sympathetically maintained pain and sympathetically independent pain, based on response to sympathetic blockade.
4. Occurs more frequently in young adults and in women.

5. Can result from an array of insults.
a. Major and minor trauma, surgery, inflammation, stroke, nerve injury, myocardial infarction, neoplasms, immobilization.
6. No correlation exists between severity of injury and intensity of CRPS signs and symptoms.
7. Course of disease can be influenced by psychologic stressors and poor coping skills.
8. Exact pathophysiologic mechanisms of CRPS remain unclear.
9. May involve both peripheral and central mechanisms.
10. Neuropeptides and other inflammatory mediators may contribute to pathophysiology.
11. Possible role of aberrant sympathetic nerve fibers, central sensitization, and continual activation of NMDA receptors in the CNS. Possible upregulation of α_2 fibers in the plasma membrane of nociceptive fibers.

B. DIAGNOSTIC CRITERIA OF CRPS
1. Regional, spontaneous pain, allodynia, or hyperalgesia not limited to the territory of a single peripheral nerve and disproportionate to a known inciting event.
2. Evidence of edema, changes in skin blood flow, or abnormal sudomotor activity in the painful region.
3. Presence of a noxious event or cause of immobilization (may be absent in 5% to 10% of pts).
4. No other condition can otherwise account for the degree of pain and dysfunction.

C. PROPOSED MODIFIED DIAGNOSTIC CRITERIA FOR CRPS (IN RESEARCH SETTINGS)
1. Continuing pain that is out of proportion to the inciting event.
2. Pt reports at least one symptom in each of the following four categories:
a. Sensory—reports of hyperesthesia, allodynia, or hyperalgesia.
b. Vasomotor—reports of temperature asymmetry or skin color changes.
c. Sudomotor—reports of hyperhidrosis, dryness, edema, or shiny skin.
d. Motor—reports of spasm, tremor, weakness, decreased range of motion, atrophy, dystonia, contractures, or dystrophic changes to hair, nails, or skin.
3. Pt displays at least one sign in two or more of the following four categories:
a. Sensory—evidence of hyperesthesia, allodynia, or hyperalgesia.
b. Vasomotor—evidence of temperature asymmetry or skin color changes.
c. Sudomotor—evidence of dryness, sweating, edema, or shiny skin.
d. Motor—evidence of spasm, tremor, weakness, decreased range of motion, atrophy, dystonia, contractures, or dystrophic changes to hair, nails, or skin.

18

CHRONIC PAIN

D. CLINICAL FEATURES

1. Both CRPS I and CRPS II can exhibit the same features.
2. Pain is described as stinging, burning, aching, shooting, squeezing, or throbbing.
3. Hyperesthesia—increased sensitivity to stimulation.
4. Hyperalgesia—exaggerated responses to stimuli that are normally painful.
5. Allodynia—pain from stimuli that normally do not produce pain.
6. Vasomotor disturbances—temperature and/or color changes.
   a. Limb feels warm, appears red.
   b. Limb feels cold, looks dusky or bluish.
7. Sudomotor changes.
   a. Hyperhidrosis (increased sweating), dryness, edema, shiny skin.
8. Motor dysfunction.
   a. Spasm, tremor, dystonia, weakness, atrophy, or contracture.
9. Trophic changes.
   a. Changes in skin, nails, or hair pattern.
10. Autonomic and radiologic testing may assist in eliminating other conditions that resemble CRPS and can aid in confirmation.

E. SEQUENTIAL CHANGES OF UNTREATED CRPS

1. Stage I—early, acute, and marked by sensory-vasomotor and sudomotor disturbances.
2. Stage II—increased pain, vasomotor disturbance, and substantial motor or trophic changes.
3. Stage III—diminished pain, significantly increased motor or trophic changes, and continued vasomotor changes.
4. These changes may not be distinct and have limited utility in guiding treatment.

F. TREATMENT

1. Treatment should be early, aggressive, and multidisciplinary.
2. Goals include restoration of function, pain relief, and psychologic improvement.
3. Pharmacotherapy with regional anesthesia and psychologic, behavioral, and physical therapy.
4. Pharmacotherapy.
   a. TCAs.
      i. Analgesic properties facilitate descending antinociceptive pathway.
      ii. Promote sleep.
      iii. Antidepressant properties.
   b. Anticonvulsants (gabapentin, pregabalin, phenytoin, carbamazepine, lamotrigine, oxcarbazepine, topiramate, tiagabine).
      i. History of efficacy in treating neuropathic pain.
      ii. Gabapentin and pregabalin offer better side-effect profiles than older anticonvulsants (phenytoin, carbamazepine).

Transdermal lidocaine.
   i.   Useful in treating focal, allodynic areas.
   ii. Protects skin from insult.
   iii. Applied for 12 hr; removed for 12 hr.
Capsaicin cream.
   i.   Applied to affected area bid to tid.
   ii. Often produces cutaneous burning sensation.
Bisphosphonates.
   i.   Help to combat patchy osteoporosis of CRPS.
   ii. Evidence supports effectiveness but not widely used.
   iii. Examples: intranasal calcitonin, IV clodronate, IV alendronate.
Opioids.
   i.   Usually employed when pain fails to respond to other modalities.
   ii. Long-acting or sustained-release type is better choice than
        short-acting type.
   iii. Consider sustained-release morphine or oxycodone, extended-
        release oxymorphone, or transdermal fentanyl.
   iv. Methadone uniquely blocks NMDA receptors; it is long-acting and
        inexpensive.
   v.   Tramadol is a weak μ-receptor agonist and inhibits serotonin and
        norepinephrine reuptake.

. Sympathetic nerve blocks have diagnostic and therapeutic value.
. Stellate ganglion block for CRPS of upper extremity.
   i.   Horner syndrome: ptosis, miosis, enophthalmos, conjunctival
        injection, nasal congestion, facial anhidrosis.
. Lumbar sympathetic block for CRPS of the lower extremity.
. Should preserve sensory and motor function.
. Observe engorgement of veins and increased temperature in blocked
  extremity.
5. Spinal cord stimulation.
. Thought to employ "gate theory."
. Stimulates large fibers, closing the gate to painful stimuli from small,
  unmyelinated A-δ and C-fibers.
. Process may promote changes in spinal or supraspinal GABA-mediated
  neurochemistry.
. Electrode stimulation at C5 to C7 for upper extremities and T8 to T10
  for lower extremities.
. It is critical that paresthesia induced by spinal cord stimulation cover
  areas of pain.
7. Peripheral nerve stimulation.
. May be effective for CRPS type II.
8. Multidisciplinary treatment.
. Depression during CRPS course is common.
. Psychotherapy, cognitive-behavioral therapy, physical therapy,
  and biofeedback are beneficial as part of comprehensive treatment
  program.

9. Functional restoration.

a. It is important to implement occupational, physical, recreational, and vocational therapies after diagnosis.

VIII. HEADACHE

A. GENERAL

1. Headache types can be divided into primary (migraine, tension, cluster) and secondary (headache as symptom of other underlying pathophysiology).

2. Differential diagnosis for headache includes rebound headache.

a. Can be seen with regular use of analgesics, caffeine, ergotamine tartrate, or triptans.

3. Primary headache disorder is highly prevalent. Tens of millions are affected in the United States; hundreds of millions are affected worldwide.

4. Lifetime prevalence is 78%; migraine prevalence alone is 20% in adult women.

5. Pathophysiology of headache still unclear.

6. Brain is relatively insensitive to pain.

a. Meninges are supplied with C fibers that project and synapse at the trigeminal nucleus caudalis located in the inferior medulla.

b. Nociceptive signals are then sent to the trigeminal subnuclei and to the thalamus.

c. From the thalamus, nociceptive input reaches the cerebral cortex, where pain is experienced and reaches consciousness.

B. MIGRAINE OVERVIEW

1. ~3 : 1 female-to-male predominance.

2. Strong familial component.

3. Neurologic, autonomic, and psychophysiologic symptoms may be components of a migraine attack.

4. Migraine classification includes three types.

a. Migraine with aura.

b. Migraine without aura.

c. Migraine variants (retinal migraine, ophthalmoplegic migraine, familial hemiplegic migraine).

5. Pathophysiology.

a. Vasogenic theory.

   i. Originally thought to be of vascular cause because vasodilation is observed; thought to cause severe throbbing pain.

   ii. Ergots (vasoconstriction) may treat the headache, whereas vasodilatory drugs, including nitrates, may trigger headaches.

   iii. Theorized that intracranial vasoconstriction triggers the aura of the migraine and that headaches result from rebound vasodilation.

ɔ. Neurogenic theory.
  i.   Now thought that primary neuronal dysfunction leads to vascular phenomena.
  ii. Event theorized to originate in the locus caeruleus, projecting to other parts of the brain, causing excessive discharge of part of the spinal nucleus of trigeminal nerve and the basal thalamic nuclei.
  iii. Positron emission tomography demonstrates increased blood flow seen in cerebral hemispheres in the cingulate, auditory, and visual cortexes and in the brainstem during attack.
  iv. Serotonin plays a role in migraine headaches.
    • A decrease in serotonin levels is observed during acute migraines, resulting in vasodilation.

C. MIGRAINE HEADACHE
1. Migraines tend to last several hours to several days.
2. Frequently severe enough to affect activities of daily living and are often exacerbated by minimal physical activity.
3. Can be unilateral or bilateral, often pulsating.
4. At least one of the following is present.
   a. N/V.
   b. Photophobia.
   c. Phonophobia.
5. Migraines with aura compose only 20% of total migraines.
6. Aura symptoms include visual disturbances (e.g., scintillating scotoma), unilateral weakness, numbness and/or paresthesias, language disturbance.
7. Chronic migraines are associated with daily pain, medication overuse, and rebound phenomenon; frequently include neuropsychiatric comorbid conditions.
8. Migraine treatment—acute attack.
   a. Mild-to-moderate attacks.
      i.   Acetaminophen.
      ii. NSAIDs or Midrin.
      iii. Isometheptene mucate (mild vasoconstrictor).
      iv. Dichloralphenazone (mild sedative).
   b. Severe attacks.
      i.   Butalbital (barbiturate with caffeine, acetylsalicylic acid, and/or acetaminophen).
      ii. Ketorolac.
      iii. Medications that contain ergotamine, dihydroergotamine, triptans, newer 5HT-receptor subtype agonists, or neuroleptics.
   c. Antiemetics metoclopramide, chlorpromazine, and prochlorperazine have demonstrated benefits for migraine pain relief in randomized, placebo-controlled trials.
   d. Opioids should be used only after alternative treatments have been exhausted.

18

CHRONIC PAIN

9. Migraine prophylactic therapy.
a. First line.
   i.   β-Blockers, NSAIDs, antidepressants, calcium channel blockers, anticonvulsants.
b. Second line.
   i.   Botulinum toxin type A injection, methysergide, phenelzine.
10. Chronic migraine therapy.
a. Should incorporate cognitive behavioral therapy, family therapy, psychotherapy.
11. Interventional treatment modalities.
a. Occipital nerve blocks are successful in some pts.
b. Botulinum toxin administration for prevention of migraine has shown to be beneficial in uncontrolled studies.
   i.   Limited data in randomized controlled studies.
   ii.   Increasingly recognized as useful in pts who have failed conventional therapy.

D. TENSION-TYPE HEADACHE
1. Most common primary headache disorder.
2. Duration—30 min to 7 days.
3. Episodic versus chronic.
4. Episodic shares certain characteristics with migraine but does not include throbbing pain, autonomic symptoms, or nausea and/or vomiting.
5. May involve pericranial muscle spasm.
6. Chronic tension headache may have features in common with chronic migraines.
7. Acute treatment.
a. NSAIDs, acetaminophen.
b. Muscle relaxants (tizanidine).
8. Prophylactic treatment.
a. TCAs are first line (amitriptyline was demonstrated to be effective in doubled-blinded, placebo-controlled studies).
b. Less preferred.
   i.   NSAIDs, atypical antidepressants, valproate.

E. CLUSTER HEADACHE
1. Least common headache type.
2. Afflicts males more than females, 3:1.
3. 1 to 3 hr in duration.
4. Always unilateral and periorbital, severe, sharp pain.
5. Occurs in series (clusters) for weeks to months, with periods of remission extending to several years.
6. Lacrimation, nasal congestion and drainage, ptosis, or miosis may accompany headache.

7. Behavior during attack may be manic and histrionic, with agitation and pacing.
8. Acute treatment.
a. Oxygen inhalation, 7 to 8 L/min via face mask.
b. Triptans and ergots.
c. Indomethacin may be helpful.
9. Preventative treatment.
a. Verapamil.
b. Ergotamine tartrate.
c. Lithium.
d. Divalproex or topiramate.
e. Steroids.
f. Occipital nerve blocks.
10. Nonpharmacologic treatments have been employed for migraine, tension, and cluster headaches, including the application of pressure, heat and cold, hypnosis, relaxation training, biofeedback, and electrical stimulation. Most have unclear efficacy.

F. OCCIPITAL NEURALGIA
1. General.
a. May be either primary (idiopathic) or secondary (structural causes).
b. Affects men and women approximately equally.
c. Structural causes.
   i.   Trauma or compression of greater or lesser occipital nerves or C2–C3 nerve roots.
   ii. Cervical disk disease.
   iii. Tumor.
   iv. Cervical spine degenerative changes are a common cause of occipital neuralgia.
   v.   Frequently, no clear structural cause is discernible.
d. Third (least) occipital nerve may also be involved.
2. Symptoms.
a. Continuous aching, burning, and throbbing with intermittent exacerbations that may be sharp or shooting.
b. Location is suboccipital, with radiation to the posterior or lateral scalp.
   i.   May have complaints of pain in the temporal or frontal areas.
   ii. May spread upward from suboccipital region in "ram's horn" distribution.
   iii. Complaints of autonomic disturbances similar to migraines not uncommon.
3. Imaging.
a. When trauma or compression is suspected, diagnostic imaging is indicated, preferably MRI.
4. Medical management.
a. Gabapentin, pregabalin, NSAIDs.
b. Baclofen for spasm-related pain.

18

CHRONIC PAIN

c. Opioids may be incorporated after failure or inadequate pain control with nonopioid therapies.

5. Interventional treatment.

a. Nerve blocks of greater occipital, lesser occipital, or third occipital nerves.

b. C2 and/or C3 ganglion blocks.

c. Botulinum toxin injection.

d. Radiofrequency thermocoagulation or pulsed radiofrequency to occipital nerve.

e. Occipital nerve stimulation via implanted electrodes at C1 to C3.

6. Surgical treatment.

a. Microvascular nerve decompression.

b. Dorsal cervical rhizotomy.

c. Neurolysis of the greater occipital nerve.

d. Radiofrequency rhizotomy.

e. Selective C2 and/or C3 rhizotomy emerging as an option.

G. PDPH

1. General.

a. May develop after dural puncture.
   i. Lumbar puncture.
   ii. Spinal anesthesia.
   iii. Inadvertent puncture during epidural placement ("wet tap").
   iv. Incidence of accidental dural puncture as high as 3%.

b. PDPH occurs in up to 70% of pts after dural puncture.

c. Not all postpartum headaches are due to dural puncture.

d. PDPH is caused by leakage of CSF through dura.

2. Symptoms.

a. Creates low CSF volume, traction, pain.

b. Classically, headache is frontal or occipital and occurs 12 to 24 hr after procedure.

c. Exacerbated by upright position and improves when pt is supine.

3. Risk factors.

a. Female gender, prior history of headache, younger age.

b. Positioning during procedure is not demonstrated to affect risk.

c. No evidence that bed rest after procedure decreases incidence of headache.

4. Treatment.

a. Conservative treatment recommended during first 24 hr.

b. Bed rest and oral analgesics, including short-acting opioids.

c. When conservative treatment fails:
   i. Oral and IV caffeine, epidural saline (associated with high recurrence), epidural blood patch (EBP).
   ii. Vasopressin, theophylline, sumatriptan, and adrenocorticotropic hormone have been reported as effective therapies.

d. IV caffeine.

i. 500 mg caffeine in 1000 mL NS; infuse over 1 hr, usually in the morning.
ii. An additional 1000 mL NS is given over 1 hr.
iii. May repeat if headache remains unresolved.
iv. Caffeine is a cerebral vasoconstrictor.
v. Advise pts of side effects of caffeine, including anxiety, sleep disturbance, palpitations, dysrhythmias, seizures.
vi. No proven adverse effects to newborn via transfer to breast milk.

e. EBP.
i. A more definitive treatment for prolonged PDPH.
ii. Autologous blood injected into epidural space at or near the site of original dural puncture.
iii. Achieves volume replacement and dural tamponade and ultimately seals the leak.
iv. Postulated increase in CSF pressure and cerebral vasoconstriction.
v. Most practitioners use 15 to 20 mL of autologous blood drawn under sterile conditions.
vi. Greater volume of blood increases success rate and adverse effects.
  • Adverse effects include back pain, lower extremity paresthesias, and fever.
vii. More than one EBP may be required.
viii. Lasting relief obtained with first EBP in 60% to 75% of cases.
ix. Effectiveness of EBP decreases if puncture occurred with large-bore needle.
x. Repeat EBP successful in nearly all cases; success rates reported at ~90%.

IX. OPIOIDS IN CHRONIC NONMALIGNANT PAIN

A. GENERAL

1. Opioids can treat pain reliably and effectively without a "ceiling effect."
2. Clear benefit (analgesia, functional status) must justify long-term use.
3. Pain diagnosis must be clearly established.
4. Committing to long-term opioid therapy.
a. Structured, goal-directed therapy.
b. Other treatment options should be thoroughly explored and maximized.
c. Focus on functional improvement, minimizing adverse effects, and decreasing reliance on medications.
d. Opioid therapy preferred as adjunct to primary therapies.
e. Choose long-acting opioids (sustained-release morphine, transdermal fentanyl) unless pain is episodic.
f. Pt must understand complications and risks.
g. Careful monitoring necessary.
h. Signed opioid agreement is optimal.

18

CHRONIC PAIN

B. DOSE TITRATION

1. Start at a low dose; increase as quickly as tolerated for analgesia.
2. More frequent visits and close communication may be necessary.
3. If unable to obtain satisfactory analgesia or if unacceptable side effects, discontinue or rotate to another opioid.

C. DOSE MAINTENANCE

1. Once effective regimen is established, maintain stable dose.
2. Provide prescriptions for at least 1 mo and engage in regular follow-up.

D. IV OPIOID CONVERSION TO LONG-ACTING AND SHORT-ACTING FORMULATIONS

1. Determine the amount of IV opioid consumed in 24-hr period.
2. Convert to 24-hr dose of oral morphine (Table 18.1).
3. Calculate equianalgesic dose of new opioid.
4. Give ~75% of the 24-hr dose in long-acting form and 25% of the dose in short-acting form.
5. Divide by desired frequency of administration for long-acting and short-acting forms (Tables 18.2 and 18.3).

E. COMPLICATIONS

1. Complications include unacceptable side effects, loss of efficacy (tolerance), hormonal effects, immune effects, physical dependence, and problematic opioid use.

TABLE 18.1

OPIOID EQUIVALENCY TABLE

Opioid	Type	Relative Potency
Codeine	Oral	200
	Parenteral	130
Fentanyl	Oral	N/A
	Parenteral	0.1
Hydromorphone	Oral	7.5
	Parenteral	1.5
Levorphanol	Oral	4
	Parenteral	2
Meperidine	Oral	300
	Parenteral	75
Methadone	Oral	10
	Parenteral	5
Morphine	Oral	30
	Parenteral	10
Oxycodone	Oral	20
	Parenteral	N/A

From the Sidney Kimmel Comprehensive Cancer Center at Johns Hopkins. Hopkins Opioid Program: http://www.hopweb.org/, with permission.

TABLE 18.2

ORAL OPIOIDS

Opioid	Half-Life (hr)	Onset (hr)	Duration (hr)	Relative Potency	Initial Dose (mg)	Dosing Interval (hr)
Codeine (Tylenol #3)	3	0.25–1.0	3–4	20	30–60	4
Hydromorphone (Dilaudid)	2–3	0.3–0.5	2–3	0.6	2–4	4
Hydrocodone* (Vicodin)	1–3	0.5–1.0	3–6	3	5–7.5	4–6
Oxycodone† (Percocet)	2–3	0.5	3–6	3	5–10	6
Levorphanol (Levo-Dromoran)	12–16	1–2	6–8	0.4	4	6–8
Methadone (Dolophine)	15–30	0.5–1.0	4–6	1	5	6–8
Propoxyphene (Darvon)‡	6–12	1–2	3–6	30	100	6
Tramadol (Ultram)	6–7	1–2	3–6	30	50	4–6
Morphine solution§ (Roxanol)	2–4	0.5–1	4	1	10	3–4

*Preparations also contain acetaminophen (Vicodin, others).
†Preparations may contain acetaminophen (Percocet) or aspirin (Percodan).
‡Some preparations contain acetaminophen (Darvocet).
§Used primarily for cancer pain.
(Adapted from Morgan GE, Mikhail MS: Clinical Anesthesiology. New York: McGraw-Hill, 2006.)

18

CHRONIC PAIN

2. Side effects.
a. Sedation.
b. Respiratory depression.
c. N/V.
d. Constipation.
e. Pruritus.
f. Dysphoria or cognitive dysfunction.
g. Hyperalgesia.

F. **DIMINISHED EFFICACY**
1. Some pts may obtain acceptable analgesia without dose escalation.
2. Others require increasing doses.
3. Tolerance develops to both analgesic effects and side effects (constipation usually persists, though).
4. Mechanisms appear to be linked to NMDA-receptor cascade.
5. What is presumed to be tolerance may be opioid-induced hyperalgesia, also linked to NMDA-receptor cascade.
6. Escalating opioid dose may either improve analgesia (tolerance) or exacerbate pain (opioid-induced hyperalgesia).

G. **HORMONAL EFFECTS**
1. Opioids affect the hypothalamic-pituitary-adrenal axis and hypothalamic-pituitary gonadal axis.
2. Occurrence of secondary increase in prolactin, which is regulated by endogenous dopamine.

TABLE 18.3
PROPERTIES AND DOSING OF ORAL OPIOID PREPARATIONS

Medication	Initial Dosage	Dosing Interval	T_{max} Peak Plasma Concentration	Duration of Action
Morphine sulfate controlled-release tablets (MS Contin)	15 mg	q 12 hr	2.5 hr	12 hr
Morphine sulfate extended-release capsules (Avinza)	30 mg	q 24 hr	9.5 hr	24 hr
Morphine sulfate extended-release capsules (Kadian)	20 mg	q 12–24 hr	8.6 hr	12–24 hr
Oxycodone controlled-release tablets (Oxycontin)	10 mg	q 12 hr	2.7 hr	8–12 hr
Oxymorphone immediate-release tablets (Opana IR)	10 mg	q 6 hr	0.5 hr	4–6 hr
Oxymorphone extended-release tablets (Opana ER)	5 mg	q 12 hr	2–3 hr	12 hr
Oral transmucosal fentanyl citrate (Actiq)	200 mcg	q 6 hr	20–40 min	3–4 hr
Transdermal fentanyl patch (Duragesic)	12.5 mcg/hr	q 72 hr	27.5 hr	72 hr
Transmucosal (buccal) fentanyl tablet (Fentora)	100 mcg	q 30 min X1, then q 4 hr	47 min	3–4 hr

3. Levels of plasma cortisol, follicle-stimulating hormone, luteinizing hormone, testosterone, and estrogen all decrease.
4. Testosterone treatment often improves energy in male pts.

H. IMMUNE EFFECTS
1. Evidence that opioids alter immune function in animals and humans.
2. Occurs with long-term more than short-term exposure.
3. Pain itself can produce immunosuppression.
4. Pts on long-term opioid therapy with inadequate pain relief are at greatest risk.

X. SUBSTANCE USE DISORDERS AND CHRONIC OPIOID USE
A. ADDICTION
1. Chronic disease with neurobiologic, social, and genetic factors.
2. Pt may exhibit impaired control over drug use, compulsive use, continued use despite harm, and craving.

B. PHYSICAL DEPENDENCE
1. Physiologic state of adaptation to a drug or class of drugs in which a withdrawal syndrome occurs in response to abrupt cessation or reduction of dose.

C. TOLERANCE
1. State of adaptation in which larger doses are required to produce the desired drug effect.
2. Tolerance may occur in time and tends to plateau.
3. Pts can then be maintained on a stable dose.
4. If dose escalation is required, regular evaluation is important.
5. Tolerance phenomenon may reflect change in or progression of disease versus addiction versus opioid-induced hyperalgesia.
6. Rotation to another opioid may provide more effective relief at an equianalgesic dose with fewer adverse effects.

D. PSEUDOADDICTION
1. Appearance of drug-seeking behavior caused by unrecognized undertreatment of pain.
2. Iatrogenically induced by inadequate treatment of pain.
3. Providing sufficient dose of opioid for analgesia will abolish symptoms.
4. Undergoing screening by a psychologist before beginning long-term opioid is often beneficial.
5. Clear, realistic goals for improvement of function should be outlined.
6. Diligent monitoring of analgesia, function, and adverse effects is important.
7. Effective pain management should yield functional improvement.
8. Worsening dysfunction should be evaluated for substance use disorder (abuse or addiction).

E. PRESCRIPTION DRUG ABUSE
1. Prescription drug abuse has increased significantly in last decade.
2. Prescription drug diversion represents a substantial problem.
3. The Drug Enforcement Agency (DEA) is now more aggressive in prosecuting physicians and pharmacists.
4. Regulatory scrutiny must not prevent appropriate treatment of pain.
5. Obtain careful and thorough medical, family, social, and psychiatric (including substance use disorder) histories.
6. Physical exam should evaluate mood, interest, grooming, signs of intoxication or withdrawal.
7. Signs of abuse include repeated loss of prescriptions, multiple prescription providers, self-escalation of dosage, multiple drug "allergies," frequent calls and visits to the office.
8. Pill counts during each visit for opioid prescription refills and urine drug testing are important for compliance and illicit drug monitoring.

18

CHRONIC PAIN

9. Pseudoaddiction must be ruled out.
10. Mental health professionals should be consulted if substance use disorder (abuse or addiction) is suspected.

XI. CANCER PAIN AND PHARMACOTHERAPIES

A. SCOPE OF PROBLEM
1. Pain prevalence ranges from 14% to 100% among cancer pts.
2. Up to 50% of cancer pts with pain may remain undertreated.
3. 33% of cancer pts in active therapy have chronic and severe pain.
4. 60% to 90% of pts with advanced stages of cancer are affected by pain.
5. 46% of terminal cancer pts die with inadequate pain treatment.

B. SOURCES OF CANCER PAIN
1. Direct invasion of tumor into nerves, bones, soft tissue, ligaments, and fascia, and visceral pain through distention and obstruction.
2. 25% of pain can be attributed to cancer-related treatments.

C. TYPES OF PAIN
1. Clinicians may describe cancer pain as acute, chronic, nociceptive (somatic), visceral, or neuropathic.
2. Somatic pain.
a. Direct injury to bones, tissue, tendons.
b. Aching or dull; very focal.
c. Examples.
    i.   Metastatic bone pain.
    ii. Postsurgical incisional pain.
    iii. Musculoskeletal inflammation and spasm.
3. Visceral pain.
a. Organ damage or tumor infiltration, compression or distortion of organs.
b. Pressure-like sensations, internal squeezing, or crampiness.
c. Vague and diffuse and may be associated with nausea, vomiting, and sweating.
4. Neuropathic pain.
a. Caused by tumor infiltration of peripheral nerves, plexi, roots, or spinal cord.
b. May be secondary to surgery, chemotherapy or radiation, or other drug-induced neuropathy or neuritis.
c. Sensory changes caused by injury to the central and/or peripheral nervous systems.
d. Burning, shooting, pins and needles, electrical or numb, and tends to radiate over dermatomal distributions.

D. BARRIERS TO TREATING PAIN
1. Psychosocial factors.
a. Fear of opioid addiction and dependence, fear of adverse effects of medications.

2. Physician concerns.

a. Opioid documentation woes, frequent opioid prescription refills, onerous telephone calls, and exposure to intense regulatory scrutiny from the provision of opioids.

3. Pt concerns.

a. 80% of pts cite fear of addiction to pain medications.

b. 85% believe that side effects of pain medications cannot be controlled.

c. 50% fear annoyance from the physician if they complain of pain.

d. 60% feel that pain medication should be reserved for severe pain; otherwise, it might be ineffective when needed.

E. CANCER PAIN "LADDER"

1. The "three-step analgesic ladder" (see Figure 18.2), developed by the World Health Organization (WHO) in 1986, provides a concrete tool for physicians worldwide to use in combating cancer pain with oral medications.

a. Begin with a nonopioid (e.g., acetaminophen, ibuprofen) and progress from weaker to stronger opioids (step 1 to step 3) for incremental pain severity.

b. Consider adjuvant medications (e.g., TCAs, antiepileptics) at any step of the ladder.

c. It is estimated that 70% to 90% of cancer pain is relieved when clinicians apply the WHO ladder appropriately.

F. PRIMARY THERAPIES

1. Directed at the source of the cancer pain and may enhance function, longevity, and comfort.

2. Analgesic agents are often required in addition to these therapies.

3. Vertebroplasty.

a. Injection of methylmethacrylate into a pain-sensitive vertebral body under radiographic guidance. Stabilizes bony metastasis by solidifying the lesion.

4. Radiofrequency tumor ablation.

a. May provide pain relief for liver cancer, pelvic tumor recurrences, pancreatic cancer, vertebral metastases, and renal and adrenal tumors.

5. Surgery.

a. Relief of painful symptoms from hollow-organ obstruction, neural compression, and unstable bony structures.

6. Radiotherapy.

a. Offers pain reduction associated with bone metastases, epidural neoplasm, and headaches caused by cerebral metastases.

7. Chemotherapy.

a. It is believed that an inverse relationship exists between cancer shrinkage from chemotherapy and analgesia, though no data support specific analgesic benefits of chemotherapy.

18

CHRONIC PAIN

8. Antibiotics.

a. When pain is a manifestation of infection, antibiotics can serve an analgesic role (e.g., pelvic abscesses, cellulitis).

G. ADJUVANT THERAPIES (CO-ANALGESICS)

1. Nonopioids that confer analgesic effects in certain medical conditions but are mainly used to treat conditions not involving pain.

2. Corticosteroids.

a. Inhibit prostaglandin synthesis and reduce neural tissue edema.

b. Dexamethasone—drug of choice, given its low mineralocorticoid effect and reduced risk of Cushing syndrome.

c. Doses range from 1 to 2 mg bid to 100 mg/day, followed by tapered doses in cases of acute and severe pain.

d. The standard dose of dexamethasone is 16 to 24 mg/day and can be administered once daily because of its extended half-life.

3. Topical LAs.

a. Painful lesions of the mucosa and skin may respond to lidocaine preparations.

4. Antidepressants.

a. For neuropathic pain; offer analgesic effects independent of their antidepressant effects.

b. The strongest level of evidence for analgesic efficacy exists for the TCAs and, specifically, the tertiary amines (e.g., doxepin, amitriptyline).

c. The secondary amines (e.g., nortriptyline, desipramine) have more favorable adverse-effect profiles (e.g., sedation, anticholinergic effects, and dysrhythmias).

5. Anticonvulsants.

a. For neuropathic pain—ease shooting, stabbing, burning, and electric-like sensations associated with a dysfunctional nervous system.

b. Gabapentin is considered a first-line agent for treating neuropathic pain. Randomized controlled trials (RCTs) support its analgesic effect, safety, good tolerability, and absence of drug-drug interactions.

c. Pregabalin offers good analgesia, rapid titration schedule, and increased tolerability.

6. Bisphosphonates.

a. As a group, these substances inhibit osteoclast activity, adhere strongly to bone, demonstrate a long half-life, and can effectively reduce bone pain.

7. Radiopharmaceuticals.

a. For painful and diffuse metastatic bone disease.

b. Deposit radiation directly to the affected region of the bone.

c. The most commonly used and best-studied radiopharmaceutical is strontium-89.

H. NONOPIOID THERAPY AND OVER-THE-COUNTER AGENTS

1. The WHO analgesic ladder recommends nonopioids beginning at step 1. These medications are useful in the management of mild-to-moderate pain.

2. Acetaminophen.

a. Analgesia and antipyretic activity without peripheral antiinflammatory activity.

b. Often combined with short-acting opioids if initial therapy is unsuccessful.

c. Combination products provide opioid dose sparing and limit opioid-induced adverse effects (e.g., sedation, N/V, constipation, dry mouth, cognitive dysfunction).

d. Risk of acetaminophen hepatotoxicity at sustained doses of 3 to 4 g/day in adults.

3. NSAIDs.

a. Reduce inflammatory pain caused by cancer, such as metastatic bone pain and soft-tissue infiltration.

b. Like acetaminophen, NSAIDs offer the benefit of an opioid-sparing effect.

c. The adverse effects of NSAIDs (e.g., GI and renal) and especially a pt's coexisting condition (e.g., thrombocytopenia, neutropenia) should be considered when selecting a particular medication.

d. Inhibit the COX enzyme that converts arachidonic acid to prostaglandins.

   i. Prostaglandins mediate renal plasma flow, gastric mucosal protection, platelet aggregation, and pain and inflammation.

e. The COX-2 selective agents have the same effectiveness as the nonselective agents with less risk of GI damage and bleeding.

I. OPIOID THERAPY

1. For symptomatic treatment of severe cancer pain.

2. Very effective analgesics, titrate easily, and offer a favorable risk/benefit ratio.

3. Bind to specific receptors (μ, κ, δ) located in the central and peripheral nervous systems.

4. Tramadol.

a. Step 2 on WHO ladder.

b. Centrally acting analgesic that shares properties of both opioids and TCAs.

   i. Binds weakly to the μ opioid receptor, inhibits the reuptake of serotonin and norepinephrine, and promotes neuronal serotonin release.

c. Not listed as a scheduled drug by the DEA.

   i. Has low abuse liability.

   ii. Is associated with low risk of respiratory depression.

d. Adverse effects resemble those of opioids; potential for serotonin syndrome with selective serotonin reuptake inhibitors, monoamine oxidase inhibitors, or TCAs.

5. Morphine.

a. Step 3 on WHO ladder.

b. The most commonly used opioid for treating severe cancer pain.

c. Widely available, cost-effective, and has multiple formulations (e.g., oral, rectal, IV, intranasal, epidural, SQ, intrathecal, sustained-release).

d. Metabolized in the liver, producing morphine-3-glucuronide (M3G) and morphine-6-glucuronide (M6G).

　　i. M3G is inactive; M6G is an active metabolite that exceeds morphine in potency and half-life.

e. Both metabolites are excreted by the kidneys.

　　i. Pts with renal dysfunction may experience prolonged morphine effects.

f. Renal impairment.

　　i. Consider small doses of immediate-release morphine and/or reducing the dosing frequency.

6. Codeine.

a. Step 2 on WHO ladder; used for mild-to-moderate pain.

b. Available as a combination product with acetaminophen or aspirin.

c. Metabolized by liver.

　　i. 90% of its metabolites are primarily excreted as inactive forms in the urine.

　　ii. Only ~10% of codeine is demethylated (converted) to morphine, which accounts for its analgesic properties.

d. Avoid using codeine in pts with renal failure because its active metabolites accumulate and can cause significant adverse effects.

7. Hydromorphone.

a. Step 3 on WHO ladder.

b. Semisynthetic derivative of morphine that is approximately six times more potent.

　　i. Binds to both μ and, to a lesser degree, δ opioid receptors.

c. Shares equivalency with morphine in analgesic efficacy and adverse effects.

d. Available in oral, parenteral, intraspinal preparations.

e. Appears to have active, nonanalgesic metabolites that may cause neuroexcitatory effects (myoclonus, allodynia, seizures, confusion) at high doses or in the setting of renal failure.

8. Fentanyl.

a. Step 3 on WHO ladder.

b. Initially used as an intraoperative anesthetic, evolved into a transdermal, controlled, systemic-delivery formulation for treating cancer pain.

c. Transdermal patch.

　　i. Alternative to oral opioids, especially when cancer or adverse treatment effects preclude the oral administration of analgesics.

d. Fentanyl is 100 times more potent than morphine and is very lipid soluble.
   i. Easy passage through the skin and mucous membranes.
e. Recommended dosing is q 72 hr, although some pts report an attenuated analgesic response by third day and request a shortened dosing interval to q 48 hr.
f. Formulations.
   i. IV.
   ii. Transdermal.
   iii. Oral (lollipop, lozenge, buccal tablet).
   iv. Epidural.
   v. Intrathecal.

9. Oxycodone.
a. Step 2 or 3 on WHO ladder.
b. Binds to both the μ and κ opioid receptors and is often used in combination with acetaminophen, aspirin, and ibuprofen as a short-acting analgesic.
c. Immediate-release (e.g., capsule, liquid, tablet) and controlled-release forms available.
d. The liver metabolizes oxycodone to small amounts of oxymorphone (the only active metabolite), and oxymorphone accumulates in renal failure, along with the parent drug.
e. Clinicians should prescribe oxycodone cautiously and should carefully monitor symptoms of toxicity in pts with renal compromise.
f. Compares favorably with morphine in relieving moderate-to-severe cancer pain with fewer hallucinations, less pruritus, and less nausea.

10. Meperidine.
a. Step 3 on WHO ladder.
b. Binds predominantly to the μ opioid receptor and is used most often as an intraoperative analgesic.
c. Small, single doses are effective for postoperative shivering.
d. May produce an anticholinergic response in the form of tachycardia and acts as a weak LA.
e. Oral and parenteral formulations are available for clinical use.
f. Most clinicians avoid meperidine for the treatment of chronic pain and cancer pain owing to its short duration of action and concerns over metabolic toxicity.
g. Use no longer than 48 hr in doses that do not exceed 600 mg/day.
h. Metabolized to normeperidine, which is eliminated by both the liver and the kidney; therefore hepatic or renal dysfunction can lead to metabolite accumulation.
i. Normeperidine toxicity manifests as shakiness, muscle twitches, myoclonus, dilated pupils, and seizures.
j. Renal failure greatly elevates the risk of normeperidine neurotoxicity; therefore clinicians should avoid its use in pts with kidney disease.

18

CHRONIC PAIN

11. Buprenorphine.

a. Step 3 on WHO ladder.

b. Partial agonist at the μ opioid receptor and an antagonist at the κ and δ receptors.

c. High affinity for, and slow dissociation from, the μ receptor.

   i. May produce less analgesia than a full μ agonist.

d. 25 to 50 times more potent than morphine.

e. Available in parenteral, sublingual, transdermal preparations.

f. Provides improvement in pain and quality of life and stable dosing among pts with cancer pain.

g. Requires no dose adjustment in pts with renal failure.

12. Methadone.

a. Step 3 on ladder.

b. Long-acting μ and δ opioid receptor agonist.

c. Causes monoamine reuptake inhibition and has NMDA antagonist properties, based on animal studies.

d. Similar efficacy and comparable adverse-effect profile as morphine.

e. Significant variability in plasma half-life among individuals.

f. Firmly binds to extravascular binding sites and releases slowly back into plasma, resulting in a characteristically long half-life.

g. Plasma half-life is 24 hr; analgesic half-life is only 4 to 6 hr.

h. Potential for delayed toxicity (e.g., respiratory depression) from drug accumulation in tissues.

i. Repeat administration coupled with a prolonged half-life increases the risk of overdose.

j. Available in oral, rectal, parenteral formulations.

k. Be aware of possible QT prolongation and torsades de pointes if pt is taking >300 mg daily or with concurrent use of antidepressants, severe hypokalemia or hypomagnesemia, and CHF.

l. Despite hazards, valuable analgesic among gravely ill pts.

m. The liver transforms methadone to inactive metabolites that are excreted in the urine and mainly in the bile (feces). Renal dysfunction does not seem to impair clearance of the drug.

13. Oxymorphone.

a. Step 3 on ladder.

b. Metabolite of oxycodone.

   i. Analgesic effects are mediated through μ and δ opioid receptors.

c. The half-life of the immediate-release formulation of oxymorphone (~7 to 9 hr) exceeds that of many short-acting formulations of opioids, including morphine, oxycodone, and hydromorphone.

d. Consider 6-hr dosing for the immediate-release formulation.

e. Available in oral (e.g., immediate-release, sustained-release), parenteral, and rectal formulations.

f. Renally excreted and accumulates in renal failure.

XII. INTERVENTIONAL PAIN TREATMENTS FOR CANCER PAIN
A. A "FOURTH STEP" IN THE WHO ANALGESIC LADDER
1. Nearly 50% of pts reach the final tier, step 3, and yearn for another step to enhance their quality of life.
2. Opioid therapy can cause limiting adverse effects, such as constipation, nausea, fatigue, delirium, and confusion.
3. Persistent adverse effects reported in 1 of 4 treatment days with WHO-recommended medications.
4. Some pts fail to respond to opioids or co-analgesics.
5. This fourth step in the ladder includes advanced interventional approaches for pain relief.

B. INTERVENTIONAL TECHNIQUES
1. Needed in 14% to 20% of cancer pts owing to intractable pain despite use of WHO ladder.
2. Epidural and intrathecal infusion therapies.
3. Sympathetic ganglion blocks and neurolysis.
a. Celiac plexus, superior hypogastric plexus, and ganglion impar.
4. Implantable drug delivery systems (IDDS).
5. Neuraxial neurolytic interventions.

C. EPIDURAL INFUSION THERAPY
1. Percutaneous epidural analgesia can provide substantial relief for thoracic, abdominal, pelvic, and leg pain, and for upper extremity, neck, and shoulder pain.
2. Insert catheters, tunnel SQ, attach filters, and connect to medication bag.
3. Infection, catheter dislocation, and obstruction are more frequent with long-term (>1 mo) epidural therapy than with long-term intrathecal infusions.
a. 55% complication rate with epidural infusion.
b. 5% complication rate with intrathecal infusion.

D. INTRATHECAL INFUSION THERAPY
1. Tunneled and externalized intrathecal catheters are used for short- or long-term treatment for malignant pain.
2. Safely used for 1 to 2 mo and even as long as 1.5 yr.
3. Data suggest that externalized intrathecal catheters are safer than epidural catheters if required for >3 wk of treatment.
4. Compared with epidural catheters, externalized intrathecal catheters require smaller drug dose and volume.
a. Allows more compact external infusion devices and longer periods before refilling of medication bag.

18

CHRONIC PAIN

E. CHEMICAL NEUROLYSIS

1. Intentional injury to a nerve or group of nerves by chemical (alcohol or phenol) methods, with the intent to relieve pain.
2. Effects usually persist for 3 to 6 mo.
3. Applied in discrete clinical conditions in which pts suffer from refractory cancer pain and previous approaches have failed.
4. Can provide effective analgesia and life-enhancing benefits.
5. Incomplete relief may occur because of adhesions, tumor, or nerve regeneration.

F. SYMPATHETIC GANGLION BLOCKS AND NEUROLYSIS

1. Neurolytic celiac plexus block (NCPB).
a. Pt indications.
   i.   Pain from pancreatic tumors, hepatic metastases or primary tumors, or other primary intraabdominal tumors.
b. Anatomy.
   i.   Network of retroperitoneal ganglia located beneath diaphragmatic crus, anterolateral to aorta, and inferior to origin of celiac artery at superior border of L1.
   ii. Greater, lesser, least splanchnic nerves contribute to the plexus.
c. Function.
   i.   Receives pain signals from nerves innervating the pancreas, liver, gallbladder, stomach, spleen, kidneys, intestines, and adrenals.
d. Techniques.
   i.   Transcrural.
        • Pt is positioned prone with fluoroscopy or CT guidance.
        • Left needle is inserted 4 cm lateral to midline directed to anterolateral aspect of aorta.
        • Right needle 5 to 10 cm lateral to midline is directed between IVC and aorta.
        • Needles lie anterior to diaphragmatic crus.
   ii. Retrocrural.
        • Chosen for extensive preaortic tumor spread, which limits adequate neurolytic agent spread.
        • Pt is prone and fluoroscopy or CT guidance is used.
        • Bilateral needles are inserted inferior to twelfth rib, 7.5 cm lateral to midline, and walked off the T12 vertebral body.
        • Proper needle positioning indicates that solution is traveling superiorly and posteriorly around splanchnic nerves and posterior to the diaphragmatic crura.
        • Smaller volumes of agents are usually injected.
   iii. Transaortic.
        • Single-needle technique.
        • Pt is prone and CT guidance is used.
        • Needle is inserted 4 to 7 cm left of midline below twelfth rib and directed through aorta.

- First loss of resistance reflects posterior aortic wall, and arterial blood is seen on stylet removal.
- Second loss of resistance is felt after anterior aortic wall is passed.
- Spread of solution is anterior to the crura and along preaortic tissue planes.

iv. Anterior.
- Pt is supine with CT or ultrasound guidance.
- Needle is inserted inferior to xiphoid and directed to preaortic region of celiac plexus, avoiding liver, bowel, pancreas, and superior mesenteric and celiac arteries.

e. Complications.
  i. Paraplegia may occur in 1% of pts who undergo retrocrural approach.
  ii. Pain at injection site, backache, hematuria from renal injury, pneumothorax, impotence.
  iii. Transient hypotension and diarrhea.

f. Efficacy.
  i. RCT comparing NCPB to medication showed 90% efficacy at 1 wk with reduced opioid consumption and adverse effects until death.
  ii. Better side-effect profile compared with opioid therapy.
  iii. Meta-analysis showed 70% to 90% of pts with partial to complete pain relief at time of death, even if occurring >3 mo after the NCPB.

2. Superior hypogastric plexus (SHP) block and neurolysis.

a. Pt indications.
  i. Pain due to gynecologic, colorectal, or genitourinary cancer.
b. Anatomy.
  i. Composed of a neuronal network of visceral afferent fibers traveling in the sympathetic trunk and traveling with parasympathetic fibers.
  ii. Located retroperitoneally and anterior to the sacral promontory at the L5 to S1 level.
c. Function.
  i. Transmits sensory information from the bladder, rectum, prostate, testes, vagina, uterus, ovaries, and descending and sigmoid colon.
  ii. SHP also sends sensory fibers to nerves that innervate perineum, anus, penis, scrotum, and clitoris.
d. Techniques.
  i. Posterior approach.
- Pt is prone and L4–L5 interspace is identified.
- Area 5 to 7 cm bilateral to midline at L4-L5 interspace is identified, and a 22-G, 7-in needle is inserted toward midline.
- Each needle is guided to anterolateral aspect of L5 vertebral body.
- Needle tips are advanced just beyond anterolateral border of L5-S1 junction.

18

CHRONIC PAIN

- LA and neurolytic are injected sequentially following proper contrast spread.
- Can use either fluoroscopic guidance or CT imaging.

ii. Transdiskal approach.
- Pt is placed prone and L5-S1 level is identified with either fluoroscopy or CT imaging.
- Fluoroscope is directed 15 to 25 degrees obliquely and angled cephalad.
- A 22-G, 7-in needle is inserted through disk and into retroperitoneal space.
- Contrast verifies proper spread outside of the disk.
- LA and neurolytic agent are then injected.
- Needle is flushed before removal, and antibiotics are given before procedure.

iii. Anterior approach.
- Fluoroscopy and CT can be used.
- Fluoroscopy.
- Pt is supine and in 15-degree Trendelenburg position.
- A 22-G, 6-in needle is inserted at midline ~2 to 3 cm inferior to umbilicus and aimed toward L5 vertebral body.
- Needle tip is advanced to inferior two thirds of L5.
- Contrast, LA, and neurolytic injected.
- CT.
- Pt is placed supine.
- 20- to 23-G, 4- to 5-in needle is inserted at midline between umbilicus and pubis.
- Needle tip is positioned anterior to left iliac vein and inferior to aortic bifurcation.
- Contrast, LA, and neurolytic agent are injected.
- Systemic antibiotics should be considered.

e. Complications.
  i. Rare.
  ii. Bladder puncture.
  iii. Retroperitoneal hematoma.
  iv. Nerve root injury.
  v. Mechanical or chemical injury to lumbar plexus and genitofemoral nerve.
  vi. Acute hypotension.
  vii. Localized tenderness, diskitis (transdiskal approach).
  viii. Bowel, small intestine injury (anterior approach).

f. Efficacy.
  i. Among 227 pts, 72% reported effective pain control and significant decrease in opioid consumption after neurolytic block. At 6-mo follow-up, 69% had continued pain relief.

ii. RCT comparing SHP neurolysis to opioids reported significant decrease in cancer pain intensity, opioid consumption, and drug-related side effects, and an enhanced quality of life.

3. Ganglion impar block.

a. Pt indications.

    i. Sustained visceral or sympathetically maintained perineal pain from cancer (e.g., anal or rectal).

b. Anatomy.

    i. The ganglion impar is a single, semicircular, retroperitoneal structure located midline at the sacrococcygeal junction, anterior to the lower part of the first coccygeal body.

    ii. Contains gray rami communicantes that travel to sacral and coccygeal nerves.

    iii. Represents termination of the sympathetic chain.

c. Function.

    i. Contains visceral afferent fibers that innervate perineum, distal rectum, anus, distal urethra, distal third of vagina, and vulva.

d. Techniques (all use fluoroscopic guidance).

    i. Anococcygeal.
- Pt is placed in lateral decubitus position, knees bent, and anococcygeal ligament palpated inferior to coccyx.
- Bent 60-degrees 22-G, 3.5-in needle is inserted through anococcygeal ligament directed cephalad and away from rectum.
- Needle tip is placed at sacrococcygeal junction.
- Contrast, LA, and neurolytic agent are injected sequentially.

    ii. Trans-sacrococcygeal.
- Pt is placed in lateral decubitus position with knees flexed.
- 22-G, 3.5-in needle is inserted through sacrococcygeal ligament and into retroperitoneal space.
- Contrast, LA, and neurolytic are injected.

    iii. Intercoccygeal.
- 22-G, 2-in needle is inserted through space between first and second coccygeal bones.
- Contrast, LA, and neurolytic agent are injected.

    iv. Coccygeal transverse.
- Pt is placed prone or lateral.
- A bent 22-G, 3.5-in needle is directed inferior to transverse process of coccyx and advanced superiorly and medially toward sacrococcygeal junction.
- Contrast, LA, and neurolytic are injected.

e. Complications.

    i. No reported complications in literature.

    ii. Theoretical risks.
- Rectal perforation.
- Periosteal injection.

- Epidural spread.
- Sacral nerve root injury.
- Motor, sexual, bowel, bladder dysfunction from accidental neurolytic spread.

f. Efficacy.
  i. Prospective studies report good efficacy of neurolysis of the ganglion impar for intractable perineal cancer pain.

G. IMPLANTABLE DRUG-DELIVERY SYSTEMS

1. Small, hockey puck–sized, electronic pump that delivers drug(s) to the intrathecal space through a catheter.
2. Pump is implanted SQ in the anterior abdominal wall and catheter-tunneled across flank to intrathecal space.
3. Reservoir that contains the drug is refilled through a port accessed by a needle inserted through the skin.
4. Pump is programmed externally with device that controls dose.
5. Intrathecal catheter trial with drug(s) is performed to assess pain relief and side effects.
a. Elements of pain, function, and mood are all assessed.
6. Selection criteria for IDDS therapy.
a. Chronic, intractable cancer pain.
b. Ineffective systemic treatment or intolerable side effects from systemic agents.
c. Favorable response to a screening trial (e.g., >50% decline in pain).
d. Life expectancy generally ~3 mo.
7. Technique.
a. Performed in the OR.
b. Pt lies in lateral decubitus position for access to lumbar spine and midportion of right or left abdominal quadrant.
c. Fluoroscopy is used.
d. Catheter is inserted into intrathecal space and advanced to lower thoracic spine.
e. SQ pocket is made in abdomen.
f. Intrathecal catheter is tunneled SQ from the spine to the abdomen and connected to pump.
g. Pump is filled with medication, and wounds are closed.
h. Pump can infuse various agents.
i. Opioids.
  i. First line includes morphine (strongest evidence) and hydromorphone, and second line includes fentanyl.
  ii. Ziconotide.
    - N-type, voltage-sensitive calcium channel blocker; first-line agent.
    - Cognitive and psychiatric changes may occur.
  iii. Clonidine.
    - α_2 agonist with analgesic efficacy.
    - Often used as dual agent with opioids or LAs.

iv. LAs.
- Bupivacaine first-line or second-line agent for cancer pain and used synergistically with opioids.
- Ropivacaine is considered a fifth-line agent.

8. Complications.
a. Pump malposition.
b. Wound infection.
c. Hardware malfunction.
d. Nausea and emesis, pruritus, urinary retention.

9. Efficacy.
a. RCT of cancer pts with IDDS versus medical management showed greater pain reduction and fewer side effects with IDDS; improved survival at 6 mo among IDDS pts.

H. NEURAXIAL NEUROLYTIC BLOCKS (INTRATHECAL AND EPIDURAL)
1. Chemical neurolysis via intrathecal or epidural route considered only in advanced, irreversible, and progressive illness (e.g., cancer).
2. Selectively interrupt sensory transmission while sparing motor function in the affected area.

3. Selection criteria.
a. Terminal cancer pain.
b. Unilateral pain localized to adjacent dermatomes of trunk, thorax, or abdomen.
c. Failure of previous analgesic modalities.

4. Anatomy and function.
a. Dorsal root carries sensory fibers.
b. Ventral root carries motor and sympathetic fibers.
c. Blocks selectively injure dorsal roots and rootlets between spinal cord and dorsal root ganglion.
d. Predictable segmental sensory loss occurs.
e. Epidural blocks are alternatives to intrathecal blockade; however, degree of pain relief may be less intense, and spread of agent is more difficult to control.

5. Technique (intrathecal).
a. Neurolytic agent selection depends on pt's ability to tolerate positioning, as baricity of agent determines flow of material in the CSF.
   i. Alcohol.
      - Hypobaric (rises) relative to CSF and is painful on injection.
   ii. Phenol.
      - Hyperbaric (falls) relative to CSF and contains analgesic properties.
b. Consider prognostic LA spinal block to confirm correct level.
c. Positioning.
   i. Lateral decubitus or sitting and angled 45 degrees toward the prone or supine direction, depending on agent selected.
   ii. Alcohol.

18

CHRONIC PAIN

- Pt is placed in lateral position with affected side uppermost.
  iii. Phenol.
    - Pt is placed with painful side dependent.
d. Subarachnoid space is entered under fluoroscopy, with 20- to 22-G spinal needle inserted at vertebral interspace.
e. Alcohol or phenol is injected in 0.1-mL increments to total of 0.5 to 0.7 mL per one to two dermatomal levels.

6. Complications.
a. Loss of touch and position sense, rare meningitis, PDPH.
b. Loss of motor function from spread to ventral rootlets.
c. Transient muscle weakness of extremities and rectal and urinary sphincters.
d. Agent specific.
   i. Phenol.
     - Vascular affinity may cause rare spinal artery thrombosis.
     - Higher viscosity requires larger-bore needle, with increased risk of PDPH.
   ii. Alcohol.
     - More painful injections.

7. Efficacy.
a. Intrathecal neurolysis produced 78% to 84% favorable response in cancer pts with somatic pain; only 19% to 24% of pts with visceral pain had positive responses.
b. Similar analgesic outcomes for alcohol and phenol.
c. Epidural neurolysis with phenol or alcohol produced pain relief in 80% of cancer pts, with maximum duration of >3 mo.

REFERENCES

Ahmedzai S, Brooks D: Transdermal fentanyl versus sustained-release oral morphine in cancer pain: preference, efficacy, and quality of life. The TTS-Fentanyl Comparative Trial Group. J Pain Symptom Manage 1997; 13:254–261.

Ananthan S, Khare NK, Saini SK, et al: Identification of opioid ligands possessing mixed micro agonist/delta antagonist activity among pyridomorphinans derived from naloxone, oxymorphone, and hydromorphone [correction of hydropmorphone]. J Med Chem 2004; 47:1400–1412.

Backonja M, Beydoun A, Edwards KR, et al: Gabapentin for the symptomatic treatment of painful neuropathy in patients with diabetes mellitus: A randomized controlled trial. JAMA 1998; 280:1831–1836.

Baker L, Lee M, Regnard C, et al: Evolving spinal analgesia practice in palliative care. Palliat Med 2004;18:507–515.

Bang SM, Park SH, Kang HG, et al: Changes in quality of life during palliative chemotherapy for solid cancer. Support Care Cancer 2005; 13:515–521.

Bonica J: The Management of Pain, vol. 1. Philadelphia: Lea & Febiger, 1990.

Bonica JJ, Buckley FP, Moricca G, Murphy TM: Neurolytic blockade and hypophysectomy. In: Bonica JJ, Loeser JD, Chapman CR, et al (eds). The Management of Pain, pp 2015–2020. Philadelphia: Lea & Febiger, 1990.

Bulka A, Plesan A, Xu XJ, et al: Reduced tolerance to the anti-hyperalgesic effect of methadone in comparison to morphine in a rat model of mononeuropathy. Pain 2002;95:103–109.

Candido K, Stevens RA: Intrathecal neurolytic blocks for the relief of cancer pain. Best Pract Res Clin Anaesthesiol 2003;17:407–428.

Cleeland CS, Gonin R, Hatfield AK, et al: Pain and its treatment in outpatients with metastatic cancer. N Engl J Med 1994; 330:592–596.

Cousins M, Dwyer B, Bigg D: Chronic pain and neurolytic blockade. In: Cousins MJ, Bridenbaugh PO (eds): Clinical Anesthesia and Management of Pain, 2nd ed. Philadelphia: JB Lippincott, 1988.

Crul BJ, Delhaas EM: Technical complications during long-term subarachnoid or epidural administration of morphine in terminally ill cancer patients: A review of 140 cases. Reg Anesth 1991; 16:209–213.

de Leon-Casasola OA: Critical evaluation of chemical neurolysis of the sympathetic axis for cancer pain. Cancer Control 2000; 7:142–148.

de Lissovoy G, Brown RE, Halpern M, et al: Cost-effectiveness of long-term intrathecal morphine therapy for pain associated with failed back surgery syndrome. Clin Ther 1997;19:96–112; discussion 84–85.

de Oliveira R, dos Reis MP, Prado WA: The effects of early or late neurolytic sympathetic plexus block on the management of abdominal or pelvic cancer pain. Pain 2004;110:400–408.

Eisenberg E, Carr DB, Chalmers TC: Neurolytic celiac plexus block for treatment of cancer pain: A meta-analysis. Anesth Analg 1995; 80:290–295.

Fourney DR, Schomer DF, Nader R, et al: Percutaneous vertebroplasty and kyphoplasty for painful vertebral body fractures in cancer patients. J Neurosurg 2003;98(1 Suppl):21–30.

Gerbershagen HU: Neurolysis. Subarachnoid neurolytic blockade. Acta Anaesthesiol Belg 1981;32:45–57.

Gutstein HB, Akil H: Opioid analgesics. In: Brunton LL, Lazo JS, Parker KL (eds): Goodman & Gilman's the Pharmacological Basis of Therapeutics, 11th ed, p 571. New York: McGraw-Hill, 2006.

Hagen NA, Swanson R: Strychnine-like multifocal myoclonus and seizures from extremely high dose opioids: Treatment strategies. J Pain Symptom Manage 1997;14:51–58.

Hershey L: Meperidine and central neurotoxicity. Ann Intern Med 1983; 98:548–549.

18

CHRONIC PAIN

Ischia S, Polati E, Finco G, et al: 1998 Labat Lecture. The role of the neurolytic celiac plexus block in pancreatic cancer pain management: Do we have the answers? Reg Anesth Pain Med 1998;23:611–614.

Jadad AR, Browman GP: The WHO analgesic ladder for cancer pain management. Stepping up the quality of its evaluation. JAMA 1995; 274:1870–1873.

Kreek MJ, Schecter AJ, Gutjahr CL, et al: Methadone use in patients with chronic renal disease. Drug Alcohol Depend 1980;5:197–205.

Makin AJ, Wendon J, Williams R: A 7-year experience of severe acetaminophen-induced hepatotoxicity (1987–1993). Gastroenterology 1995;109:1907–1916.

McQuay HJ, Tramèr M, Nye BA, et al: A systematic review of antidepressants in neuropathic pain. Pain 1996;68:217–227.

Meuser T, Pietruck C, Radbruch L, et al: Symptoms during cancer pain treatment following WHO-guidelines: A longitudinal follow-up study of symptom prevalence, severity and etiology. Pain 2001;93:247–257.

Miguel R: Interventional treatment of cancer pain: The fourth step in the World Health Organization analgesic ladder? Cancer Control 2000; 7:149–156.

National Institutes of Health (NIH): NIH state of the science statement on symptom management in cancer: Pain, depression, and fatigue. NIH Consens State Sci Statements 2002:1–29.

Nitescu P, Hultman E, Appelgren L, et al: Bacteriology, drug stability and exchange of percutaneous delivery systems and antibacterial filters in long-term intrathecal infusion of opioid drugs and bupivacaine in "refractory" pain. Clin J Pain 1992;8:324–337.

Oh CS, Chung IH, Ji HJ, et al: Clinical implications of topographic anatomy on the ganglion impar. Anesthesiology 2004;101:249–250.

Pace MC, Passavanti MB, Grella E, et al: Buprenorphine in long term control of chronic pain in cancer patients. Front Biosci 2007; 1:1291–1299.

Penn RD, Paice JA, Gottschalk W, et al: Cancer pain relief using chronic morphine infusion. Early experience with a programmable implanted drug pump. J Neurosurg 1984;61:302–306.

Plancarte R, Amescua C, Patt RB, et al: Superior hypogastric plexus block for pelvic cancer pain. Anesthesiology 1990;73:236–239.

Plancarte R, de Leon-Casasola OA, El-Helaly M, et al: Neurolytic superior hypogastric plexus block for chronic pelvic pain associated with cancer. Reg Anesth 1997;22:562–568.

Portenoy RK, Miransky J, Thaler HT, et al: Pain in ambulatory patients with lung or colon cancer. Prevalence, characteristics, and effect. Cancer 1992;70:1616–1624.

Ripamonti C, Zecca E, Bruera E: An update on the clinical use of methadone for cancer pain. Pain 1997;70:109–115.

Simon LS, Lipman AG, Caudill-Slosberg M, et al: Guideline for the Management of Pain in Osteoarthritis, Rheumatoid Arthritis, and Juvenile Chronic Arthritis. Glenview, IL: American Pain Society, 2002.

Sjoberg M, Appelgren L, Einarsson S, et al: Long-term intrathecal morphine and bupivacaine in "refractory" cancer pain. I. Results from the first series of 52 patients. Acta Anaesthesiol Scand 1991; 35:30–43.

Sjoberg M, Karlsson PA, Nordborg C, et al: Neuropathologic findings after long-term intrathecal infusion of morphine and bupivacaine for pain treatment in cancer patients. Anesthesiology 1992;76:173–186.

Smith TJ, Staats PS, Deer T, et al. Randomized clinical trial of an implantable drug delivery system compared with comprehensive medical management for refractory cancer pain: Impact on pain, drug-related toxicity, and survival. J Clin Oncol 2002;20:4040–4049.

Smitt PS, Tsafka A, Teng-van de Zande F, et al: Outcome and complications of epidural analgesia in patients with chronic cancer pain. Cancer 1998;83(9):2015–2022.

Swofford JB, Ratzman DM: A transarticular approach to blockade of the ganglion impar (ganglion of Walther). Reg Anesth Pain Med 1998; 23(Sup 1):103.

Wallace M, Yaksh TL: Long-term spinal analgesic delivery: A review of the preclinical and clinical literature. Reg Anesth Pain Med 2000; 25:117–157.

Ward SE, Miller-McCauley V, Mueller C, et al: Patient-related barriers to management of cancer pain. Pain 1993;52:319–324.

Zech DF, Grond S, Lynch J, et al: Validation of World Health Organization Guidelines for cancer pain relief: A 10-year prospective study. Pain 1995;63:65–76.

18

CHRONIC PAIN

Appendix A
Code-Call and Airway
Management Duties

One of the roles of the anesthesia call team is airway management for pts experiencing respiratory failure; this may or may not be associated with a cardiac arrest or "code." During a cardiac arrest, the anesthesia team, which usually includes an experienced anesthesia resident and an attending physician (whenever possible) are responsible for airway management, and an internal medicine team directs the medical management of the code if the pt has hemodynamic compromise or requires cardiopulmonary resuscitation. Many of the calls are primarily for respiratory distress or failure for which intubation is necessary. In these cases, the anesthesia team is responsible for securing the airway safely while providing adequate anesthesia based on the situation.

DUTIES OF THE ANESTHESIA TEAM AT A CODE CALL

On arriving at the code call, the anesthesia provider(s) should introduce themselves and their role and then move to the head of the bed and assess the pt:

- **A** – Does the pt have a patent airway?
- **B** – Is the pt breathing, oxygenating, and ventilating effectively? If not, is appropriate and effective support being provided via bag-mask ventilation?
- **C** – Is the pt's cardiac status compromised?
- **D** – Is the pt's mental status decreased?
- **E** – Ensure that pt's vital signs are being monitored: audible pulse oximetry, ECG, and frequent BP measurements (every minute).

After assessing the pt:

1. Confirm that oxygen is connected to the Ambu bag and turned to 15 L/min.
2. Assess ability to effectively bag-mask ventilate.
3. If the pt is alert and oriented, perform a quick airway assessment, including Mallampati classification and dentition.
4. Have a discussion with the primary team regarding intubation.
5. Confirm availability of all needed equipment with **SOAP**:
   a. **S**uction.
   b. **O**xygen.
   c. **A**irway equipment (preferred laryngoscope blade, ETT, oral airways, LMAs, Eschmann intubating stylet, and other desired emergency equipment if difficult airway).
   d. **P**harmacology and personnel (anesthesia attending physician, respiratory therapist, IV access).

6. If the pt is in cardiorespiratory arrest, it is reasonable to attempt a direct laryngoscopy and intubation without induction drugs. If intubation is unsuccessful, continue with bag-mask ventilation.
7. Formulate a plan for securing the airway and a backup plan if pt has a potential for or known difficult airway.
8. If the pt is not in cardiorespiratory arrest, make an assessment of the pt's specific needs for pharmacology on induction, including:
   a. Choice of induction drug and dose (consider hypotension, increased ICP, bronchospasm, need for slow titration of drug).
   b. Choice of rapid-sequence induction versus routine induction (consider pt's ability to oxygenate during nonventilated period, full stomach precautions, contraindications to succinylcholine).
9. Once the decision has been made to intubate the trachea, reconfirm reliable IV access and free-flowing fluid and obtain additional access if necessary. Designate a nurse or another anesthesia provider to administer medications and direct him or her as to order of administration and dosing.
10. Once the airway is secure, confirm $ETCO_2$ and adequate oxygenation and ventilation.
11. Transfer care to available respiratory therapist as appropriate.
12. Once the pt has a secure and effective airway, the anesthesia team may assist in obtaining IV access or other invasive monitoring access. If no medicine providers are present at the code, it is the responsibility of the anesthesia provider to institute BLS and/or ACLS and direct the staff.

Appendix B
Trauma Setup

I. MACHINE

A. TURN ON MACHINE AND MONITORS, PERFORM ROUTINE MACHINE CHECK, AND CONFIRM THAT ALL VOLATILE AGENT CYLINDERS ARE FULL.

B. PREPARE 7.0 AND 8.0 ETT (SMALLER FOR PEDIATRIC TRAUMA ROOM) WITH LUBRICATED STYLETS AND SYRINGES ATTACHED; CHECK CUFFS FOR LEAKS.

C. CHECK MAC 3, MAC 4, AND MILLER 2 OPERATING ROOM 3 BLADES AND HANDLES FOR LIGHTS.

D. CONFIRM IMMEDIATE AVAILABILITY OF ALL AGE-APPROPRIATE LMA SIZES, ESCHMANN STYLET.

E. HAVE NONINVASIVE MONITORS SET UP ON OPERATING ROOM TABLE (PULSE OXIMETER, BP CUFF, AND ECG).

F. CONFIRM THAT INVASIVE MONITOR CABLES ARE ATTACHED TO TRANSDUCERS WITH FULL, PRESSURIZED FLUSH BAGS.

G. CHECK SUCTION; SHOULD HAVE TWO SET UP AND TURNED ON.

H. CONFIRM THAT OG TUBE, HUMIDIVENT, AND TEMPERATURE PROBE ARE EASILY ACCESSIBLE.

I. HAVE SILK TAPE AND EYE TAPE READY ON MACHINE.

II. VASCULAR ACCESS AND FLUIDS

A. IV FLUIDS
1. Two 1-liter bags of NS with blood infusion tubing ("pumper"), extension tubing, and extra stopcock.
2. One 1-liter bag with blood infusion tubing run through fluid warmer with extension tubing and extra stopcock.

B. CENTRAL VENOUS ACCESS
1. The following should be available on a Mayo stand, unopened, for easy access.
a. 16-G, single-lumen, central venous access kit.
b. Separately packaged long and short catheter sheath introducers (Cordis) and single-lumen introducer catheter (SLIC).
c. Large, sterile occlusive dressing.

d. Triple-gang infusion set.
e. Whole-body drape.
f. Sterile gown.
g. Two sets of sterile gloves.

C. PERIPHERAL IV SUPPLIES
1. 14-, 16-, and 18-G peripheral IV catheters.
2. Tourniquet.
3. Gauze.
4. Alcohol and chlorhexidine bullets.
5. Small occlusive dressing.
6. Plastic tape.

D. ARTERIAL CATHETER SUPPLIES
1. Arrow catheters and 20-G angiocatheters.
2. Small wire.
3. 100-mL saline syringe flushed through 9-inch tubing with stopcock.
4. Chlorhexidine.
5. Small occlusive dressing.
6. Sterile towels.
7. Lundy board and 2-inch paper tape for hand positioning.
8. Sterile gauze.

III. DRUGS

A. ALL DRUGS SHOULD BE LABELED CLEARLY WITH DATE AND TIME OF EXPIRATION IF DRAWN INTO THE SYRINGE BY THE ANESTHESIA PROVIDER.

B. FOR SAFETY PURPOSES, EMPTY SYRINGES SHOULD NOT BE PRELABELED WITH DRUG NAMES UNTIL THE ACTUAL TIME AT WHICH THE DRUG IS DRAWN INTO THE SYRINGE.

C. INDUCTION AGENTS
1. Propofol—two 20-mL vials.
2. Etomidate—one 10-mL vial.
3. Scopolamine 0.4 mg.

D. OPIATES AND SEDATIVES
1. To be signed out under patient's name and ID number.

E. NMB AND REVERSAL AGENTS
1. Succinylcholine—two 10-mL syringes (20 mg/mL).
2. Vecuronium—one 10-mL syringe (1 mg/mL).
3. Neostigmine—one 5-mL syringe (1 mg/mL).
4. Glycopyrrolate—one 5-mL syringe (0.2 mg/mL).

F. VASOACTIVE DRUGS
1. Epinephrine—one 10-mL syringe of 1:10,000 (0.1 mg/mL) and one 10-mL syringe of 1:100,000 (0.01 mg/mL).
2. Labetalol, metoprolol, and esmolol vials.
3. Atropine—one 1-mL syringe (1 mg/mL).
4. Phenylephrine—two 10-mL syringes (0.1 mg/mL).
5. Ephedrine—one 10-mL syringe (5 mg/mL).

G. ANTIBIOTICS
1. Appropriate antibiotics per institutional policy, specific surgery, and patient allergies.

H. ANTIEMETICS
1. Bicitra—30-mL container at bedside.
2. Ranitidine, dolasetron, and metoclopramide vials.

I. MISCELLANEOUS
1. Sodium bicarbonate—one vial.
2. Calcium chloride—one vial.
3. Lidocaine 2%—5-mL syringe.
4. Lacri-Lube ointment.
5. Lidocaine jelly for OG placement.

Appendix C
Resident Checklist for Adult Cardiac Setup

1. Medications

Emergency Drugs
- [ ] Epinephrine
- [ ] NTG
- [ ] Phenylephrine
- [ ] Ephedrine
- [ ] Succinylcholine
- [ ] Calcium
- [ ] Esmolol
- [ ] Heparin—exact dose (generally 300 units/kg, calculated and confirmed with perfusionist)

Anesthesia Drugs
- [ ] Midazolam
- [ ] Fentanyl
- [ ] Pancuronium
- [ ] Optional: etomidate, propofol, ketamine

Bypass Pump Drugs
- [ ] Phenylephrine
- [ ] Lidocaine
- [ ] $MgSO_4$
- [ ] Midazolam
- [ ] Fentanyl
- [ ] Pancuronium

Antibiotics
- [ ] Cefazolin or, if pt is penicillin allergic, vancomycin

2. Anesthesia Machine
- [ ] Adult laryngoscopes
- [ ] ETT—8.0 with competent cuff (if pt is small, have 7.0 or 7.5 ETT)
- [ ] ETT stylet
- [ ] Oral airways
- [ ] LMA adult sizes
- [ ] Eschmann intubating stylet
- [ ] Temperature probes × 2
- [ ] Gastric tube
- [ ] Functioning pacemaker
- [ ] Working suction with Yankauer tip

Continued

3. Monitors
☐ Key in pt's weight and height if pulmonary artery catheter is planned.
☐ Arterial catheter supplies, with Lundy board.
☐ Zero all transducers, pressurize saline flush bag, and turn transducer stopcocks so that flush fluid does not drip from tubing.
☐ Transesophageal echocardiography (TEE) probe, machine and gel if TEE is planned.

4. Infusion Pump Pole
☐ Prime carrier fluid (normal saline) through tubing.
☐ Obtain infusion medications from pharmacy:
    ☐ Epinephrine
    ☐ NTG
    ☐ Aminocaproic acid (Amicar)
    ☐ Insulin
☐ Other infusion medications should be discussed with attending prior to setup (e.g., norepinephrine, milrinone, vasopressin, fentanyl, nicardipine).

5. OR Table
☐ Head ring or padding + sheets for head support, if necessary
☐ Elbow padding
☐ Shoulder roll
☐ ECG monitor on bed
☐ Noninvasive blood pressure cuff
☐ SpO_2 cable (with extension)
☐ Defibrillation pads for redo cases
☐ Armboards for bed
☐ Holders for surgical screen

6. IV Fluids
☐ Fluid warmer with Y-type transfusion primed with normal saline.
☐ For inpatients, peripheral IV setup.

7. Blood Products
☐ Confirm blood product availability before bringing pt to OR

Appendix D
Resident Checklist for Pediatric Cardiac Setup

1. Medications
Emergency Drugs in Syringes
- ☐ Atropine
- ☐ Epinephrine
- ☐ Phenylephrine
- ☐ Ephedrine
- ☐ Succinylcholine
- ☐ Calcium
- ☐ Heparin—exact dose (usually 300 units/kg for bypass cases), confirmed with perfusionist

Anesthesia Drugs
- ☐ Midazolam
- ☐ Fentanyl
- ☐ Pancuronium
- ☐ Propofol

Pump Drugs
- ☐ Phenylephrine
- ☐ Lidocaine
- ☐ $MgSO_4$
- ☐ Fentanyl
- ☐ Pancuronium

Others
- ☐ Cefazolin
- ☐ Decadron

2. Anesthesia Machine
Age and size appropriate:
- ☐ Laryngoscope blades
- ☐ ETT—estimated size + one-half size larger and one-half size smaller
- ☐ Stylet and oral airways
- ☐ Paper tape cut to cover eyes
- ☐ Brain oximeter probes × 2
- ☐ WORKING SUCTION with Yankauer and ETT size-appropriate suction catheters available in cart
- ☐ Pacemaker

Continued

3. Invasive Monitors
☐ Zero transducers, pressurize bag.
☐ If transesophageal echocardiography (TEE) is requested, have echo gel and appropriate-sized TEE probe.

4. Infusion Pump
☐ Normal saline carrier fluid primed through tubing and carefully de-aired.
☐ Program pumps and set on standby.
    ☐ Epinephrine
    ☐ Milrinone
    ☐ Fentanyl
☐ Other medications (vasoactive infusions, antifibrinolytics, etc., per discussion with attending)

5. OR Table
☐ Forced air warmer with blanket on bed
☐ Foam head ring or padding
☐ Shoulder roll, size appropriate for pt
☐ ECG monitor on bed
☐ NIBP cuff: size appropriate for pt
☐ SpO_2 cable and 2 probes
☐ Defibrillator pads for redo cases
☐ Holders on bed for surgical screen
☐ Clamps for drapes

6. IV and Arterial Catheter Supplies
☐ Arterial catheter supplies and arm board
☐ 24-G catheters for infants; 22-G catheters for other children; small wire
☐ 2.5 Fr, 2.5 cm arterial catheter kit
☐ Peripheral IV fluid on buretrol with stopcock and extension tubing (use small-bore extension tubing for infants; check with attending for fluid type) carefully de-aired.

7. Blood Products
☐ Confirm blood product availability before bringing pt to OR

Appendix E
Common Anesthesia and
Critical Care Drugs and Doses

Geoffrey Boyd, JD, BsPharm, and Jin Sun Cho, MD
Edited by Eugenie S. Heitmiller, MD

E

Drug	Route; Indication	Pediatric Dose	Adult Dose (>50 kg)	Comments
Acetaminophen	PO; pain	10–15 mg/kg/dose q 4–6 hr	500–1000 mg q 4 hr	Max dose:
	PR; pain	20–40 mg/kg initial dose only; then 10–15 mg/kg/dose q 4–6 hr	650 mg q 4–6 hr	Infant: 60 mg/kg/day Older child: 90 mg/kg/day Adult: 4 g/day
Adenosine	IV, IO; ACLS	0.1 mg/kg/dose; max 6 mg/dose; may repeat at 0.2 mg/kg/dose q 1–2 min × 2 doses	Initial: 6 mg, ↑ to 12 mg max q 1–2 min × 2 doses	Rapid IV push with flush
	IV; SVT	0.1 mg/kg/dose; may ↑ by 0.05–0.1 mg/kg/dose q 1–2 min × 2 doses		
Aminocaproic acid	IV loading dose	100–200 mg/kg over 1 hr	4–5 g over 1 hr	
	IV infusion	10–33 mg/kg/hr	1 g/hr (50 mL/hr)	
Amiodarone	IV, IO; pulseless VT/VF	5 mg/kg rapid IV bolus; may repeat up to 15 mg/kg	300 mg rapid IV bolus; may repeat with 150 mg; max dose: 2.2 g/day	
	IV; hemodynamically stable tachycardia	5 mg/kg over 20–60 min; repeat up to max daily dose of 15 mg/kg or 300 mg		
Atropine	IV, IO; bradycardia	0.02 mg/kg; minimum, 0.1 mg; repeat once after 5 min	0.5–1 mg IV q 3–5 min to max total dose of 3 mg	Max dose:
	ETT; bradycardia	0.03 mg/kg; minimum, 0.1 mg; flush with 5 mL NS and follow with five ventilations; repeat once after 5 min	1–2 mg dilute to max 10 mL sterile water or NS	Young children: 0.5 mg/dose Adolescents: 1 mg/dose
	IM, PO	0.02–0.03 mg/kg	0.4–0.6 mg	

Bupivacaine	Epidural anesthesia—bolus doses		
	Caudal	Single dose 1 mL/kg of 0.25%	10–20 mL of 0.25% (partial motor block);
	Lumbar epidural	Single dose 0.5 mL/kg of 0.25%	0.5% (moderate to total motor block)
	Thoracic epidural	Single dose 0.3 mL/kg of 0.25%	Repeat dose with ½–⅔ initial dose q 60–90 min
	Epidural analgesia— continuous infusion	0.1–0.2 mg/kg/hr (<10 kg) 0.2–0.4 mg/kg/hr (>10 kg) as a 0.1%, 0.125%, or 0.25% solution	Max dose: 2 mg/kg without epinephrine 3 mg/kg with epinephrine
			Epidural, continuous infusion, 6.25–18.75 mg/hr as a 0.0625%–0.125% solution
			Max infusion rate: 0.2 mg/kg/hr (<10 kg) 0.4 mg/kg/hr (>10 kg)
Butorphanol	IV, intranasal; pain	10–20 mcg/kg	IV: 1 mg q 3–4 hr Nasal: 1 mg, followed by a second dose in 60–90 min; then q 3–4 hr
	Pruritus	30–50 mcg/kg q 4–6 hr	30–50 mcg/kg q 4–6 hr
Calcium chloride	IV, IO—slow push; administer via CVC	10–20 mg/kg (10% solution) q 10 min	10–20 mg/kg (10% solution) q 10 min; usually 0.5–1 g/dose
Calcium gluconate	IV; hyperkalemia, hypocalcemia	15–30 mg/kg	500 mg–2 g	Rate not to exceed 200 mg/min
Chloral hydrate	PO; sedation	50–100 mg/kg	0.5–1 g	Max dose: 2 g/dose
Cisatracurium	IV bolus; NMB	0.1–0.2 mg/kg, 0.03 mg/kg redose	Initial, 0.15–0.2 mg/kg; maintenance, 0.03 mg/kg	
	IV infusion; NMB	1–4 mcg/kg/min	Initial, 3 mcg/kg/min; thereafter, 1–2 mg/kg/min	

Continued

COMMON ANESTHESIA AND CRITICAL CARE DRUGS   F

Drug	Route; Indication	Pediatric Dose	Adult Dose (>50 kg)	Comments
Clonidine	Epidural infusion; postoperative or cancer pain	0.5 mcg/kg/hr	30 mcg/hr, titrate up to 40 mcg/hr	
	IV; hypertension	2–6 mcg/kg alone 0.625–1.25 mcg/kg with anesthesia	150 mcg	
	PO; hypertension	5–10 mcg/kg/day in two or three divided doses	Initial treatment for acute hypertension, 0.1 mg q 1 hr up to max 0.6 mg; maintenance, 0.1–0.3 mg bid	
	PO; narcotic withdrawal	1 mcg/kg q 4–6 hr	0.1–0.2 mg q 4 hr prn for 7 days	
	PO; premedication Transdermal; hypertension	4 mcg/kg, 1.5 hr before induction	0.1 mg/day transdermal patch q 7 days	
Daclizumab (Zenapax)	IV; transplant antirejection	1 mg/kg	1 mg/kg	
Desmopressin (DDAVP)	IV, SQ; diabetes insipidus	>12 yr: 2–4 mcg/kg in two divided doses	2–4 mcg/kg/day in two divided doses	1 mcg Desmopressin is equivalent to 4 IU of vasopressin, and 1 mL of intranasal solution has an antidiuretic activity of 400 IU of vasopressin Comparable Antidiuretic dose of the injection is ~1/10 the

Drug	Indication / Route	Dose	Dose	Comments
	Nasal spray; diabetes insipidus (one compression delivers 0.1 mL [10 mcg])	<12 yr: 5-30 mcg (0.05-0.3 mL) (use rhinal tube for doses <10 mcg)	10-40 mcg/day (0.1-0.4 mL) either as a single dose or two or three divided doses	
	IV; hemophilia A or von Willebrand disease, and factor VIII levels >5%	0.3 mcg/kg infused slowly over 15 min	0.3 mcg/kg infused slowly over 15 min	
Dexamethasone	IV; allergic reaction	0.08-0.3 mg/kg/day in divided doses q 6-12 hr	0.5-9 mg/day	Max dose: 2 mg/kg/day
	IV; ↑ ICP treatment	1-2 mg/kg; then 0.25-0.35 mg/kg q 6 hr	Initial: 10 mg; then 4 mg q 6 hr	
	IV; PONV	0.05-0.5 mg/kg, up to 8 mg	4-8 mg	
	IV; stridor or croup	0.25-0.5 mg/kg, up to 10 mg, q 6 hr		
	IV; extubation or airway edema	0.1-0.3 mg/kg/day divided q 6 hr	IV, 0.5-1 mg/kg/day; IM, divided q 6 hr	
Dexmedetomidine (Precedex)	IV	1 mcg/kg load over 10 min; then 0.2-0.7 mcg/kg/hr	1 mcg/kg load over 10 min, followed by infusion 0.2-0.7 mcg/kg/hr	Not indicated for use >24 hr
Dextrose (25%)	IV; hypoglycemia	0.5 mg/kg (2 mL/kg)	10-25 g at 3 mL/min	Check serum glucose When concentrated dextrose infusion is abruptly withdrawn, administer 5% or 10% dextrose to avoid reactive hypoglycemia
	Dextrose and insulin for hyperkalemia	2 mL/kg + 0.1 unit of insulin per kilogram	30-50 g + 10 units of insulin	
Dobutamine	IV infusion; ↓ cardiac output, heart failure	2-20 mcg/kg/min	2.5-20 mcg/kg/min	

COMMON ANESTHESIA AND CRITICAL CARE DRUGS

Continued

Drug	Route: Indication	Pediatric Dose	Adult Dose (>50 kg)	Comments
Dolasetron	IV; PONV	0.35 mg/kg; max dose: 12.5 mg	12.5 mg	
Dopamine	IV infusion	Initial, 2–5 mcg/kg/min; titrate to effect up to 30 mcg/kg/min max	Initial, 2–5 mcg/kg/min; titrate to effect up to 50 mcg/kg/min max	
Ephedrine	IV	0.2–0.3 mg/kg	12.5–25 mg	
Epinephrine	IV, IO; pulseless arrest, symptomatic bradycardia	10 mcg/kg bolus; repeat q 3–5 min	1 mg IV/IO; repeat q 3–5 min	
	ETT; pulseless arrest	30 mcg/kg for ≤28 days of age 100 mcg/kg for >28 days of age	2–2.5 mg ETT if IV/IO access is delayed or cannot be established	
	IV, IO bolus; hypotensive shock, anaphylaxis, β-blocker overdose	0.1 mg/kg (0.1 mL/kg of 1:1000) q 3–5 min	0.05–1 mg IV bolus	
	IV, IO infusion; hypotensive shock, anaphylaxis, β-blocker overdose	0.1–1 mcg/kg/min (consider higher dose if needed)	2–20 mcg/min	
	IM; anaphylaxis	0.01 mg/kg (0.01 mL/kg) 1:1000 IM in thigh q 15 min prn Autoinjector: 0.3 mg (≥30 kg) IM or Child Jr autoinjector: 0.15 mg (10–30 kg) IM	0.3 mg (0.3 mL of 1:1000) IM; may be repeated if severe anaphylaxis persists	
	SQ; asthma	0.01 mg/kg (0.01 mL/kg) 1:1000 SQ q 15 min	0.2–0.5 mg (0.2–0.5 mL of 1:1000) SQ q 2 hr as required; in severe attacks, may repeat dose q 20 min for max three doses	

Drug	Route/Indication	Dose	Dose	Comments
	IV; croup	0.25–0.5 mL racemic solution (0.25%) mixed in 3 mL NS or 3 mL 1:1000		
Epinephrine, racemic	Nebulize 2.5% solution	0.25–0.5 mL in 3 mL NS		
Esmolol	IV bolus	0.5–1 mg/kg	0.5–2 mg/kg	
	IV infusion	0.5 mg/kg IV load over 2 min; then, 25–300 mcg/kg/min	0.5 mg/kg IV load over 1 min; then 25–300 mcg/kg/min	
Etomidate	IV; induction	0.3 mg/kg (0.2–0.6 mg/kg) over 30–60 sec	0.3 mg/kg IV (0.2–0.6 mg/kg) over 30–60 sec	Pain on injection
Fentanyl	IV bolus; pain	0.5–1 mcg/kg	25–50 mcg	
	IV infusion; pain and sedation	1–3 mcg/kg/hr	1–3 mcg/kg/hr	
	IV bolus; adjunct to GA	2–3 mcg/kg	2–3 mcg/kg	
	IV infusion; adjunct to GA	3–5 mcg/kg/hr	1–5 mcg/kg/hr	
	IV PCA basal infusion	0.5–1 mcg/kg/hr	25–200 mcg/hr	
	EPCA bolus	0.2–0.25 mcg/kg/dose	50–100 mcg	
	EPCA infusion	0.4–0.5 mcg/kg/hr	25–50 mcg/hr; EPCA infusion contains 2 mcg of fentanyl per milliliter	
	Intranasal; pain	1–2 mcg/kg		Undiluted, drops in nose
Flumazenil	IV; reversal of benzodiazepines	0.01 mg/kg (up to 0.2 mg) over 15 sec q 1 min × 4	0.2 mg over 15 sec q 1 min × 4	Max total dose 0.05 mg/kg or 1 mg, whichever is lower
Fosphenytoin	IV infusion	10–20 mg/kg load over 10–20 min	10–20 mg/kg load IV or IM; maintenance, 4–6 mg/kg/day; max infusion rate, 150 mg/min	

Continued

COMMON ANESTHESIA AND CRITICAL CARE DRUGS

Drug	Route; Indication	Pediatric Dose	Adult Dose (>50 kg)	Comments
Furosemide	IV bolus	0.5–2 mg/kg	20–40 mg over 1–2 min	Give bolus slowly; ototoxic
	IV infusion	0.1–0.4 mg/kg/hr	not >4 mg/min	
Gabapentin	PO; partial seizure	Initial: 3–5 mg/kg three times per day; Maintenance: 3–4 yr: titrate upward over 3 days to 40 mg/kg/day; 5–12 yr: 25–35 mg/kg/day (divided into three doses)	300 mg three times per day; may increase up to 1800 mg/day (divided into three doses)	
	PO; postherpetic neuralgia, neuropathic pain	5 mg/kg on day 1; increase to bid on day 2; increase to tid on day 3	300 mg on day 1; increase to bid on day 2; increase to tid on day 3; may increase dosage up to 1800 mg/day (divided into three doses)	
Glucagon	IV, IM, SQ; hypoglycemia	<20 kg: 20–30 mcg/kg/dose or 0.5 mg/dose; >20 kg: 1 mg	1 mg; may repeat after 20 min if needed	
Glycopyrrolate	IV; cardiac dysrhythmia	4 mcg/kg up to 0.1 mg	0.1–0.2 mg/dose	Do not use in infants <1 mo (contains benzyl alcohol)
	IV, IM; antisialagogue	4–10 mcg/kg	4–10 mcg/kg	
	PO; antisialagogue	40–100 mcg/kg/dose	40–100 mcg/kg/dose	
	IV; block cholinergic effects of neostigmine	0.2 mg for each 1 mg neostigmine or 5 mg pyridostigmine	0.2 mg for each 1 mg neostigmine or 5 mg pyridostigmine	
Granisetron	IV	10–40 mcg/kg/dose	10 mcg/kg or 1 mg	
Haloperidol	IV, IM, PO; psychosis	0.05–0.15 mg/kg/day in two or three divided doses	0.5–10 mg	Contraindicated for Parkinson disease

Drug	Route; indication			Comments
Heparin	IV bolus; vascular procedures	50–100 units/kg	5000 units	
	IV; CPB	300 units/kg	300 units/kg	
	IV infusion; thrombosis, DIC	10–25 units/kg/hr	10–25 units/kg/hr	Adjust infusion by 2–4 units/kg/hr prn
				Follow ACT/PTT
Hydrocodone	PO; analgesia	0.1–0.2 mg/kg q 4–6 hr (do not exceed 6 doses/day)	5–10 mg four times per day	
Hydromorphone	IV; analgesia	15 mcg/kg/dose q 4–6 hr	0.2–0.6 mg q 2–3 hr prn	
	PO; analgesia	50–100 mcg/kg/dose q 6 hr	2–8 mg q 3–4 hr prn	
	IV PCA, bolus	3–5 mcg/kg/dose	0.1–0.2 mg/dose	
	IV PCA, basal infusion	3–5 mcg/kg/hr	0–0.5 mg/hr	
	Epidural PCA, bolus	0.1 mcg/kg/dose	1–1.5 mg/dose	
	Epidural PCA, infusion	0.2–0.3 mcg/kg/hr	0.04–0.4 mg/hr	
Hydroxyzine	IM, PO; pruritus	0.5–1.0 mg/kg q 4–6 hr	25 mg three or four times per day	
	IM, PO; anxiety	50–100 mg daily in divided doses	50–100 mg four times per day	
	PO; sedation	0.6 mg/kg/dose	50–100 mg	
	IM; sedation	0.5–1 mg/kg/dose	25–100 mg	
Ibuprofen	PO, PR	<12 yr: 5–10 mg/kg q 6–8 hr; max: 400 mg/dose >12 yr: 200–400 mg q 4–6 hr; max dose: 1200 mg/day	200–400 mg q 4–6 hr; max dose: 1200 mg/day	
Insulin (regular or aspart)	SQ	0.5–1 unit/kg/day	0.5–1 unit/kg/day	Titrate per blood glucose levels
	Infusion	0.1 unit/kg/hr	0.1 unit/kg/hr	
Isoproterenol	IV; heart block	0.1–1 mcg/kg/min	2–10 mcg/min	
Ketamine	IV; analgesia	0.25–0.5 mg/kg	0.25–0.5 mg/kg	
	IV; anesthetic induction	1–2 mg/kg	1–4.5 mg/kg	
	IM; induction	5–10 mg/kg	6.5–14 mg/kg	

Continued

Drug	Route; Indication	Pediatric Dose	Adult Dose (>50 kg)	Comments
Ketorolac	IV	0.5 mg/kg	<65 yr: 30 mg single or q 6 hr >65 yr: 15 mg single or q 6 hr	Max dose: Pediatric: 15 mg IV, 30 mg IM
	IM	1 mg/kg	<65 yr: 60 mg single or 30 mg q 6 hr >65 yr: 30 mg single or 15 mg q 6 hr	<65 yr: 120 mg IV, IM >65 yr: 60 mg IV, IM
Labetalol	IV bolus; hypertension	0.2–1 mg/kg bolus	Initial dose of 20 mg (0.25 mg/kg) by slow injection over 2 min; repeat injections of 40 or 80 mg at 10-min intervals as indicated; max dose: 300 mg; max effects occur within 5 min of injection	
Lidocaine	IV, IO; ventricular dysrhythmia	1 mg/kg; max bolus dose 100 mg	50–100 mg (0.7–1.4 mg/kg) IV over 2–3 min; may repeat in 5 min up to 300 mg in any 1-hr period	
	IV infusion	20–50 mcg/kg/min	1–4 mg/min (14–57 mg/kg/min)	
Magnesium sulfate	IV; hypomagnesemia	25–75 mg/kg over 30 min	1–2 g over 15–60 min	Slow infusion
Mannitol	IV infusion; ↑ ICP	1–2 g/kg	0.25–2 g/kg	Do not use if crystals are visible
	IV infusion; diuresis	0.25–2 g/kg	50–100 g or 300–400 mg/kg	Use filter for solutions >20% mannitol
Meperidine (Demerol)	IV; postoperative shivering	0.5–2 mg/kg (up to 25 mg)	25 mg	

Continued

Methadone	IV, PO	0.1–0.2 mg/kg PO q 6 hr; max: 10 mg/dose	2.5–10 mg (may also be given IM or SQ) q 3–4 hr
Methylprednisolone	IM; asthma	1–2 mg/kg; then 0.5–2 mg/kg q 6 hr	40–80 mg/day
	IV; cord protection	30 mg/kg bolus over 15 min, followed by a 45-min pause; then continuous infusion 5.4 mg/kg/hr for 23 hr	30 mg/kg bolus over 15 min, followed by a 45-min pause; then continuous infusion 5.4 mg/kg/hr for 23 hr
	IV; adrenal supplement	1–2 mg/kg	1–2 mg/kg
Metoclopramide	PO; GERD	0.1 mg/kg three or four times daily	10–15 mg up to four times daily
	IV; PONV	0.25 mg/kg/dose q 6–8 hr	10–20 mg q 4–6 hr
Milrinone	IV; ↓ cardiac output	50 mcg/kg over 15 min; maintenance, 0.5 mcg/kg/min	50 mcg/kg over 20 min, followed by continuous infusion of 0.5 mcg/kg/min for minimum of 4 hr
Morphine	IV; pain	0.05–0.1 mg/kg increments	2–10 mg
	Epidural; pain	10–30 mcg/kg	5-mg epidural injection in lumbar region; additional incremental doses of 1–2 mg at appropriate interval
Nalbuphine	IV, IM, SQ; pain	0.1 mg/kg	10 mg q 3–6 hr; max dose: 20 mg/dose, 160 mg/day
Naloxone	IV, IM, SQ	1–10 mcg/kg	0.4–2 mg q 2–3 min
Naproxen	PO	5–7 mg/kg q 8–12 hr	200–400 mg, followed 200 mg q 8–12 hr; max dose: 600 mg/day

COMMON ANESTHESIA AND CRITICAL CARE DRUGS E

Drug	Route; Indication	Pediatric Dose	Adult Dose (>50 kg)	Comments
Neostigmine	IV; NMB reversal	0.03–0.07 mg/kg	0.5–2 mg	Administer atropine or glycopyrrolate before neostigmine to counteract cholinergic effects
Nicardipin	IV infusion	Initial: 0.5–5 mcg/kg/min Maintenance: 1–4 mcg/kg/min Max dose: 5 mcg/kg/min	Initial: 5 mg/hr; titrate 2.5 mg/hr q 5–15 min Maintenance (after reaching BP goal): 3 mg/hr Max dose: 15 mg/hr	At the recommended doses, dihydropyridines are specific to peripheral vascular calcium channels. At higher doses, negative inotropy may occur
Nitroglycerin	IV infusion	0.5–20 mcg/kg/min	0.5–20 mcg/kg/min	
Nitroprusside	IV infusion	Initial: 0.3 mcg/kg/min; titrate every few min to desired effect; usual dose, 3 mcg/kg/min IV	Initial: 0.3 mcg/kg/min; titrate every few min to desired effect; usual dose, 3 mcg/kg/min	Max dose: 10 mcg/kg/min
Norepinephrine	IV infusion	Initial: 0.1 mcg/kg/min IV; titrate to desired effect Maintenance: 0.05–0.3 mcg/kg/min	Initial: 8–12 mcg/min Maintenance: 2–4 mcg/min	
Novoseven (recombinant factor VII)	IV; acquired factor VII deficiency IV; factor VII deficiency	70–90 mcg/kg over 2–5 min q 2–3 hr 15–30 mcg/kg over 2–5 min q 4–6 hr	70–90 mcg/kg over 2–5 min q 2–3 hr 15–30 mcg/kg over 2–5 min q 4–6 hr	For acute hemorrhage, dose may be repeated in 1 hr if response is inadequate. Once constituted, the drug is good for 4 hr—i.e., once opened, save the $10,000 vial for potential second dose

Continued

Ondansetron	IV; PONV	<40 kg: 0.1 mg/kg; max: 4 mg >40 kg: 4 mg	4 mg
	Oral disintegrating tablets	4–8 mg	16 mg
Oxybutynin	PO	0.1 mg/kg	5–10 mg
Oxycodone	PO	0.1 mg/kg q 4–6 hr	5–30 mg q 4–6 hr
Pancuronium	IV bolus	0.04–0.1 mg/kg	0.04–0.1 mg/kg
PGE₁	IV infusion	0.05–2 mcg/kg/min	
Phenobarbital	IV; seizure	15–25 mg/kg load; then 4–6 mg/kg/day PO	100–320 mg slow injection repeated up to a max total dose of 600 mg/day or 50–100 mg PO × 2–3 daily
Phentolamine	IV bolus; hypertensive episode, pheochromocytoma	0.05–0.1 mg/kg (max 5 mg/dose) given 1–2 hr before procedure; repeated prn q 2–4 hr	5 mg given 1–2 hr before procedure; repeated prn q 2–4 hr
	IV infusion	2–20 mcg/kg/min	
Phenylephrine	IV bolus	5–10 mcg/kg	0.2 mg (0.1–0.5 mg); initial dose not to exceed 0.5 mg; do not repeat dose more often than q 10–15 min
	IV infusion	0.1–0.5 mcg/kg/min	Initial: 100–180 mcg/min continuous IV infusion; once BP is stabilized, decrease rate to 40–60 mcg/min to maintain BP
Potassium	IV	0.5–1 mEq/kg over 1–2 hr	Serum K <2 mEq/L: 20–40 mEq/hr
	Infusion	0.3–0.5 mEq/kg/hr	Serum K >2.5 mEq/L: 10–15 mEq/hr

COMMON ANESTHESIA AND CRITICAL CARE DRUGS E

Drug	Route; Indication	Pediatric Dose	Adult Dose (>50 kg)	Comments
Prednisone	PO; preoperatively for asthma prophylaxis	1 mg/kg qd × 3 days prior to surgery	40 to 60 mg PO in 1 or 2 divided doses for 3 days prior to OR	
Procainamide	IV bolus; ventricular dysrhythmia	2–6 mg/kg q 5 min up to 15 mg/kg; then	20 mg/min until dysrhythmia is suppressed; then	Watch QRS
	IV infusion	20–80 mcg/kg/min	1–4 mg/min	
Prochlorperazine (Compazine)	PO, IM, PR; antiemetic	0.1–0.15 mg/kg q 6–8 hr	5–10 mg IM; may repeat q 3–4 hr if needed;	
		Max dose:	25 mg PR twice daily;	
		9–13 kg: 7.5 mg/day	5–10 mg as a slow IV injection or infusion, at a rate not to exceed 5 mg/min; max dose:	
		14–18 kg: 10 mg/day		
		19–39 kg: 15 mg/day	40 mg/day	
Promethazine (Phenergan)	IV, IM, PO, PR; N/V	0.25–1 mg/kg PO, PR q 4–6 hr	12.5–25 mg PO, PR, IM, IV q 4–6 hr	<2 yr: beware respiratory depression
Propofol	IV	2.5–3.5 mg/kg	2–2.5 mg/kg	
	Infusion	125–300 mcg/kg/min	100–200 mcg/kg/min	
Propranolol	IV; Tet spell (tetralogy of Fallot)	0.15–0.25 mg/kg		
	IV; dysrhythmia	0.01–0.1 mg/kg	1 mg IV, may repeat q 5 min to 5 mg total	
Protamine	IV	1 mg for each 100 U heparin	1 mg for each 100 units of heparin	Effective dosage may be increased by use of antithrombolytics
Ranitidine	PO; aspiration pneumonia prophylaxis	2 mg/kg divided q 12 hr	150–300 mg	

Remifentanil	IV; aspiration pneumonia prophylaxis	1–2 mg/kg/day	5–50 mg
	IV bolus	0.5–1 mcg/kg	0.5–1 mcg/kg
	IV infusion; sedation	0.02–0.1 mcg/kg/min	0.05–0.3 mcg/kg/min
	IV infusion; GA	Initial: 0.25 mcg/kg/min; maintenance: 0.025–1.3 mcg/kg/min; supplemental doses: 1 mcg/kg q 2–5 min prn	Initial: 0.5–1 mcg/kg/min Maintenance: 0.025–2 mcg/kg/min Supplemental doses: 1 mcg/kg q 2–5 min prn
Rocuronium	IV	0.5–1.2 mg/kg	0.5–1.2 mg/kg
	IM	1–1.8 mg/kg	
	Infusion	4–16 mcg/kg/min	5–12 mcg/kg/min
Ropivacaine	Regional	1–5 mg/kg	Field block: 5–200 mg Major nerve block: 75–300 mg
	Caudal or epidural	⅔ of initial dose after 90–120 min	75–150 mg
Scopolamine	IV, IM, SQ; preoperative sedation	6 mo–3 yr: 0.1–0.15 mg 3–6 yr: 0.2–0.3 mg	0.32–0.65 mg three or four times per day
	SQ; N/V	6 mcg/kg/dose	0.6–1 mg
	Transdermal patch; PONV		1 patch behind ear at least 1 hr before surgery	Keep in place for 24 hr after surgery
Sodium bicarbonate	IV	1–2 mEq/kg or per ABG	1 mEq/kg
Succinylcholine	IV; depolarizing NMB for intubation	1–2 mg/kg	0.5–1.5 mg/kg
	IV; to break laryngospasm		0.1–0.2 mg/kg
	IM	3–4 mg/kg	3–4 mg/kg

Continued

COMMON ANESTHESIA AND CRITICAL CARE DRUGS E

Drug	Route; Indication	Pediatric Dose	Adult Dose (>50 kg)	Comments
Sufentanil	IV; GA	10–25 mcg/kg, additional doses up to 25–50 mcg for maintenance	Primary anesthetic agent: 8–30 mcg/kg IV; then 0.5–10 mcg/kg Analgesic adjunct to balance GA: 1–8 mcg/kg IV; 75% given before intubation, then incrementally as 10–50 mcg	
Terbutaline	SQ; asthma	≤12 yr: 5–10 mcg/kg, may repeat once after 15 min >12 yr: 0.25 mg, may repeat once after 15 min	0.25 mg, may repeat once after 15 min; max dose: 0.5 mg/4 hr	
	IV infusion; severe asthma	Bolus 10 mcg/kg over 10 min; then infusion 0.2 mcg/kg/min, increasing dose as needed by 0.2 mcg/kg/min		
	IV infusion; preterm labor			
Thiopental	IV; induction	Neonate: 3–4 mg/kg 1–6 mon: 5–8 mg/kg IV 1–15 yr: 5–6 mg/kg IV	0.25 mg q 20 min-3 hr Slow induction: 25–50 mg Rapid induction: 210–280 mg (3–4 mg/kg)	Hold for HR >120 beats/min
	IV (increment)	1 mg/kg	25–50 mg	
Tigan	PO	100–200 mg three or four times daily	200–300 mg three or four times daily	

Drug	Route; Indication		
Vasopressin	IV infusion; vasopressor for hypotension	0.05–2 milliunits/kg/min	0.01–0.04 units/min
	IV, IO bolus; cardiac arrest	0.5 unit/kg/dose	40 units
	IV; diabetes insipidus	Bolus: 0.1 unit/kg/dose Infusion: 0.5 milliunits/kg/min	
	SQ, IM; diabetes insipidus	0.1 unit/kg/dose	5–10 units SQ or IM repeated two or three times daily prn
Vecuronium	IV bolus	0.1 mg/kg	0.08–0.1 mg/kg
	IV infusion	1.5–2.5 mcg/kg/min	0.8–1.2 mcg/kg/min
Verapamil	IV	0.1–0.2 mg/kg	5–10 mg (0.075–0.15 mg/kg)

ABG, Arterial blood gases; *ACLS*, advanced cardiac life support; *ACT*, activated clotting time; *BP*, blood pressure; *CPB*, cardiopulmonary bypass; *CVC*, central venous catheter; *DIC*, disseminated intravascular coagulopathy; *EPCA*, epidural patient-controlled analgesia; *ETT*, endotracheal tube; *GA*, general anesthesia; *GERD*, gastroesophageal reflux disease; *HR*, heart rate; *ICP*, intracranial pressure; *IM*, intramuscular; *IO*, intraosseous; *IV*, intravenous; *max*, maximum; *NMB*, neuromuscular blockade; *NS*, normal saline; *N/V*, nausea and vomiting; *PCA*, patient-controlled analgesia; *PGE₁*, prostaglandin E₁; *PO*, by mouth; *PONV*, postoperative nausea and vomiting; *PR*, per rectum; *PTT*, partial thromboplastin time; *SQ*, subcutaneous; *SVT*, supraventricular tachycardia; *Tet spell*, tetralogy of Fallot, characterized by sudden cyanosis and syncope; *VT/VF*, ventricular tachycardia/ventricular fibrillation.

COMMON ANESTHESIA AND CRITICAL CARE DRUGS

Appendix F
Abbreviations

A

μA	microampere
A-a	alveolar-arterial
AAA	abdominal aortic aneurysm
ABA	American Board of Anesthesiology
ABG	arterial blood gas
ABO	blood group system of groups A, AB, B, O
ACE	angiotensin-converting enzyme
ACGME	Accreditation Council for Graduate Medical Education
ACLS	advanced cardiac life support
ACTH	adrenocorticotrophic hormone
AIDS	acquired immunodeficiency syndrome
AMA	American Medical Association
APS	Acute Pain Service
ARDS	acute respiratory distress syndrome
ARF	acute renal failure
ASA	American Society of Anesthesiologists
AV	atrioventricular
AVM	arteriovenous malformation

B

BBB	blood-brain barrier
bid	*bis in die* (twice per day)
BiPAP	bilevel positive-airway pressure
BIS	bispectral index
BJR	Bezold-Jarisch reflex
BLS	basic life support
BMR	basal metabolic rate
BP	blood pressure
BSA	body surface area
BUN	blood urea nitrogen

C

CA-1,2,3	clinical anesthesia year
CABG	coronary artery bypass
CAD	coronary artery disease
cAMP	cyclic adenosine monophosphate
CaO_2	arterial oxygen content
CBC	complete blood count
CBF	cerebral blood flow
CBY	clinical base year
$Cc'O_2$	pulmonary capillary O_2 content
CDC	Centers for Disease Control and Prevention
CHD	congenital heart disease
CHF	congestive heart failure

CMS	Centers for Medicare and Medicaid Services
CMV	cytomegalovirus
CN	cranial nerve
CNS	central nervous system
CO	cardiac output
COPD	chronic obstructive pulmonary disease
CPAP	continuous positive airway pressure
CPB	cardiopulmonary bypass
CPP	cerebral perfusion pressure
CPR	cardiopulmonary resuscitation
CPT	Current Procedural Terminology
CRF	chronic renal failure
CRMD	cardiac rhythm management device
CRNA	Certified Registered Nurse Anesthetist
CRRT	continuous renal replacement therapy
CRT	cardiac resynchronization therapy
CSF	cerebrospinal fluid
CT	computed tomography
CV	cardiovascular
$C\bar{v}O_2$	mixed venous O_2 content
CVC	central venous catheter
CVP	central venous pressure
CVR	cerebrovascular resistance
CXR	chest x-ray study

D

DDAVP	1-deamino(8-D-arginine) vasopressin
DEA	Drug Enforcement Administration
DIC	disseminated intravascular coagulopathy
DLT	double-lumen tube
DNR	do not resuscitate
DVT	deep vein thrombosis
$\dot{D}O_2$	oxygen delivery
$\dot{D}O_2I$	oxygen delivery index

E

E. coli	Escherichia coli
EBP	epidural blood patch
ECG	electrocardiogram
ECMO	extracorporeal membrane oxygenation
ECT	electroconvulsive shock therapy
ED	emergency department
EDP	end-diastolic pressure
EDV	end-diastolic volume
EEG	electroencephalogram
EF	ejection fraction
ELISA	enzyme-linked immunosorbent assay
EMI	electromagnetic interference
epi	epinephrine
ERAS	Electronic Residency Application Service

ESWL	extracorporeal shock-wave lithotripsy
ETCO$_2$	end-tidal carbon dioxide
ETT	endotracheal tube

F

F	French
FENa	fractional excretion of sodium
FEV$_1$	forced expiratory volume in one second
FFP	fresh frozen plasma
Fio$_2$	fraction inspired oxygen
FOB	fiberoptic bronchoscope
FRC	functional residual capacity
FVC	forced vital capacity

G

G	gauge
GA	general anesthesia or anesthetic
GABA	gamma-aminobutyric acid
GERD	gastroesophageal reflux disease
GFR	glomerular filtration rate
GI	gastrointestinal

H

H&P	history and physical
Hb	hemoglobin
Hb$_e$Ag	hepatitis B early antigen
Hct	hematocrit
HF	heart failure
HFJV	high-frequency jet ventilation
HIPAA	Health Insurance Portability and Accountability Act
HIV	human immunodeficiency virus
HR	heart rate
HTN	hypertension

I

ICH	intracerebral hemorrhage
ICP	intracranial pressure
ICU	intensive care unit
ID	identification
IgG	immunoglobulin G
IJ	internal jugular
IM	intramuscular or intramuscularly
INR	International Normalized Ratio
ITP	idiopathic thrombocytopenic purpura
IV	intravenous or intravenously
IV IgG	intravenous immunoglobulin G
IVC	inferior vena cava
IVP	intraventricular pressure
IVPCA	IV pt-controlled analgesia

F

ABBREVIATIONS

L

LA	left atrium *or* left atrial
LA	local anesthesia *or* anesthetic
LFCN	lateral femoral cutaneous nerve
LIM	line isolation monitor
LMA	laryngeal mask airway
LMWH	low-molecular-weight heparin
LR	lactated Ringer solution
LV	left ventricle *or* left ventricular
LVEDP	left ventricular end-diastolic pressure
LVH	left ventricular hypertrophy

M

M3G	morphine-3-glucuronide
M6G	morphine-6-glucuronide
mA	milliampere
MAC	minimum alveolar concentration
MAOI	monamine oxidase inhibitor
MAP	mean arterial pressure
MET	metabolic equivalent of the task
MI	myocardial infarction
MR	mitral regurgitation
MRI	magnetic resonance imaging
MRSA	methicillin-resistant *Staphylococcus aureus*
MS	mitral stenosis

N

NG	nasogastric
NICU	neonatal intensive care unit
NIPPV	negative inspiratory positive-pressure ventilation
NMB	neuromuscular block or blocking
NMDA	*N*-methyl-D-aspartate
NO	nitrous oxide
NPO	*nil per os* (nothing by mouth)
NRMP	National Residency Match Program
NS	normal saline
NSAID	nonsteroidal antiinflammatory drug
N/V	nausea and vomiting
NYHA	New York Heart Association

O

OB	obstetrics
OG	orogastric
OIG	Office of Inspector General
OLV	one-lung ventilation
OR	operating room
ORT	Operation Restore Trust (ORT)
OSA	obstructive sleep apnea

P

PAC	pulmonary artery catheterization
$Paco_2$	arterial CO_2 tension
PACU	postanesthesia care unit
PAO_2	alveolar O_2 tension
PaO_2	arterial O_2 tension
PAP	mean pulmonary artery pressure
P_B	barometric pressure (760 mm Hg)
PCA	pt-controlled analgesia
PCEA	pt-controlled epidural analgesia
PCWP	pulmonary capillary wedge pressure
PD	Parkinson disease
PDA	patent ductus arteriosus
PDPH	postdural puncture headache
PEA	pulseless electrical activity
$P\bar{E}co_2$	mixed expired CO_2 tension
PEEP	positive end-expiratory pressure
PEP	postexposure prophylaxis
PFT	pulmonary function test
P_{H_2O}	H_2O vapor tension (47 mm Hg)
PICC	peripherally inserted central catheter
PICU	pediatric intensive care unit
PMD	primary medical doctor
PO	*per os* (by mouth)
PONV	postoperative nausea and vomiting
PPHN	persistent pulmonary hypertension
PPV	positive-pressure ventilation
PR	per rectum
prn	*pro re nata* (as needed)
pt	patient
PT	prothrombin time
PTT	partial thromboplastin time
PTU	propylthiouracil
PTX	pneumothorax
PVC	premature ventricular contraction
$P\bar{V}O_2$	mixed venous O_2 tension
PVR	pulmonary vascular resistance

Q

$\dot{Q}s/\dot{Q}t$	intrapulmonary shunt fraction

R

RA	regional anesthesia
RAE	Ring-Adair-Elwyn
RBC	red blood cell
RCT	randomized controlled trial
RD	respiratory depression
REM	Roentgen equivalent man
RR	respiratory rate
RSI	rapid-sequence induction
RV	right ventricle *or* right ventricular

S

SaO_2	arterial O_2 saturation percentage
SCD	sudden cardiac death
SCM	sternocleidomastoid muscle
SI	sacroiliac
SQ	subcutaneous
SSEP	somatosensory-evoked potential
$\bar{S}O_2$	mixed venous O_2 saturation percentage
SVR	systemic vascular resistance

T

T&A	tonsillectomy and adenoidectomy
TEE	transesophageal echocardiography
TIA	transient ischemic attack
tid	*ter in die* (three times per day)
TIVA	total IV anesthesia
TOF	train of four
TOF	tetralogy of Fallot
TPN	total parenteral nutrition
TRH	thyrotropin-releasing hormone
TSH	thyroid-stimulating hormone
TTE	transthoracic and transesophageal color-flow Doppler echocardiography
TURBT	transurethral resection of bladder tumor
TURP	transurethral prostatectomy

U

UOP	urine output
URI	upper respiratory infection
US	ultrasound

V

V_D	dead space gas volume
VF	ventricular fibrillation
$\dot{V}O_2$	O_2 consumption (minute)
$\dot{V}O_2I$	O_2 consumption index
VRE	vancomycin-resistant enterococci
VT	ventricular tachycardia
V_T	tidal volume

W

WBC	white blood cell
WHO	World Health Organization

Index

Page numbers followed by f indicate figures; t, tables; b, boxes.

INDEX